THE PROBLEM OF DARK-CUTTING IN BEEF

CURRENT TOPICS IN VETERINARY MEDICINE AND ANIMAL SCIENCE

VOLUME 10

Other titles in this series

Volume 1
Control of Reproduction in the Cow
edited by J.M. Sreenan

Volume 2
Patterns of Growth and Development in Cattle
edited by H. de Boer and J. Martin

Volume 3
Respiratory Diseases in Cattle
edited by W.B. Martin

Volume 4
Calving Problems and Early Viability of the Calf
edited by B. Hoffmann, I.L. Mason and J. Schmidt

Volume 5
The Future of Beef Production in the European Community
edited by J.C. Bowman and P. Susmel

Volume 6
Diseases of Cattle in the Tropics: Economic and Zoonotic Relevance
edited by M. Ristic

Volume 7
Control of Reproductive Functions in Domestic Animals
edited by W. Jöchle and D.R. Lamond

Volume 8
The Laying Hen and its Environment
edited by R. Moss

Volume 9
Epidemiology and Control of Nematodiasis in Cattle
edited by P. Nansen, R.J. Jørgensen and E.J.L. Soulsby

Series ISBN: 90-247-2429-5

THE PROBLEM OF DARK-CUTTING IN BEEF

A Seminar in the EEC Programme of Coordination of Research on Animal Welfare, organised by D.E. Hood and P.V. Tarrant, and held in Brussels, October 7-8, 1980

Sponsored by the Commission of the European Communities, Directorate-General for Agriculture, Coordination of Agricultural Research

Edited by

D.E. Hood and P.V. Tarrant

Meat Research Department,
An Foras Taluntais,
Dunsinea Research Centre, Castleknock, Co. Dublin, Ireland

MARTINUS NIJHOFF PUBLISHERS
THE HAGUE / BOSTON / LONDON

for

THE COMMISSION OF THE EUROPEAN COMMUNITIES

Distributors

for the United States and Canada
Kluwer Boston, Inc.
190 Old Derby Street
Hingham, MA 02043
USA

for all other countries
Kluwer Academic Publishers Group
Distribution Center
P.O. Box 322
3300 AH Dordrecht
The Netherlands

This volume is listed in the Library of Congress Cataloging in Publication Data

ISBN 978-94-011-8702-2 ISBN 978-94-011-9528-7 (eBook)
DOI 10.1007/978-94-011-9528-7

Publication arranged by
Commission of the European Communities,
Directorate-General Scientific and Technical Information and Information Management

EUR 7328 EN

Softcover reprint of the hardcover 1st edition 1981

Manuscript Preparation by
Janssen Services, 33a High Street, Chislehurst, Kent BR7 5AE, UK

CONTENTS

PREFACE

This publication contains the proceedings of a seminar 'The problems of dark-cutting in beef' held by the Commission of the European Communities (CEC) at the Commission in Brussels on 7 and 8 October 1980. As part of the CEC programme of coordination of agricultural research, this meeting was organised in the framework of the beef and animal welfare activities by Dr. D.E. Hood and Dr. P.V. Tarrant, Meat Research Department, An Foras Taluntais, Dunsinea, Castleknock, Dublin, Ireland. The proceedings, edited by the organisers assisted by Janssen Services, 33a, High Street, Chislehurst, Kent, UK, provide an authoritative text-book on this important aspect of meat technology.

Reduction of pre-slaughter stress and improvement in carcass and meat quality is becoming increasingly important in the international meat trade. This results in particular from growing consumer concern about the welfare of meat animals during the pre-slaughter period and from specific meat packaging and marketing requirements. Technical development of the beef processing industry is dependent on a uniformly high level of meat quality in the raw material.

The CEC wishes to thank all those who took responsibility in the organisation and running of this seminar, who prepared papers, posters and who participated in the seminar discussions.

INTRODUCTION

This seminar was originally planned by the Carcass and Meat Quality Expert Group under the aegis of the CEC Beef Research Programme. This Group has given stress-related problems in meat a high priority for future research. The original idea was to hold a seminar on stress in meat animals with particular reference to meat quality. The meeting was to be held in Dublin but due to budgetary restrictions a change in venue became necessary. The scope of the original proposal was later restricted to a consideration of the more specific problems of dark-cutting in beef as a widely recognised though perhaps ill-defined phenomenon which would stand more critical examination and appraisal.

In parallel with a concern for meat quality aspects there has been increasing emphasis in recent years within the Community and elsewhere on animal welfare. The topic of the seminar falls readily also within the scope of this area since dark-cutting is a specific example of the effect of stress in beef animals, where an animal is slaughtered at a time when muscle glycogen is low. This results in the production of high pH meat which in turn produces an undesirable dark colour and poor keeping-quality. These objectives then form the basis for the seminar which we have organised during the next two days. They are: to examine scientifically the phenomenon of dark-cutting in beef in all its aspects including the aetiology of the condition, possible heritability characteristics, identification and prevention, microbiology, eating quality and technological potential. Superimposed on this are consideration of the live animal, animal behaviour, stress and welfare.

An important element of the seminar is the interaction which should follow from the multi-disciplinary content and the widely differing backgrounds of the participants. From this point of view discussion periods are most important and as much time as possible has been allotted for this purpose. Review papers will be presented at six main plenary sessions and other contributed papers at a poster session.

D.E. Hood

SESSION I

QUALITY ASPECTS

Chairman: J. Wismer-Pedersen

THE OCCURRENCE, CAUSES AND ECONOMIC CONSEQUENCES OF DARK-CUTTING IN BEEF - A SURVEY OF CURRENT INFORMATION.

P.V. Tarrant
Meat Research Department, Agricultural Institute,
Dunsinea, Castleknock, Co. Dublin, Ireland.

ABSTRACT

In the preparation of this seminar on stress in cattle and dark-cutting in beef, information was collected from a wide background by means of a survey to determine the present position and recent developments in this area. Questionnaires (see Appendix 1) were sent to senior scientists in meat research laboratories. Twenty-seven completed questionnaires were returned from nineteen countries[1]*. Respondents were asked to present the situation as it exists in their own countries.*

The results represent informed scientific opinion based on research findings and practical experience of the problem in the meat industry. They provide a reasonable estimate of the extent of the problem, in terms of incidence and type of cattle affected, the principle characteristics of the condition and its impact on the meat industry.

In presenting the results, responses are frequently identified on a national basis. This was found to add considerably to the usefulness of the data. However, it is necessary to emphasise that the information presented in any particular case does not necessarily represent the national position, but rather a prevailing situation within each country. In assessing the results, all replies were given an equal weighting.

[1] Australia, Belgium (2), Britain, Bulgaria, Canada, Czechoslovakia, Denmark, France, Finland, West Germany, Ireland, The Netherlands, New Zealand, Norway, Poland (2), South Africa, Sweden, The United States (Maryland, Illinois, Missouri, Wyoming, Texas (2), Oregan) and Yugoslavia.

The principal results of the survey follow and the detailed results are presented in Appendix 2.

Question: What sectors of the beef trade have problems associated with dark-cutting?

The sectors of the beef trade most widely considered to have problems associated with dark-cutting are the carcass sector, vacuum-packed primal sector and retail fresh beef sector. All the other sectors of the trade which were listed in the questionnaire, (see Appendix 1) were occasionally considered to have problems with dark-cutting beef.

Question: What category of animal is affected?

Young bulls are universally considered to be affected by dark-cutting, whereas opinions regarding the other sex categories were divided. In steer-producing countries, in general, all categories of cattle were considered to be affected. In countries with substantial bull beef production, dark-cutting is predominantly associated with young bulls and other categories were not frequently thought to be affected.

Question: Is there a breed effect?

There is a lack of information concerning the effect of breed on the incidence of dark-cutting in beef.

Question: Can you estimate the incidence of dark-cutting?

Estimates of incidence varied. The incidence was most frequently estimated at 1 - 5 per cent for steers and heifers, 6 - 10 per cent for cows and 11 - 15 per cent for young bulls.

Question: What muscles are most liable to be affected?

M. Longissimus dorsi was universally considered to be one of the muscles most liable to be affected. Other muscles were much less frequently cited. These tended to be the major hindquarter muscles more often than forequarter muscles.

Question: What ultimate pH values (measured in M. l. dorsi) *would indicate dark-cutting to you?*

Beef quality deteriorates when the ultimate pH value is equal to, or above, 5.8. The precise value at which a carcass is deemed 'dark-cutting' depends largely on processing and marketing factors and is in the range pH 5.8 - 6.3. Values above this range are always associated with an unacceptable degree of dark, firm, dry (DFD) beef.

Question: Is there a seasonal effect? If your answer is 'yes', please indicate in which months dark-cutting is most likely.

A majority of respondents reported a seasonal effect. These respondents were mainly from the traditional steer-producing regions. There was considerable agreement concerning which months are most frequently associated with incidence or intensity of DFD. In the northern hemisphere, these are September to January, inclusive, and the month of April.

Please suggest three causes of dark-cutting in your country in order of importance.

Mismanagement of cattle before slaughter, resulting in physiological stress and exhaustion, was the most frequently suggested cause of dark-cutting in beef. In particular, the practice of penning cattle together in mixed lots at the abbatoir, and unsuitable transport conditions, were often cited. The other causes suggested concerned climatic conditions, nutrition, pathological conditions, genetic factors and stress in general.

Question: What do you think are the main objections to dark-cutting beef?

There was general agreement that abnormal colour and spoilage characteristics are the main reasons for objecting to DFD beef. The appearance, consistency and organoleptic characteristics of the meat are also considered to be objectionable.

Question: Is there an economic penalty for dark-cutting beef at any stage in the marketing chain? If so, what is the economic loss relative to a normal carcass or meat cut?

A majority of replies indicated that there is an economic penalty. The economic loss relative to normal meat was most frequently put at 10 per cent. Much higher losses were occasionally reported.

Question: Is there down-grading of carcasses on a national, regional or local classification or grading scheme?

Down-grading of dark-cutting carcasses at beef classification or grading is fairly common and was reported by 44 per cent of respondents.

Question: Are there other economic consequences?

Rejection of DFD beef at various stages of the marketing chain was the principle area of concern. Cost of disposal of DFD beef and substituting normal meat, loss of reputation for quality and down-grading of non-affected cuts were also cited as additional economic consequences.

CONCLUSIONS

The survey confirms that dark-cutting is a persistent condition in cattle, occurring in all categories of cattle and in all countries surveyed. Conclusions relevant to the subjects of meat quality and animal welfare can be drawn and these will be considered separately.

Meat quality

The results of the survey show that dark-cutting beef is rejected by the meat industry and by the consumer on the basis of a number of serious quality faults. These are such as to exclude its use in normal fresh meat products. The frozen beef trade is a possible outlet. However, the reduced organoleptic characteristics of the product raise the question whether such meat can be diverted into frozen beef outlets, particularly the home freezer market, without long-term repercussions.

The estimated incidences (Table 4, Appendix 2) show that the condition is of considerable proportions in many of the countries surveyed. The reported high variability in the daily incidence makes detection and control by industry more difficult. For example, the seasonal effect in Ireland is estimated to cause a four-fold increase in the average incidence and this is made up of a highly variable daily incidence.

Young bulls were, predictably, reported to have the highest incidence. The meat industry itself has control over the major causes of dark-cutting in these animals, which concern pre-slaughter management procedures. Proper control of penning and handling procedures at abattoirs would greatly reduce the incidence in young bulls and other cattle from intensive production systems. As it is often economically more favourable to produce beef from bulls rather than steers, it is clearly important for the industry to minimise meat quality defects in bull beef.

The acceptability of beef of abnormal ultimate pH is greatly influenced by production and trading circumstances. There is scope for the preparation of a comprehensive pH standard for use in quality control and quality assessment. Measurement of ultimate pH is widely practised and pH standards vary considerably, to meet particular production and marketing circumstances. A suitable pH standard for use within the European Community would take into account the type of carcass under examination and the process and market for which it is intended. In this context it is important to emphasise the wholesomeness of dark-cutting beef, despite its technological and organoleptic disadvantages.

Substantial economic penalties were widely reported. These may serve as an impetus towards developing practical procedures aimed at reducing the incidence and improving the methods of detection. Suitable procedures should be developed for utilising DFD beef. Any attempt to market DFD as normal beef should be discouraged in the long-term interests of the industry.

Animal Welfare

The dark-cutting condition is relevant to animal welfare because it results from exposure to stress and is indicative of physical exhaustion before slaughter. The condition is unknown in well-fed and rested animals. Some categories of cattle are more likely to be affected than others. This may be due to inherent sex characteristics as in the case of young bulls. Alternatively, in the case of cows, it may be due to lower standards of care before slaughter.

The difficulty of inducing dark-cutting experimentally, e.g. by fasting, exercise or similar stressors, has been reported in the literature. It follows that the observed incidence of dark-cutting underestimates the number of cattle exposed to stress before slaughter. The observed incidence of dark-cutting represents only the most severely stressed animals.

From the point of view of animal welfare, young bulls should be considered apart from the other categories of cattle. The high incidence of dark-cutting in these animals is associated with the sex characteristics of an excitable temperament and aggressive or sexual activity. These activities are more pronounced in a novel environment and, although stressful, represent normal animal behaviour. Dark-cutting in these animals does not necessarily indicate ill treatment before slaughter.

Dark-cutting was attributed to severe environmental stress factors, sometimes potentiated by genetic factors. The causes reported in the survey are obviously the most common ones. In practice, any situation which results in substantial depletion of muscle glycogen reserves will cause dark-cutting if the animal is slaughtered before recovery takes place. The mechanisms of muscle glycogen depletion are (a) the performance of heavy muscular work resulting in an increased intra-cellular energy demand, (b) adrenergic activation of glycogenolysis by increased adrenaline concentration in the circulation, and (c) long-term depletion of glycogen reserves as a consequence of inanition.

Because of the frequency with which mismanagement of cattle before slaughter was cited as a cause of dark-cutting, the results suggest that there is a need for further information concerning procedures for handling and transport of cattle. Standards must be agreed upon and made available to cover the various situations which exist in the industry. The construction of pens and their method of use would appear to require particular attention. The recommended holding time for the different categories must be clarified, together with procedures for allowing exhausted cattle to recover before slaughter.

The results suggest that the climate and other seasonal factors are important in the aetiology of the dark-cutting condition. Exposure to the elements and inadequate nutrition obviously occur, particularly in extensive beef production systems, and the consequences are apparent in the carcass. Alleviation of animal suffering due to seasonal factors is a more difficult proposition than is the case with pre-slaughter factors.

ACKNOWLEDGEMENTS

Information was kindly provided by the following persons: Dr. A.J. Bailey, United Kingdom; Dr. H.F. Bernholdt, USA; Ir. H. de Boer, the Netherlands; O.S. Braathen, Norway; Mrs. L. Buchter, Denmark; Canada Packers Ltd., Canada;

Ir. M. Casteels, Belgium; Dr. B. Chrystall, New Zealand; Dr. E. Cosentino, Italy; Dr. C.L. Davey, New Zealand; Dr. T.R. Dutson, USA; Dr. R.A. Field, USA; Eng. Geraldo Cia, Brazil; Dr. Maria Gorna, Poland; Dr. H.B. Hedrick, USA; Ing. J. Jedlička, Czechoslavakia; Dr. D.E. Hood, Ireland; Prof. Dr. E. Kallweit, Federal Republic of Germany; Dr. W.H. Kennick, USA; Dr. A.W. Kotula, USA; Dr. K. Krzywicki, Poland; Dr. G. Monin, France; Dr. R. Naudé, South Africa; Prof. Dr. N. Nestorov, Bulgaria; Prof. F.P. Niinivaara, Finland; Prof. Dr. H. Pfeiffer, German Democratic Republic; E. Puolanne, Finland; Dr. S. Rahelic, Yugoslavia; H. Ruderus, Sweden; Prof. Dr. L. Schön, Federal Republic of Germany; Dr. G.C. Smith, USA; Prof. N.M. Tulloh, Australia; Prof. Dr. J. van Hoof, Belgium; Dr. D.J. Walker, Australia; Dr. Maria Vada, Hungary.

APPENDIX 1

QUESTIONNAIRE DARK-CUTTING IN BEEF

Please tick (thus ✓) the box on the questionnaire that best expresses your opinion of the situation in your country or region. Where appropriate more than one box may be ticked. Please give additional information which you consider to be relevant to this subject.

Please give the country or general region to which your answers apply:

---

1. What sector(s) of the beef trade in your country or region has (have) problems associated with dark-cutting:

☐	☐	☐	☐	☐	☐	☐
Carcass trade	Vac-pack fresh beef primals	Retail fresh beef	Ground beef	Cured/ salted products	Fermented products	Other (please specify

COMMENT:

---

2. What category of animal is affected:

☐	☐	☐	☐	☐	☐
Steer (castrate) ♂	Heifer (virgin) ♀	Cow (lactating) ♀	Young bull (entire) ♂	Other (specify)	All categories

COMMENT:

---

3. Is there a breed effect?

☐	☐	☐
Yes	No	Don't know

If 'yes', what breeds are most susceptible:

4. Can you estimate the incidence of dark-cutting:

	0	1-5%	6-10%	11-15%	16-20%	20%+	Don't know
Steer							
Heifer							
Cow							
Young bull							
All categories							

ADDITIONAL COMMENTS:

5. What muscles are most liable to be affected:

☐ *M. biceps femoris*
☐ *M. psoas major*
☐ *M. gluteus medius*
☐ *M. adductor*
☐ *M. semimembranosus*
☐ *M. semitendinosus*
☐ *M. longissimus dorsi*
☐ *M. triceps brachii*
☐ *M. trapezius*
☐ *M. infraspinatus*
☐ *M. supraspinatus*

Other muscles or meat cuts, please specify:

6. What ultimate pH values (measured in *M. l. dorsi)* would indicate dark-cutting to you:

	☐	☐	☐	☐	☐	☐	☐	☐
pH	5.7	5.8	5.9	6.0	6.1	6.2	6.3	6.4

COMMENT:

7. Is there a seasonal effect:

☐ Yes ☐ No ☐ Don't know

If your answer is 'yes', please indicate in which months dark-cutting is most likely:

J	F	M	A	M	J	J	A	S	O	N	D

8. Please suggest three causes of dark-cutting in your country in order of importance:

(1)

(2)

(3)

9. What do you think are the main objections to dark-cutting beef:

	Very important	Important	Not important
Dark colour			
Faster spoilage			
Firm, dry consistency			
Other (specify)			

10. Is there an economic penalty for dark-cutting beef at any stage in the marketing chain:

☐ Yes ☐ No ☐ Don't know

If 'yes', what is the economic loss relative to a normal carcass (or meat cut):

☐ 10% ☐ 20% ☐ 30% ☐ 40% ☐ 50%

---

11. Is there down-grading of dark-cutting carcasses on a national, regional or local classification or grading scheme:

☐ Yes ☐ No ☐ Don't know

---

12. Are there other economic consequences (please specify):

APPENDIX 2

ANALYSIS OF REPLIES

Question: What sector(s) of the beef trade in your country or region has (have) problems associated with dark-cutting?

TABLE 1

SECTORS OF THE BEEF INDUSTRY REPORTED TO HAVE PROBLEMS WITH DARK-CUTTING IN BEEF

Sector	Number (%) of times specified
Carcass trade	24 (89)
Vacuum-packed primal cuts	16 (59)
Retail fresh beef	15 (56)
Ground beef	4 (15)
Cured/salted products	2 (7)
Fermented products	1 (4)
Others	0

Twenty-seven replies were received, each reply specifying one or more than one of the sectors listed. The results are shown in Table 1.

All sectors listed can be affected, although problems are most frequently encountered in the valuable carcass and fresh meat sectors, where the bulk of trading actually occurs.

All replies, except those from New Zealand, South Africa and Sweden, reported problems in the carcass sector. In Sweden the routine measurement of carcass pH is reported to be gaining interest and could, in future, mean that the carcass trade there will also be increasingly concerned about dark-cutting.

In the vacuum-pack sector, problems were reported by two-thirds of the respondents*. Additionally, in Denmark, it was noted that bull beef is not usually vacuum-packed but, where it is, the industry has been recommended to sort out high pH meat before packing.

Over half of the replies received specified problems in the retail fresh meat sector**. Difficulty in retailing abnormally dark beef in supermarkets was commented on in four replies.

Problems associated with dark-cutting were reported to occur in the ground beef trade, in cured and salted products, and in fermented products.

The following additional comments were received. From France and Yugoslavia it was noted that export markets are more sensitive to problems associated with DFD beef than are internal or local markets. Thus, marketing factors have an important influence on the acceptability of meat of a particular quality. It was also observed (New Zealand) that DFD is not an obvious problem in the frozen, manufacturing beef sector. From Czech-oslovakia it was observed that a proportion of DFD beef is advantageous in the production of fresh sausages.

Question: What category of animal is affected?

Twenty-seven replies were received, each specifying one or more of the listed categories (Table 2).

The overall result confirms that young bulls are universally considered to be affected (replies specifying 'young bulls' plus 'all categories' amounted to 92 per cent of the total

* Australia, New Zealand, Canada, the USA (Maryland, Illinois, Missouri, Oregon), France, West Germany, The Netherlands, Britain, Ireland, Finland, Norway, Sweden and Poland.

** Australia, South Africa, Canada, The USA (Maryland, Illinois, Missouri, Wyoming), France, The Netherlands, Belgium, Britain, Ireland, Finland, Norway and Bulgaria.

TABLE 2

TYPE OF CATTLE WHICH MAY BE AFFECTED

Category	Number (per cent) of replies specifying each category:		
	Total	Group 1[a]	Group 2[b]
Steer	8 (30)	8 (62)	0
Heifer	9 (33)	6 (46)	3 (21)
Cow	6 (22)	4 (31)	2 (14)
Young bull	19 (70)	6 (46)	13 (93)
All categories	6 (22)	5 (38)	1 (7)

[a] Group 1 consists of replies from countries producing steer beef: Australia, New Zealand, South Africa, USA, Canada, Britain and Ireland.

[b] Group 2 consists of replies from countries with substantial production of bull beef: Belgium, Denmark, Netherlands, France, West Germany, Norway, Sweden, Finland, Czechoslovakia, Poland, Yugoslavia and Bulgaria.

received). However, opinion concerning all the other categories was divided; replies are split into two groups for the purpose of analysis (see Table 2). Group 1 consists of thirteen replies from countries where steer production is traditionally practised and Group 2 consists of fourteen replies from countries with substantial or exclusive production of bull beef. It was the unanimous opinion in Group 1 that steers are affected by dark-cutting. Replies specifying 'steers' plus 'all categories' totalled 100 per cent. In Group 2, young bulls were unanimously associated with dark-cutting and steers were not considered to be affected (no reply specified 'steers' and only one specified 'all categories'). Many respondents in Group 1 considered that all of the listed categories of cattle are affected, whereas in Group 2 opinion tended to be polarised towards the single category of young bulls. Thus, production practices influence the perception of the problem. Where there is a high incidence of dark-cutting among young bulls, the incidence in other categories may pass unnoticed, particularly in the absence of substantial steer production.

Comments were made concerning detection of dark-cutting meat in cow carcasses. It was noted from New Zealand that DFD meat may go unnoticed in carcasses destined for manufacturing. It was also pointed out that DFD is more difficult to detect in older animals (due to the naturally darker colour of the meat).

Question: Is there a breed effect? If so, what breeds are most susceptible?

Twenty-seven replies were received, and the results are shown in Table 3.

TABLE 3

IS DARK-CUTTING ASSOCIATED WITH BREED?

Yes	8 (30 per cent)
No	5 (18 per cent)
Don't know	14 (52 per cent)

The majority of the respondents were undecided. Affirmatives were asked to name the most susceptible breeds. Replies specified both dairy and beef breeds as follows: Charolais (Oregan); Pedi-breed *(Bos indicus)* and Brahman (South Africa); *Bos indicus* breeds (Texas); Hereford and Angus (New Zealand); Friesian/Holstein (France); Finnish Landrace (Finland); Bulgarian Red breed (Bulgaria). Simmenthal, Limousine and their crosses were also suspect (Canada). It was reported from Australia that sire or dam breed have little or no effect on the mean ultimate pH of sire or dam groups; pure breeds were not compared.

Question: Can you estimate the incidence of dark-cutting?

There were twenty-seven replies, four of which stated that no information was available at present. The remaining twenty-three contained estimates of the incidence in one or more of the beef categories listed in Table 4. As was pointed out in replies from Australia and Britain, the estimates submitted may

TABLE 4

ESTIMATED INCIDENCES OF DARK-CUTTING IN BEEF CARCASSES, SHOWING THE NUMBER OF REPLIES RECEIVED FOR EACH FREQUENCY INTERVAL TOGETHER WITH THE COUNTRIES OF ORIGIN

	0	1 - 5%	6 - 10%	11 - 15%	16 - 20%	20% +	Don't know
Steer	France	Australia[a] Canada Illinois Wyoming Texas (2) Oregon[d] Ireland	Australia[a]	Poland			South Africa[b] New Zealand[c] Britain Denmark Netherlands Sweden[e] Poland Czechoslovakia Bulgaria
	1	8	1	1			9
Heifer		Australia[a] Illinois Wyoming Texas (2) Oregon France West Germany Ireland Yugoslavia	Australia[a,f] Canada Poland Poland	Finland[g]			South Africa New Zealand Denmark Netherlands Sweden Czechoslovakia Bulgaria
		10	3	1			7

TABLE 4 (Cont/d)

	0	1 - 5%	6 - 10%	11 - 15%	16 - 20%	20% +	Don't know
Cow	West Germany Denmark Poland	France	Australia[a,f] Canada Illinois Texas (2) Britain[h]	Australia[a,f] Wyoming Finland[g]			South Africa New Zealand Ireland Netherlands Sweden Poland Czechoslovakia Bulgaria
	3	1	[6]	3			8
Young bull		Oregon Illinois Belgium Denmark[k]	West Germany Britain[j]	Canada Wyoming Texas (2) France Yugoslavia[l]	Poland	(Norway)[i] Finland[g] Poland Bulgaria	Australia South Africa New Zealand Ireland Netherlands Sweden Czechoslovakia
		4	2	[6]	1	4	7
All categories		Maryland[m] Illinois Missouri France Belgium[n] Denmark[o] Poland[p]	Australia Wyoming			Finland[g]	South Africa New Zealand Britain Ireland Netherlands Sweden Poland Czechoslovakia
		[7]	2			1	8

[a] These estimates may not equate with the Australian annual mean prevalence of dark-cutting animals.

[b] No data available at present; a survey is anticipated shortly.

[c] In general, the incidence is low. At certain times up to 30 per cent of prime beef at some plants is affected.

[d] Estimated incidence of 1 per cent or less.

[e] Large scale pH measurements are now underway, but no reliable data are yet available.

[f] Estimate based on small numbers only.

[g] Based on a sample of 13 292 carcasses of young bulls, cows and heifers, the average incidences were - heifers, 12.6 per cent; cows, 13.6 per cent; young bulls, 26.3 per cent; all categories, 21.6 per cent.

[h] A restricted investigation of dark-cutting in culled mature cows revealed about 8 per cent ≥ pH 6.0.

[i] Considerable day to day variation from zero incidence upwards.

[j] In a sample of 1 500 bulls slaughtered at two abattoirs over a twelve month period, 6 - 7 per cent ≥ pH 6.0.

[k] The incidence of DFD in young bulls varies from less than 1 per cent in some plants to somewhat higher values in other plants.

[l] Occasionally up to 50 per cent of young bulls can be affected.

[m] The estimated incidence is 2 per cent.

[n] Except in emergency slaughtered cattle, where 11 - 15 per cent of the carcasses are characterised by dark-cutting beef (all categories but more predominant in cows).

[o] The estimated incidence is less than 1 per cent.

[p] The estimated incidence is 5 - 6 per cent.

not equate closely with the national incidences of dark-cutting in beef. The results are given in Table 4, and show the number and origin of estimates in each frequency interval for the listed categories of cattle.

Examination of the median values in Table 4 shows that steers and heifers were most often cited in the 1 - 5 per cent frequency interval, cows at 6 - 10 per cent, young bulls at 11 - 15 per cent and 'all categories' at 1 - 5 per cent. The results suggest that the incidence is highest in young bulls and next highest in cows.

Estimated incidences for young bulls and cows were more variable than for the other categories listed. The reason for this is not clear but a possible explanation may lie in different pre-slaughter handling practices in different countries. The results for cows may also be influenced by the difficulties (reported above) of detecting DFD in older animals and the possibility of DFD passing unnoticed in manufacturing beef (three out of thirteen estimates put the incidence in cows at zero).

The highest reported incidences were from Finland (young bulls, 26.3 per cent; all categories, 21.6 per cent) and these were based on a comprehensive sample of 13 292 carcasses of young bulls, heifers and cows at 14 slaughterhouses. (See separate report on this subject by Puolanne and Aalto).

Question: What muscles are most liable to be affected?

Eleven muscles were listed and the number of times each muscle was specified in the twenty-four replies received to the question are shown in Table 5.

M. l. dorsi is the only muscle which was universally considered to be liable to dark-cutting. (Two replies noted that all parts of the carcass are affected, without specifying intermuscular differences). In Denmark, *M. l. dorsi* was found to

TABLE 5

MUSCLES MOST LIABLE TO BE AFFECTED BY THE DARK-CUTTING CONDITION

Muscle	Number (per cent) of replies
M. longissimus dorsi	22 (92)
M. semimembranosus	9 (38)
M. biceps femoris	8 (33)
M. semitendinosus	5 (21)
M. adductor	5 (21)
M. gluteus medius	5 (21)
M. trapezius	4 (17)
M. psoas major	2 (8)
M. triceps brachii	3 (13)
M. infraspinatus	2 (8)
M. supraspinatus	2 (8)

be the best indicator muscle for identifying DFD, because it showed a tendency to increased ultimate pH values before other muscles. When the pH in the *M. l. dorsi* was approximately 6.5, the whole carcass was usually found to be badly affected, and slightly higher pH values might be found in some of the other muscles. However, in New Zealand, it was noted that the *M. l. dorsi* is the most obviously affected since it is seen the earliest (i.e. at quartering). It was noted that no single muscle seemed to be most susceptible and certainly measurement on one muscle could not be used to predict for other muscles of the carcass.

Fourteen replies specified muscles, in addition to *M. l. dorsi*, found to be particularly liable to DFD. Hindquarter muscles (*M. semimembranosus, biceps femoris, semitendinosus, adductor, gluteus medius*) are more frequently specified (Table 5) than forequarter muscles (*M. trapezius, triceps brachii, infraspinatus* and *supraspinatus*). *M. psoas major* is an exception, as a major hindquarter muscle which is not frequently associated with dark cutting.

The muscles listed in the questionnaire were selected for size, anatomical distribution and ease of access for pH measurement. Obviously, many important meat muscles were not listed and the following were mentioned additionally in replies: *M. quadriceps femoris* and *M. quadratus* (cited once each); it was also noted that the muscles of the neck and shin habitually have the highest ultimate pH values in the carcass. No correlation was observed between origin of replies and specific muscles affected. The results confirm that certain muscles are most liable to dark-cutting. It is clear, and was noted in five replies, that all muscles are affected in severe cases of dark-cutting.

Question: What ultimate pH values (measured in M. l. dorsi) would indicate dark-cutting to you?

Twenty-seven replies were received and the results are shown in Table 6, including additional information received which is useful for interpreting the different values used.

TABLE 6

ULTIMATE pH VALUES *(M. l. dorsi)* INDICATIVE OF DARK-CUTTING

pH values	Number (per cent) of replies	Cumulative totals
5.7	0	0
5.8	2 (7)[1]	2 (7)
5.9	1 (4)[2]	3 (11)
6.0	11 (41)[3]	14 (52)
6.1	5 (19)[4]	19 (70)
6.2	6 (22)[5]	25 (93)
6.3	2 (7)[6]	27 (100)
6.4	0	27 (100)

[1] Australia[a], Oregon.

[2] Missouri.

[3] Canada, Wyoming, Texas[b], Britain, Finland[c], France[d], Ireland, Netherlands[e], Norway[f], West Germany, Poland[g].

4 New Zealand, South Africa, Illinois, Poland[h], Yugoslavia.

5 Maryland, Texas, Belgium, Denmark[i], Sweden, Czechoslovakia.

6 Belgium, Bulgaria.

a The value varies with geographical location. In the southern half of Australia, meat of pH 5.8 is judged 'darkish' by consumers. In the northern half, consumers are slightly more tolerant and usually do not complain provided meat pH is below 5.9 - 6.0.

b pH 6.0 = 'shady'; pH 6.2 = 'dark'; pH 6.4 = 'sticky'.

c Two classes are used, pH 6.00 - 6.39 indicate moderate DFD; pH > 6.40 indicate extreme DFD.

d The lower value of pH 5.9 is suggested for vacuum packaging.

e At pH values of 6.0 - 6.2 the meat is not normal, too dark, but still acceptable. At pH 6.5 the meat is extremely dark and is unacceptable. Acceptability of meat of a particular quality or pH value varies according to supply and demand, destination of the meat and local custom.

f Norway does not import beef above pH 6.0.

g A lower limit of pH 5.8 in *M. l. dorsi* is used if the quality of other cuts is being evaluated or if changes in consistency are being considered.

h The value used depends to some extent on the sex and degree of fatness of the carcass. For young bulls and steers distinct symptoms of DFD are observed at pH 6.1 and for cows at pH 6.3 - 6.4.

i For whole carcasses pH values of 6.2 and above are considered to be inferior. For experimental animals, pH 5.8 in *M. l. dorsi* causes discarding of results.

The results show that pH standards for beef carcasses vary considerably and it is clear from the additional commentary that this is mainly due to production and marketing circumstances. There is general agreement on the relation between meat pH and intrinsic characteristics such as darkness, keeping quality and consistency. Values below pH 5.8 are considered normal everywhere. At pH values of 5.8 and 5.9, beef may be rejected on the basis of lower keeping quality (for vacuum packing) and darkening of the fresh meat colour, and is unacceptable for experimental purposes. Nevertheless, only 11 per cent of respondents would actually consider such carcasses to be dark-cutting. Carcasses of pH 6.0, 6.1 and 6.2 are considered dark-cutting by a further 82 per cent of respondents. Marketing difficulties are now encountered, due to deterioration in the quality of the meat, however some outlets are available and disposal is not a major obstacle. Carcasses of pH 6.4 and above are universally rejected and the term 'extreme DFD' is often used. Such meat is unacceptable in most circumstances and may be condemned (e.g. in Belgium and the Netherlands).

There is some suggestion in the results (see Table 6) that carcasses are considered dark-cutting at lower pH values in steer-producing regions than where bulls are produced.

Question: Is there a seasonal effect? If so, please indicate in which months dark-cutting is most likely.

Twenty-six replies were received and the results are shown in Table 7.

TABLE 7
IS THERE A SEASONAL EFFECT?

	Number (per cent) of replies
Yes	14 (54)[1]
No	3 (12)[2]
Don't know	9 (35)[3]

[1] From Australia, New Zealand, Canada, Maryland, Illinois, Missouri, Wyoming, Texas (2), Ireland, France, Norway, Poland (2).

[2] From Oregon, Belgium, Finland.

[3] From South Africa, Britain, Belgium, Denmark, West Germany, Netherlands, Sweden, Czechoslovakia, Bulgaria.

A majority favoured a seasonal effect, although one-third of the respondents were undecided. It is useful to look at the geographical distribution of replies in relation to production practices. Ten of the fourteen affirmatives are from traditional steer-producing regions, while nine of the twelve which were undecided, or against seasonal effect, are regions where bull beef is produced. The expression of a seasonal effect appears to be influenced by production methods. For example, it may be expressed more strongly under extensive systems, where cattle are more exposed to climatic conditions and changes in the availability of feed. Extensive systems are commonly used in steer production but not in the production of young bulls.

Those observing a seasonal effect were asked to indicate in which months dark-cutting is most likely. All except two of the replies came from countries in the northern hemisphere. Results for the northern hemisphere are shown in Table 8.

TABLE 8

MONTHS IN WHICH DARK-CUTTING IS MOST LIKELY TO OCCUR. (RESULTS FOR THE NORTHERN HEMISPHERE).

Month	Number (per cent) of times specified	Month	Number (per cent) of times specified
Jan	4 (33)	Jul	2 (17)
Feb	2 (17)	Aug	1 (8)
Mar	3 (25)	Sep	4 (33)
Apr	6 (50)	Oct	6 (50)
May	2 (17)	Nov	6 (50)
Jun	1 (8)	Dec	4 (33)

The peak periods for dark-cutting are shown to be autumn and winter (September to January, inclusive) and spring (March and April). Seasonal differences between geographical regions would account for some of the spread observed in the data. Two replies received from the southern hemisphere specified seasonal increases in June and July (Australia), August (Australia and New Zealand) and February (New Zealand). Thus, winter is a peak period in the southern hemisphere also, and this was attributed to cold, wet weather. The February increase was thought to relate to drought conditions in late summer. Other reasons put forward to explain the seasonal effect were large daily temperature fluctuations, very hot or cold weather and seasonal changes in feeding.

Please suggest three causes of dark-cutting in your country in order of importance.

Twenty-six replies were received with a total of seventy-seven causes. These fall into six general categories which are shown in Table 9. The most frequently cited category is the pre-slaughter management of cattle. This category is subdivided into more specific areas in Table 10.

TABLE 9

CAUSES OF DARK-CUTTING IN BEEF

Category	Number of times specified	Number (per cent) times specified as the primary cause
Management before slaughter	39	19 (70)
Climate	10	3 (11)
Nutrition	11	1 (4)
Pathological or related conditions	8	0
Heredity	6	1 (4)
Stress (unspecified)	3	3 (11)

TABLE 10

SUBDIVISION OF PRE-SLAUGHTER MANAGEMENT INTO MORE SPECIFIC PROBLEM AREAS. (The number of times each area was specified as a cause of dark-cutting is shown, with the number of times specified as a primary cause in parenthesis).

FARM

↓

'HANDLING' 8 (4)

TRANSPORT 12 (5)

SALEYARD 1

PENNING { in mixed lots 12 (8); overlong 5 (2); air/water 1 }

ABATTOIR

Most of the problems at pre-slaughter are associated with penning procedures. The main problem here concerns mixing separate lots of cattle together. This was usually, but not always, with reference to young bulls (eight out of twelve citations).

Another closely related penning problem concerns the length of time cattle are held before slaughter. These two causes ('time' and 'mixing' in pens) are not independent, as dark-cutting resulting from mixing is clearly time-dependent. Concern about length of time in pens came from countries with substantial production of bull beef*. Overnight or weekend penning was generally considered to be unsuitable, and more than two hours in pens was considered unsuitable for young bulls in West Germany. Inadequate air and water supplies to pens were suggested as causes in Finland.

Problems with transport were specified as overlong distances or times in transit, bad conditions during transport and insufficient recovery time after transport. Replies citing transport were of general origin and came from all major geographical regions covered by the survey.

Bad handling of slaughter stock was also frequently cited. This is a general term which includes herding, loading, transport, unloading, penning and slaughter of cattle.

Climate was cited ten times** as a cause of dark-cutting in beef, including three times as the primary cause (Table 9). Most of these respondents also reported a seasonal effect (see Table 7) and came mainly from steer-producing regions. The specific climatic features mentioned here again are inclement weather, large daily temperature fluctuations and excessively hot or cold environmental temperatures.

* From West Germany, Denmark, Sweden, Norway, Yugoslavia.

** These replies originated from Australia, New Zealand, Illinois, Missouri, Wyoming, Texas (2), Belgium, France and Poland.

An inadequate plane of nutrition was cited as a causative factor four times*. Inadequate feeding or prolonged fasting during the immediate pre-slaughter period was also cited four times**. Wrong feeding and seasonal changes in feed were cited twice in replies from Poland. Forage-fed cattle were observed to have the highest incidence of dark-cutting (in Texas). It was, however, suggested that this could be because they are not accustomed to being handled.

Pathological conditions (disease and fever) were cited twice. Also included under this heading in Table 9 are exhaustion (cited twice), hormonal imbalance, trauma and inadequate hygiene/tendering on the farm.

Genetic factors consisted of breed (cited four times) and temperament (cited twice, including once as the primary cause).

Question: What do you think are the main objections to dark-cutting in beef?

Twenty-seven replies were received and the results are shown in Table 11.

TABLE 11

MAIN OBJECTIONS TO DARK-CUTTING. RESULTS ARE SHOWN AS THE NUMBER (PER CENT) OF REPLIES RECEIVED.

Characteristic	Very Important	Important	Not Important
Dark colour	19 (70)	6 (22)	2 (7)
Faster spoilage	13 (48)	9 (33)	4 (15)
Firm dry consistency	0	12 (44)	10 (37)
Other	2 (7)	2 (7)	2 (7)

* New Zealand, Canada, Ireland and Yugoslavia.

** Illinois, Wyoming, Texas, West Germany.

Colour and spoilage are the main objections to dark-cutting in beef. It is of interest that seven replies, all from Europe, rated spoilage at a higher level of importance than dark colour. Some other respondents did not recognise spoilage as a problem with DFD meat.

The consistency of DFD meat rated as a much less important objection than colour or keeping quality. Other objections which were mentioned concern the organoleptic and technological properties of DFD; it is tasteless or of abnormal taste, is usually very tender although not in the same way as with normal meat, is unacceptable for curing or drying, is difficult to brown during frying and is of abnormal appearance and stickiness.

Question: Is there an economic penalty for dark-cutting beef at any stage in the marketing chain?

An economic penalty was reported by a majority of respondents (Table 12), including all those from North America and EEC countries.

TABLE 12

IS THERE AN ECONOMIC PENALTY?

	Number (per cent) of replies
Yes	18 (69)
No	6 (23)
Don't know	2 (8)

Affirmatives were then asked to quantify the economic loss relative to a normal carcass or meat cut. The results are shown in Table 13. These data indicate that monetary losses are usually incurred and are quite substantial. Comments received and reproduced as footnotes to Table 13 indicate that the magnitude of losses is determined by processing and marketing factors.

TABLE 13

PER CENT ECONOMIC LOSS ATTRIBUTABLE TO DARK-CUTTING

Per cent loss	Number of replies
10	11[a]
20	4[b]
30	2[c]
40, 50	0
(Other)	3[d]

[a] From Australia[1], Canada[2], Maryland, Missouri[3], Texas, Oregon[4], Belgium, Finland, France[5], Ireland[6], Yugoslavia[7].

[b] From Missouri[3], Wyoming, Denmark[8], France[5].

[c] From Illinois, France[5].

[d] From Texas[9], Belgium[10], Netherlands[11].

[1] Probably 20 per cent if the meat is destined for the vacuum-pack export trade.

[2] Loss estimated at 7 per cent.

[3] Loss estimated at 10 - 20 per cent.

[4] Can be sold to institutional trade with very little loss but normal retail distribution causes problems.

[5] The economic loss is very variable according to how the carcass is used, and ranges from 10 - 30 per cent.

[6] The price penalty for dark muscling in Irish beef on the British market was estimated at 6.2 per cent of the ex wholesale price. In other markets losses vary from 0 - 30 per cent.

[7] The economic loss is > 10 per cent.

[8] In some rare cases the penalty can amount to a loss of approximately 20 per cent.

[9] Economic loss depends on how the carcass is disposed of.

[10] The consumer does not accept this meat and it cannot be sold. The economic loss depends on the circumstances. For fresh meat it is up to 100 per cent. It is a reason for condemnation of the meat.

[11] The economic penalty may vary, depending on the decision at meat inspection. The penalty is usually covered by the insurance.

Question: Is there a down-grading of dark-cutting carcasses on a national, regional or local classification or grading scheme?

Twenty-six replies were received and the results are shown in Table 14.

TABLE 14

DOES DOWN-GRADING OCCUR?

	Number (per cent) of replies
Yes	12 (46)[a]
No	14 (54)[b]
Don't know	0

[a] From Australia (Queensland), Canada, Maryland, Missouri, Wyoming, Texas (2), Oregon, Denmark, Finland, Yugoslavia, Bulgaria.

[b] From New Zealand, South Africa, Illinois, Belgium (2), Britain, France, West Germany, Ireland, Netherlands, Norway, Sweden, Czechoslovakia.

The practice of down-grading is most common in North America and is practically absent in the EEC countries.

Question: Are there other economic consequences?

Twelve respondents supplied additional information, which is listed in Table 15.

TABLE 15

ADDITIONAL ECONOMIC CONSEQUENCES

1. DFD beef may be rejected at:-
    - meat inspection
    - vacuum-packing (or unpacking)
    - wholesale
    - export
    - retail (supermarkets)
    - retail (vacuum packs)
2. Possible loss of reputation for the production of high quality beef.
3. Limitations on use of the product; disposal of expensive cuts as sausage meat; cost of substituting normal meat to fill orders.
4. Grading of carcasses on the basis of ultimate pH tends to down-grade non-affected cuts, introducing further losses.

DISCUSSION

<u>Lis Buchter</u> *(Denmark)*

I would like to refer to pathology and DFD. The animals which we receive and measure at the slaughterhouse have already passed veterinary inspection. This may include measurement of ultimate pH as one of the determinants of whether or not the meat is acceptable for human consumption. You found that pathological conditions were never specified as primary causes of DFD, but I feel that this is because the carcasses of diseased animals have already been taken out by the time we look at the animals.

<u>P.V. Tarrant</u> *(Ireland)*

That it a very good point. Although pathological or related conditions were not considered to be primary causes of DFD they were nevertheless quoted eight times as causes of DFD (see Table 9). These conditions included disease, fever, exhaustion, trauma and others. I agree that many carcasses affected by pathological conditions may be taken from the slaughter line and are therefore not available when ultimate pH is measured for quality control or research purposes. Consequently the incidence of DFD meat in condemned or partly condemned carcasses is not known.

<u>E. Dransfield</u> *(UK)*

Can you indicate what kind of institute or laboratory or slaughterhouse answered the questions? Were questionnaires given to research institutes, industry, abattoirs or veterinary officers?

<u>P.V. Tarrant</u>

In all cases the questionnaires were sent to senior scientists in meat research establishments. These included national meat research institutes, universities and meat industry laboratories. The response was excellent, indicating a high degree of interest in the problem, and replies were received from all but one of the countries circulated. Of 37 questionnaires distributed, 27 were completed satisfactorily and were used to compile the results. All sources of information are acknowledged at the end of the paper.

D.E. Hood *(Ireland)*

Do the results enable you to define DFD?

P.V. Tarrant

The term DFD is used to describe meat which has a value of ultimate pH which is higher than normal. The dark cutting conditions worsens progressively with increasing value of ultimate pH. The actual pH value at which meat is defined as DFD is determined by the particular muscle, type of animal (i.e. young or old) and also by the nature of the product and the marketing circumstances. In the present survey no respondents considered values below pH 5.8 to be abnormal and all respondents considered values above 6.3 to be DFD.

BEEF QUALITY, MARKETING AND THE CONSUMER

B.L. Dumont
Laboratoire de Recherches sur la viande de l'INRA,
CNRZ, 78350 Jouy-en-Josas, France.

ABSTRACT

This paper deals with the marketing consequences which arise from the heterogeneous nature of beef. 'Nature' and 'value' quality are distinguished as contributory attributes to overall acceptability. The major quality traits, colour and tenderness and their interaction with consumer attitudes are discussed. The future of beef marketing is discussed with reference to the improvement of beef quality.

INTRODUCTION

Meat which issues from cattle production - and which for ease of reference appears in the list of food products under the simple name of 'beef' - is a very heterogeneous product.

It is very heterogeneous firstly because the original material it comes from, namely the cattle, is itself heterogeneous. Cattle production consists of animals of different sex, from breeds of different purposes (milk or meat, or both), different physiological maturity and different size, which are sent to be slaughtered at different ages and after very different nutritional treatments.

In each animal heterogeneity is marked by the existence of more than 200 butchering muscles, each of them having a particular structure and composition in relation to the specific role it plays in the mobility and posture of the whole body.

Beef is the product which results from the transformation each muscle undergoes during the different operations of meat processing. These operations are also very variable. This variety of treatments acting on a heterogeneous material results in a product of an extremely diversified nature. Beef is thus a simple name which covers a very complex product.

Use made of beef by people is also variable, with respect to:

- type of cooking or processing;
- time in storage;
- eating places;
- retail outlets.

Table 1 gives a survey of the main situations which apply in each case.

From these introductory remarks it is clear that beef quality cannot be considered to be a simple question.

TABLE 1

VARIETY IN BEEF USE

Type of use	Time of storage	Consumption place	Purchase place
Intact meat for - grilling (at various - roasting internal temperatures) - braising - boiling	Variable, in fresh	- Individual (home)	Butcher's shop
Processed meats - Fresh meat ground or minced (with different ingredients) - Processed meats, such as sausages etc. - Corned beef etc.	or frozen state	- Collective (different types)	Self-service Supermarket Hypermarket

BEEF QUALITY

It is always difficult to talk about quality of products in general and especially about food quality. The first reason is that the word quality has many meanings; it can be considered in at least two ways. Firstly, the broad meaning of quality of anything depends on its intrinsic nature. Quality is collectively all the attributes which make a thing (or any object or any food) what it is. Quality, in this sense, may be precisely expressed by the values of the different traits which describe the object. This first definition of quality thus corresponds to 'nature' quality.

Most of the traits can be objectively measured so that 'nature' quality has an absolute value. In the case of beef, quality will include various traits such as colour, tenderness or fat content, etc. Each of them may be assessed by specific methods, e.g. by EEC recommended procedures for colour (McDougall, 1978) or tenderness (Joseph, 1978). From all the data obtained by assessing a sample of beef one may produce an 'identity card' for that sample which clearly shows to any experienced person the quality level of the meat. Table 2 gives examples of such a definition of beef 'nature' quality.

The meaning of the word quality referred to in discussing 'nature' quality is, however, not the most usual nor the one generally accepted by consumers. More commonly, quality is what makes a product more or less pleasant, more or less acceptable. From the consumer's point of view quality, which is basically a quantitative notion, becomes a qualitative one. For consumers, quality is linked with personal satisfaction and then as defined long ago by Hammond, quality is what consumers like best.

It is clear that what makes a product more or less satisfactory must take price into account. It seems that for most consumers - who have a limited amount of money - the price intervenes to determine the acceptability of the product. This second definition thus corresponds to 'value' quality. Such a quality is very relative because it is expressed according to a reference system for each individual. To a large extent this 'value' quality is also subjectively defined.

TABLE 2

IDENTIFICATION OF THE 'NATURE' QUALITY OF BEEF SAMPLES A AND B

Trait	Beef samples	
	A	B
Warner-Bratzler Shear-force (N)	55.1	41.1
Haem iron (μg/g)	11.6	14.3
Lipid (per cent)	3.2	5.3
pH	5.60	5.90
Water loss (Press method, per cent)	19.3	17.4

Quality factors in beef

The meaning given (unconsciously) by consumers to quality has a major economic importance because it explains the consumer's attitudes toward each product. In fact, the trade is governed by the quality of products, and precisely by the triplet: amount/quality/price.

In the case of beef a large number of traits must be considered as quality factors, acting more or less strongly on the consumer to determine first his acceptance of the meat and then his degree of satisfaction (Table 3).

TABLE 3

BEEF QUALITY TRAITS

Quality on display Quality on cooking	- Hygienic quality - Convenience aspect of the food - Amount of wastes (fat in excess) - Freshness - Eating qualities of the meat suggested by general appearance, colour, lean/fat ratio, texture etc - Shelf-life, keeping quality on domestic storage - Drip on cooking, weight loss
Quality for the eater	- Texture, tenderness - Flavour - Juiciness - Colour

The characteristics consumers are interested in, or that they can assess, largely depend on the type of beef they are using. Thus all the attributes of fresh raw meat need not be considered when buying processed meat. It is evident that texture has not the same importance in intact muscles and in ground meat. The number of quality traits is clearly higher when beef is sold as large pieces of fresh muscles.

With regard to beef quality the consumer often has two faces or is a 'double-person'. The first individual is judging quality on display and on cooking, the other is tasting meat on the plate, as a beef-eater.

Table 3 gives the list of traits to be considered as general quality traits in the case of beef meat.

The importance of colour and tenderness

According to Rhodes (1978) very little can be deduced about the eating quality of meat from visual examination of the raw portion on display. One cannot but agree with this opinion and might add that it largely depends on the skill of the observer. Nevertheless, colour has been and still is a very important factor in beef marketing. The importance of colour as an indicator of 'freshness' is probably overestimated in the consumer's mind, because it has been clearly established (see e.g. Billault et al., 1973) that there is no clear relation between colour defects and meat spoilage. Even though colour of lean is an irrational basis for consumer preference, it still remains, as pointed out by Hood (1978) that: "The psychological attractiveness of the bright-red colour makes it a fundamental criterion".

More and more consumers use their own experience to decide exactly what freshness is when they keep their beef at home in a domestic refrigerator. Habits of buying all the meat they need once a week may cause some problems due to inadequate conditions of domestic storage. For this reason, as well as for other considerations, the level of microbial contamination at the time of sale is an important quality trait. Even though the eating qualities of cooked meat are appreciated first through overall visual and olfactory impressions of the piece of beef, colour and odour seem to be of relatively minor importance, mainly because they are at least satisfactory in most cases.

Tenderness is by far the most important criterion of beef. It is only if tenderness is satisfactory that any judgement about flavour and juiciness need be performed. Tenderness is without doubt the key; it is the limiting factor in the eating quality of beef (Dumont, 1952).

THE CONSUMER

According to Baron and Carpenter (1976), who completely reviewed consumer attitudes and requirements for meat, any study in this field "must presuppose a theory or model of demand or consumer behaviour". In its simplest presentation, the hierarchy of events leading to consumption of a particular product "would separate the action into three components:

1) a need or desire to consume meat
2) the actual purchase of the meat
3) the eating of the meat".

All three components are related to beef quality.

The attitudes of consumers towards beef depend on economic considerations, psycho-physiological factors and socio-economic events.

The buyer and the eater

Dealing with consumer attitudes, tastes and preferences we must be careful in our conclusions drawn from a general economic analysis of the market. There is not necessarily a close relationship between level of consumption and true satisfaction of consumers. Economic pressures from various origins may more or less completely hide the basic trend of consumption which exists among consumers. It is clear that for a part of the population (the percentage is probably slightly different from one country to another) one cannot deduce the tastes and the preferences of consumers (i.e. of the eaters) from their buying habits (Dumont, 1979). As previously indicated the consumer is a 'double-person': the 'buyer' always precedes the 'eater'.

The world of consumers

In every country, all the people, together with their dogs and cats, represent the consumers. However, the consumer as an individual cannot be given an accurate definition. Even though each consumer is an individual being, with particular tastes and preferences, the only way we have to describe him is a statistical one.

Fortunately or otherwise, everyone is different in many aspects of his personality. In the field of psychology, and more specifically in sensory physiology, we thus observe a large range of reactions and sensitivity. In terms of beef quality this means that we may expect to find a great variety among consumers' reactions and opinions.

The great variety existing among beef consumers may be roughly demonstrated by the existence of the different types of cattle which are produced and used in the EEC: all the beef produced is consumed. This variation can be experimentally shown from studies where consumers are given samples of beef of the same cut prepared in the same way (Table 4). Whatever the variety found among consumers one must exphasise that there is a very strong general tendency for most consumers to seek a known quality each time a specific product is bought (Buchter, 1977).

Socio-economic factors

Today there are also changes in quality demands from consumers due to socio-economic factors such as:

- housewives engaged in paid activity outside the home and having less time to spend on cooking;
- housewives (and men, specially the young) having less skills or desire to spend time on cooking;
- growth in freezer ownership;
- more meat bought in self-service (super- and hypermarket).

Consumers' reactions; statistical definition of quality levels

On a given market, acceptability of one piece of beef may be reflected, in statistical terms, by the percentage of consumers satisfied or not by that type of beef. One classical

TABLE 4

VARIATION IN CONSUMERS' TASTE

Tenderness score	10	9	8	7	6	5	4	3	2	1
A			3	8	1	4	2			
B	1		3	1	5	2	2	4		
C	2		6	3	1	2	1	2		1
D		3	2	1	2	5	3	2		
Juiciness score	**10**	**9**	**8**	**7**	**6**	**5**	**4**	**3**	**2**	**1**
A			2	7	5	3		1		
B	1	2	2	2		6	1	2	2	
C	1	1	6	5	1	1	1	1	1	
D	1	4	2	4	3	2		1	1	
Flavour score	**10**	**9**	**8**	**7**	**6**	**5**	**4**	**3**	**2**	**1**
A				2	2	6	4	4		
B			2	1	5	5	1	2	2	
C			2	3	3	5	3	2		
D		2		3	6	2		2	2	1

Four cuts of beef (A, B, C and D) were judged by a consumer panel of 18 persons for tenderness, juiciness and flavour (on a ten-point scale; 1 = poorest and 10 = best) (Dumont, 1979).

example in this field is that of consumer reaction to discoloured pre-packaged beef, studied in Dublin supermarkets by Hood and Riordan (1973) (Figure 1). Table 5 gives another example of statistical definition of quality level by eater consumers, in this case on the tenderness of different muscles.

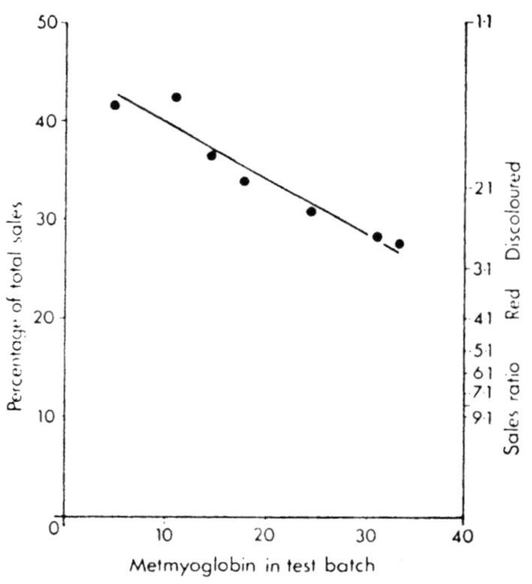

Fig. 1. Comparison of sales of round steak discoloured to various extents against bright red meat as control. (Source: Hood and Riordan, 1973).

It is <u>theoretically</u> possible to plot percentage of increased satisfaction for each quality trait in any consumer population against the variation of the objective measurement of that trait. Figure 2a illustrates a possible suggested relation between both.

Below a minimum level of quality (Q_o) the product is completely discarded by consumers and the percentage of satisfied people is nil. At the opposite end, at a level Q_m, every consumer is highly satisfied with the sample. Any further increase in quality traits does not change consumer acceptability.

TABLE 5

OPINION (AFTER EATING) ON THE USE OF DIFFERENT MUSCLES AS STEAKS

Muscle	Percentage of opinions considering tenderness as satisfactory	Percentage of opinions considering the sample as acceptable steak
M. triceps brachii caput laterale	20.7	31.0
M. extensor carpi radialis	62.1	44.8
M. semispinalis capitis	71.4	78.6
M. latissimus dorsi	51.7	58.6
M. pectoralis ascendeus (tender portion)	75.9	75.9
M. pectoralis ascendeus (tough portion)	31.0	48.3
M. rhomboideus	31.0	41.4
M. infraspinatus	96.4	100.0
M. splenius	60.7	64.3
M. supraspinatus	76.7	82.8
M. transversus abdominis	43.3	60.0
M. longissimus dorsi	88.0	92.3

(Source: Billault et al., 1970)

Figure 2b presents another possible relation between 'nature' quality and 'value' quality when an optimum level of 'nature' quality exists.

An accurate knowledge of the parameters of this curve 'value' quality/'nature' quality for different traits in different markets should greatly help us to understand what exactly consumer demand is in relation to beef quality in different countries. Such studies will sometimes be difficult to realise due to the heterogeneous nature of meat, which limits the amount of meat which can be distributed to consumers and thus limits the size of the sample of consumers who could be included in any experiment or survey.

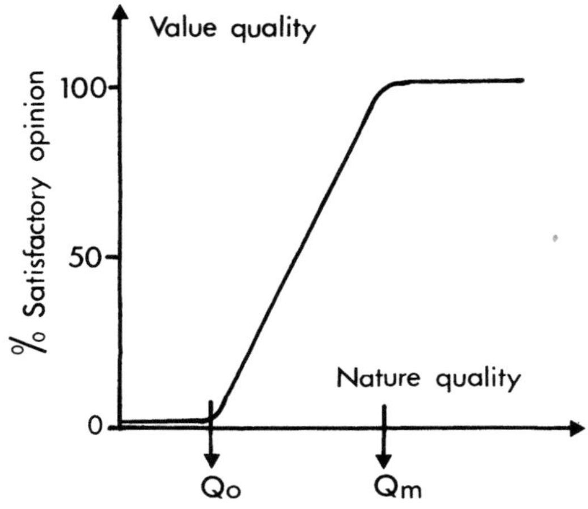

Fig. 2a. Relationship between 'nature' quality and 'value' quality: linear relation between both.

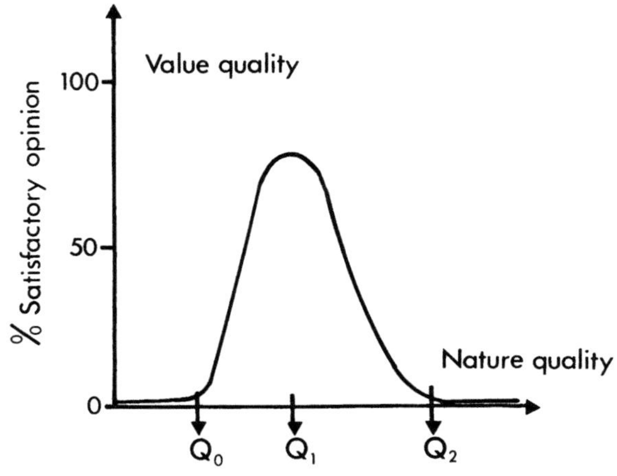

Fig. 2b. Relationship between 'nature' quality and 'value' quality: optimum level of quality.

A consumer survey must be conducted so that selection procedures ensure that they are representative of the population. For this reason a consumer survey is quite different from a laboratory panel using a small group of selected individuals.

Although such laboratory panels can be satisfactorily used to measure quality traits in a quantitative way (i.e. to measure 'nature' quality) they cannot be used to measure consumer attitudes and requirements.

BEEF MARKETING

The purchase of meat

As previously indicated, beef is now sold in many different ways, either by individual retailers, through specialist service butchers' shops, or in self-service outlets, mainly through supermarkets and hypermarkets. Wherever beef is purchased, one must consider that the selling of meat is not only an economic operation; it is also an integral part of the whole processing operation which starts with the departure of live animals from their production farms and ends when consumers have bought their meat.

The presentation of meat for purchase is a very important step. In this respect there is considerable difference between cutting in a butcher's shop for immediate sale and a centralised packaging operation where cutting is carried out some hours, or longer, before exposure for purchase. Discolouration is then especially feared due to the discrimination of consumers against it. It is also feared because the prevailing conditions in prepackaging predispose meat to oxidation, and this is often made worse by the poor temperature control in retail display cabinets.

The difference between the two methods of presentation is not only limited to the problem of colour freshness. The disappearance of the butcher means also the disappearance of advice, service and reassurance. One may suppose that consumers need such information for beef more than other types of meat because the range of different cuts is greater and their culinary uses more numerous.

In the case of prepackaged meats consumers strongly demand maximum information concerning culinary and cooking uses (Rose, 1977). The butcher can cut the piece of beef according to the weight and size required by the consumer. There is also an opportunity for dialogue between seller and buyer which is important and fruitful to both.

The future for beef marketing

To maintain and if possible to increase the demand for beef against an increasing range of pleasant, convenient, nutritious and often cheaper products it is necessary to market consumer cuts in a form that maximises convenience and guarantees the required level of quality, particularly tenderness and flavour.

Maximising convenience concerns especially those cuts or muscles which need a lot of preparation time and a large amount of skill in cooking. The meat processing industry everywhere still has a lot to do in order to satisfy the main consumer requirement for more convenience in beef.

Guarantees of quality could be considered as some protection for consumers who do not always find all the satisfaction they are looking for in the beef they eat. We can sometimes speak of consumer 'frustration' (Rhodes, 1978) which mainly stems from the fact that there is an apparently unpredictable variability in eating quality. Many people hope that meat can be sold with declarations of eating quality characteristics. Guarantees on the different quality traits of beef (Table 3) are necessary for any real marketing of beef, if one considers that marketing also means commercial strategy.

Marketing comprises the whole range of study, research and activities needed to promote a product under the best conditions. Study of the market is a very important step. In the case of beef such a study must include not only economic and statistical enquiries about consumer attitudes and requirements, but also consumers' tastes and preferences based on real purchase and real eating patterns. Such studies are necessary to define the goal to be attained; it will be determined in each case by some specific value of a 'nature' quality trait (Figure 2). The overall acceptability of the beef must also be determined from studies of the relative importance of each factor in the definition of overall quality (Figure 3).

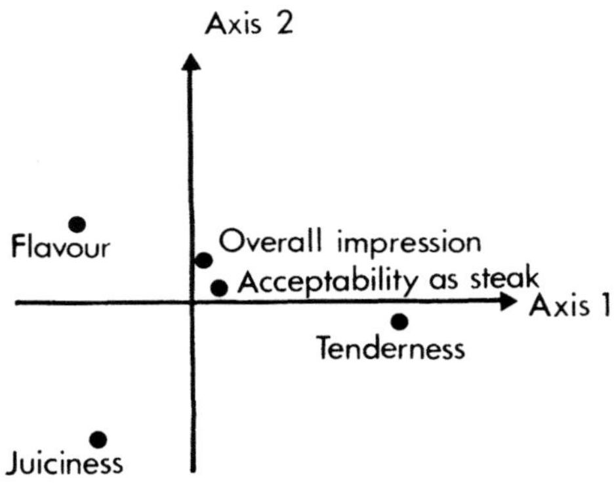

Fig. 3. Multivariate analysis of beef quality

The relative influence of tenderness, juiciness and flavour on overall impression and acceptability as steaks of beef samples have been studied by factorial analysis of correspondence. Results for acceptability and overall impression are very similar and can be considered as closely related. Both these characteristics are influenced in a rather similar way by tenderness, flavour and juiciness.
(Source: Dumont, work in progress)

Promotion and publicity are also important aspects of marketing. In this field a declaration of the quality traits of the product becomes a necessity. Some of these traits, like colour and marbling, may be directly observed by the consumer and just need some decisive additional comment. For other traits the seller may give more information derived either from objective measurements made on the product or from what is known about its history, the origin of the animal and processing of the meat.

At the moment such information is not easily available or accurate. Identification of the type of cut (even given in an anatomical way) is merely a gross indication about culinary use and recommended method of cooking. Even if it is known, the history of the animal (sex, age, breed etc.) does not offer much help due to the large variability between beef cattle of similar origin in their different quality traits, especially tenderness (Dumont, 1979; Dumont and Colleau, 1978).

In addition, meat characteristics are influenced to a great extent by slaughtering and processing procedures, so that any original quality is more or less changed during processing and only the processor knows what it was. As indicated by Rhodes (1978), the housewife complains to her retailer after she has paid for a high priced cut if she receives tough and unappetising beef instead of superior eating quality. But "she cannot obtain any satisfactory explanation because, in most cases, the retailer has no information or knowledge about the meat he has sold. Nor is it often possible for the retailer to pass the information about the product back to earlier sections of the industry because the identity of the carcass is lost in the abattoir. This situation leads to frustration in the mind of the consumer and to the rather poor image of beef that she has".

Ways of improvement

From these remarks it is clear that one can try to develop beef marketing only if good information is available and when there is strict supervision of the different factors concerned with the breeding, fattening and slaughtering of the animal; chilling and processing of the carcass.

With regard to beef quality it is specially necessary to supervise

- transport from farm to slaughter,
- slaughtering process,
- rate of chilling,
- full ageing period.

In a general way one may also suppose that we must adopt a specific technology for different cuts adapted according to their specific textural, biophysical and biochemical characteristics. The diversity of the raw material which is the whole musculature of cattle must be taken into consideration to get the best from each muscle.

In the future improvement of beef marketing will oblige meat industry people to have closer contact with the final consumer. They will also have to respect the basic principles involved in preserving meat against microbial contamination, meat toughening and discolouration. At our present state of knowledge, partial success can be achieved and it is now possible to sell beef of a rather good level of quality. Further improvements are necessary in many fields of meat processing and equipment (e.g. to improve tenderness, to develop more convenient food, etc.). But one may ask whether the major part of the improvement must not be found at first in cattle, where the double problem is to raise the general level of quality and to reduce the variability found between animals. This last point may be of the utmost importance for selling beef in hyper- or supermarkets where homogeneity of products is demanded. This is also important for marketing in general, since consistency in supply is the basis of consumer satisfaction.

CONCLUSIONS

Breeders are also directly concerned in the improvement of beef quality. The main objective in beef production has been said to maximise the efficiency of converting the available resources into lean meat. As pointed out by Cuthbertson and Harrington (1977), for each type of cattle there is an optimum point of growth under a particular system of production, at which the lean meat is produced at least unit cost. This cost is associated with a certain weight of fat and bone. Evidently it is also associated with a certain level of quality for colour, tenderness, juiciness etc. If any change from that quality level is proposed to meet consumers' requirements, there will be a correlated change in the cost of lean which will influence the final price of beef. This economic aspect of quality has always to be considered in any general programme of improvement of beef quality by breeding or feeding. The same consideration has also to be made with improvement through slaughtering and processing.

On this problem it is fundamental to bear in mind that everything invested to improve the conditions of production and processing has to be recovered on the selling price, often from only a limited part of the carcass.

REFERENCES

Baron, P.J. and Carpenter, E.M., 1976. A review of consumer attitudes and requirements for meat. University of Newcastle-Upon-Tyne, Department of agricultural marketing, report no. 23.

Billault, J., Dumont, B.L. and Le Guelte, P., 1970. Observations sur l'aptitude à l'emploi de différents muscles de jeunes bovins de races à viande. Laboratoire de recherches sur la viande de l'INRA. Bull. Techn. no. 6.

Billault, J., Drieux, H., Dumont, B.L. and Perron, P., 1973. Note sur la liaison existant entre l'aspect macroscopique (coloration) et la pollution microbienne. Rec. Méd. Vét., 149 (2): 27-34.

Buchter, L., 1977. Possibilities for fulfilling trade and consumer requirements for meat quality in present and future beef production systems. In: Patterns of growth and development in cattle. CEC Seminar, Ghent, October 11 - 13, 1977. Current topics in veterinary medicine, 2: 579-588. Martinus Nijhoff (Ed.), The Hague, 1978.

Cuthbertson, A. and Harrington, G., 1977. Targets for beef production in relation to market and consumer requirements. In: Patterns of growth and development in cattle. CEC Seminar, Ghent, October 11 - 13, 1977. Current topics in veterinary medicine and animal science, 2: 588-601. Martinus Nijhoff (Ed.), The Hague, 1978.

MacDougall, D.B., 1978. Recommended procedures for use in the measurement of meat colour. In: The future of beef production in the European community. CEC Seminar, Abano Terme, Italy, Nov. 13 - 17, 1978. Current topics in veterinary medicine and animal science, 5: 607-613. Martinus Nijhoff (Ed.), The Hague, 1979.

Dumont, B.L., 1952. La tendreté de la viande. Ann. Zootech., 1: 71-95.

Dumont, B.L., 1979. Problèmes posés par la définition et l'appréciation des qualités de la viande de boeuf. Cah. Nutr. Diétét., 14 (3): 167-179.

Dumont, B.L. and Colleau, J.J., 1978. Relations entre la qualité des carcasses et les variations intra-race du potentiel laitier des taurillons. XXIV Eur. Meet. Meat Res. Workers, Kulmbach, Germany, 4 - 8 Sept., 1978.

Hood, D.E., 1978. Technical developments in wholesaling and retailing to meet consumer demands. In: The future of beef production in the European community. CEC Seminar, Abano Terme, Italy, Nov. 13 - 17, 1978. Current topics in veterinary medicine and animal science, 5: 90-100. Martinus Nijhoff (Ed.), The Hague, 1978.

Hood, D.E. and Riordan, E.B., 1973. Discolouration in prepackaged beef: measurement by reflectance spectrophotometry and shopper discrimination. J. Fd. Technol., 8: 333-343.

Joseph, R.L., 1978. Recommended method for assessment of tenderness. In: The future of beef production in the European community. CEC Seminar, Abano Terme, Italy, Nov. 13 - 17, 1978. Current topics in veterinary medicine and animal science, 5: 596-606. Martinus Nijhoff (Ed.), The Hague, 1979.

Rhodes, D.N., 1978. Meat quality and the consumer in the future of beef production in the European community. CEC Seminar, Abano Terme, Italy, Nov. 13 - 17, 1978. Current topics in veterinary medicine and animal science, 5: 79-89. Martinus Nijhoff (Ed.), The Hague, 1979.

Rose, E., 1977. Le point de vue du consommateur sur la commercialisation de la viande bovine. Pour une filière viande bovine plus efficace. Symposium Paris, Jan. 10 - 13, 1977. Marchés et produits agricoles. OCDE - Paris, 1977.

DISCUSSION

J. Wismer-Pedersen *(Denmark)*

Thank you, Dr. Dumont, for your very interesting paper on a question which concerns us all: the question of what we mean by meat quality.

I was very interested in your conception of 'nature' quality and 'value' quality. However, will the relationship between them not vary according to the gastronomic traditions of different consumer groups?

B.L. Dumont *(France)*

I think so. Our laboratory is in rather a good position to compare opinions about aspects of quality, such as the acceptable level of tenderness. We have many visitors from all over the world; we can arrange to give them samples and compare their reactions. Under these conditions, we find there is a very wide variation in the acceptable level of tenderness. For instance, the acceptable level of meat tenderness for an American meat research worker is different to that of an Argentinian or Russian meat research worker.

There is a difference of opinion about meat quality around the world. If you look at my Figure 2a, it represents the percentage of satisfaction inside a geographic group - within one country - and even within a certain age group. If we experimented with different types of people, there would be a similar shape, but the value of Qo and Qm would not be the same. This is very important.

I feel there is a very large difference between purchasing meat in a butcher's shop and the supermarket. As I said in my report, when the function of the butcher is suppressed, many other things are suppressed also, both problems and advantages. The advantage of butchers in the meat industry is that, knowing the consumer, he can give each one the cut most suited to him/her.

The best cut for me may not be the best cut for you. However, in the supermarket one is obliged to accept an average quality. This is a problem for the supermarket, but the butcher does not have the same type of problem because among his consumers he can probably find someone who will accept some tough muscle as well as those who will accept only very tender muscle.

E. Dransfield *(UK)*

The meat quality group of the EEC is currently studying this in connection with the beef coordination programme. Meat samples from the same carcasses were sent to different institutes to be assessed in their different laboratories. The findings were that basically each institute, in the different EEC countries, came to a decision about overall quality in a similar way. Judgement was mainly on tenderness or texture, with flavour and juiciness playing a smaller part. In general, they came to a similar decision about overall eating quality despite using very different methods of preparation. For instance, cooking in France is much less than in the UK, but, given the same piece of meat, they came to a similar decision.

B.L. Dumont

I do not think this would be true if you considered a greater range of people, especially people who are used to eating meat only a very short time after slaughter - people who are accustomed to eating meat that has not aged, as is the case with many people in South America. They accept less tender meat than Americans and Europeans.

E. Dransfield

This was considered in the experiment insofar as the samples tasted by the five participating countries came from each of eight European countries. These eight countries sent meat which they felt to be typical of their meat production - their local consumption. Therefore, this included the variation that would be present at local level.

SESSION II

MUSCLE METABOLISM AND ANIMAL PHYSIOLOGY

Chairman: J. Wismer-Pedersen

MUSCLE METABOLIC TYPE AND THE DFD CONDITION

G. Monin

Station de Recherches sur la Viande,
INRA Theix, 63110 Beaumont, France.

ABSTRACT

This paper examines the relationships between metabolic or contractile types and muscle reaction to stress, as related to the DFD condition in carcasses of ruminants (sheep and cattle). Results discussed here originate principally from research work carried out at INRA for some years with respect to ovine muscle, and from the literature with respect to bovine muscle.

INTRODUCTION

Meat quality is related to both the intrinsic characteristics of muscles in the living animal and the treatments experienced by the animals and carcasses during the slaughter process. This is clearly illustrated in the dark-firm-dry (DFD) or dark-cutting (DC) meat condition: this condition results mainly from preslaughter stress, and it manifests itself with high inter-muscle variability (Tarrant, 1976; Sornay and Legras, 1978).

Stress induces hormonal changes in living animals; the effects of these on the tissues largely vary with the metabolic characteristics of the latter. Skeletal muscles exhibit a wide range of metabolic activities, which therefore influence their reaction to stress (see Lister, 1979). Metabolic activities - glycolytic or oxidative - define the so-called metabolic type of muscles (white or red); speed of contraction, reflected in myofibrillar ATPase activity, defines the contractile type (slow-twitch or fast-twitch). This paper examines the relationships between metabolic or contractile types and muscle reaction to stress, as related to the DFD condition in carcases of ruminants (sheep and cattle). Results discussed here originate principally from research work carried out at INRA for some years with respect to ovine muscle, and from the literature with respect to bovine muscle.

I - DEFINITION OF MUSCLE METABOLIC TYPE

For many years, it has been known that there are different metabolic types of muscles (Ranvier, 1874). However this concept has become really clear only during the past ten years. Most muscles are composed of fibres of various types, associated in variable proportions. The number of existing metabolic types varies according to different authors. As far as we are concerned, we accept the classification proposed by Ashmore and Doerr (1971). According to these authors, there are two basic fibre types: α fibres, i.e. fast-twitch fibres with high glycolytic activity, and β fibres, i.e. slow-twitch fibres with low glycolytic activity. α fibres contain variable oxidative activity, which allows a distinction between α white (αW) fibres with low oxidative capacity, and α red (αR) with high oxidative capacity, although there is really a continuum in oxidative activities between αR and αW fibres. β fibres always contain intermediate or high oxidative activities and are therefore called βR. In our opinion this classification takes better account of the continuum in metabolic activities within α fibres than the three group classification of Peter et al. (1972): fast-twitch glycolytic, fast-twitch oxidative glycolytic and slow-twitch oxidative myofibres. Of course the two classifications are very similar from a practical point of view.

Such accurate terminology cannot generally be applied to the whole muscles, most of which are composed of a mixture of myofibres of the three types αR, αW and βR. However, in many muscles of various species, myofibres of one type are predominant. It is therefore possible to distinguish fast-white muscles predominantly composed of αW fibres, fast-red muscles predominantly composed of αR fibres, and slow-red muscles predominantly composed of βR fibres. It follows from the characteristics of individual myofibres that fast-white muscles have high myofibrillar ATPase and glycolytic but low oxidative activities; fast-red muscles have high myofibrillar ATPase, high glycolytic and high oxidative activities; slow-red muscles have low myofibrillar ATPase and glycolytic but intermediate to high oxidative activities. Peter et al. (1972) were able to verify these properties of the three types of muscle in the guinea pig. This gives rise to a biochemical way of assessing the predominant metabolic type of individual muscles, which we used in studies on ovine muscles. Myofibrillar ATPase and various glycolytic and oxidative activities (Briand et al., 1980) were measured in eleven ovine muscles. By plotting a glycolytic or myofibrillar ATPase activity against an oxidative one, it is possible to assess the metabolic type of the muscles (Figure 1).

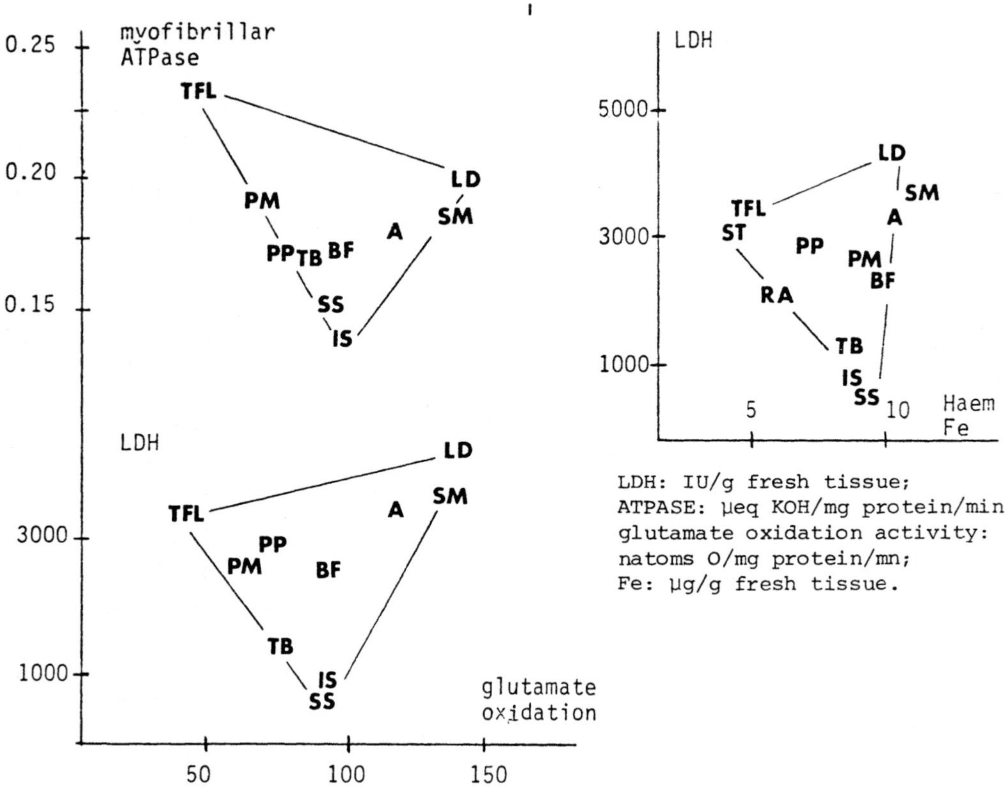

LDH: IU/g fresh tissue;
ATPASE: µeq KOH/mg protein/min;
glutamate oxidation activity: natoms O/mg protein/mn;
Fe: µg/g fresh tissue.

Fig. 1. Diagrammatic representation of metabolic type in ovine muscles.

ABBREVIATIONS

A: *M. adductor*; BF: *M. biceps femoris*; D: *M. diaphragma*; GM: *M. gluteus medius*; IS: *M. infraspinatus*; LD: *M. longissimus dorsi*; M: *M. masseter*; PM: *M. psoas major*; PP: *M. pectoralis profundus*; RA: *M. rectus abdominis*; S:*M. sternomandibularis*; SM: *M. semimembranosus*; SS: *M. supraspinatus*; ST: *M. semitendinosus*; T: *M. trapezius*; TBL: *M. triceps brachii caput laterale*; TB2: *M. triceps brachii caput longum*; TFL: *M. tensor fasciae latae*.

The muscles which were examined were seen to be roughly grouped on every diagram in the shape of a triangle, the corners of which are occupied by muscles of a characteristic metabolic type: so, TFL and ST can be classified as fast-white, SS and IS as slow-red, and LD and SM as fast-red muscles. It is noteworthy that fast-red muscles are more glycolytic than fast-white ones and more oxidative than slow-red ones. This agrees well with histochemical observations: in ovine muscles, αR fibres have a higher oxidative activity as assessed by succinate dehydrogenase (SDH) staining than βR fibres (Suzuki, 1971; Lacourt, personal communication). The same thing was shown by Peter et al. (1972) for the guinea pig. Another interesting observation is that the distribution of the muscles in the diagrams is very similar whatever the couple of variables used to assess metabolic type. So in practice it is possible to choose the more convenient system, as for instance lactate dehydrogenase (LDH) haem/iron, which can be easily and accurately measured even on frozen samples.

In cattle the situation is quite different (Figure 2). Preliminary results obtained by measuring enzyme activities in sixteen muscles of three cows are reported here. An inverse relationship between ATPase or glycolytic activities and oxidative activities or haem iron is found: points representing muscles on the diagrams are roughly grouped on lines instead of in triangles as in ovine muscles. This is due to the fact that αR myofibres, in bovine muscles, have a lower ATPase activity than αW myofibres, and a lower oxidative capacity than βR myofibres (Ashmore and Doerr, 1971). So αR fibres really appear to be intermediate between αW and βR fibres, and probably fast-red muscles are biochemically intermediate between fast-white and slow-red muscles. Thus it is difficult to make a distinction between predominantly fast-red and the other types of muscles using only the assessment of glycolytic or myofibrillar ATPase activity and oxidative activity. There is a need to look for more accurate biochemical criteria in order to estimate the predominant metabolic type in bovine muscles.

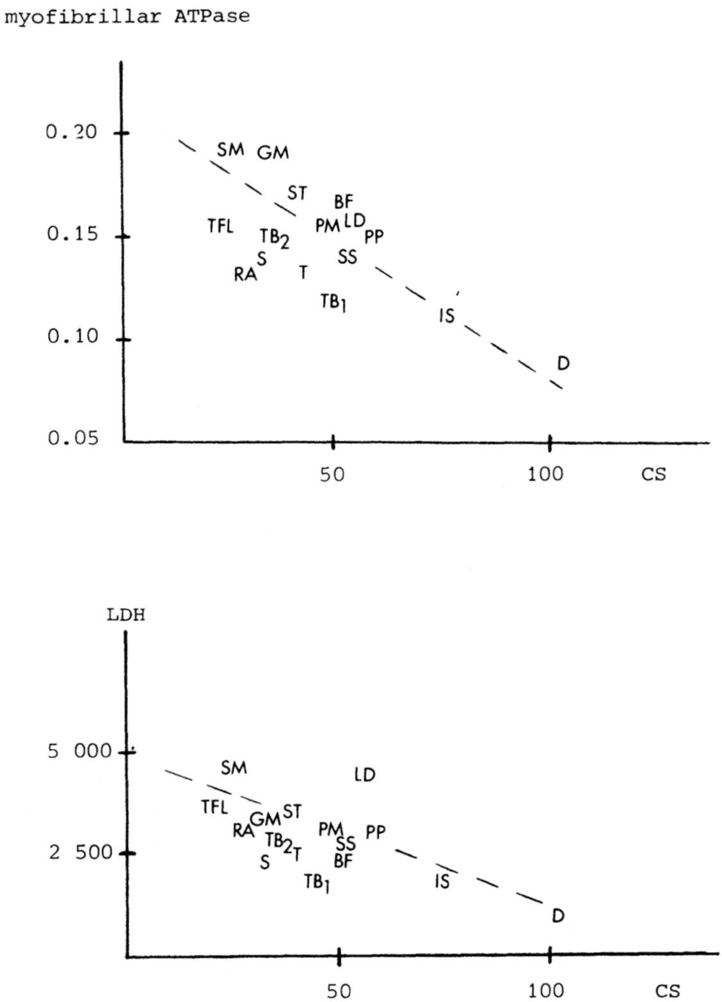

Fig. 2. Diagrammatic representation of metabolic type in bovine muscles. CS: citrate synthetase, IU/ g protein; ATPase: μeq KOH/mg protein/ mn; LDH: IU/g soluble protein.

II - RELATIONSHIP BETWEEN METABOLIC TYPE AND MEAT ULTIMATE pH

In ovine muscles, there is an obvious relationship between muscle metabolic type and meat pH after the completion of *rigor mortis*. In Figure 3 the ultimate pH of eleven muscles from sheep killed at rest or after transport stress is reported. Values of pH are arranged in order of increasing magnitude. It can be seen that in animals killed at rest, the fast-red LD and SM, as well as A (close to the fast-red muscles, see Figure 1) have the lowest pH, and that the slow-red IS and SS show a rather high pH. Fast-white ST muscle, and intermediate BF and PM have intermediate pH. RA appears exceptional in having a very high pH. The pH increase due to preslaughter stress is greater in the slow-red IS and SS muscle and in the fast-white ST muscle than in the other muscles (except RA). This is even better illustrated by the results of an experiment using two groups of three animals each which were obviously particularly sensitive to transport stress and shown in Figure 4.

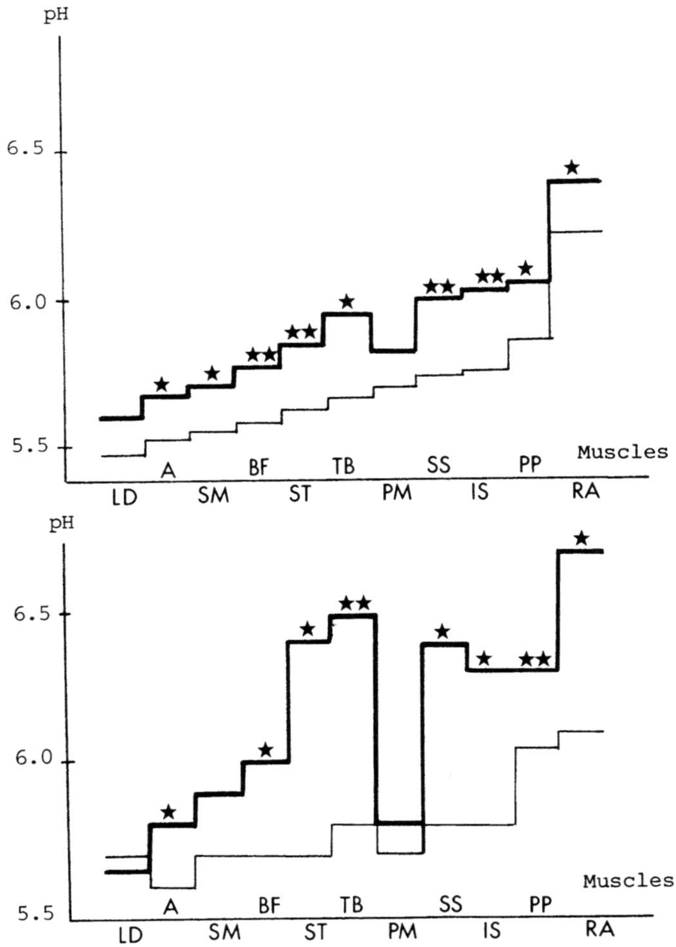

Fig. 3 and 4. Ultimate pH in muscles of lambs killed or at rest or after transport stress. Fig. 3: n = 50 lambs in each group. Fig. 4: n = 3 lambs in each group. * $P < 0.05$ ** $P < 0.01$
——— rested ▬▬▬ transported

In normal bovine muscles there is an inverse relationship between ultimate pH and myofibrillar ATPase activity: the muscles with high ATPase tend to have lower ultimate pH (Figure 5). Examination of the results of Hunt and Hedrick (1977a) shows that normal muscles with a high proportion of red fibres (assessed by relative area on histochemical slides) tend to have higher ultimate pH, although differences in pH between muscles were small in their study. These authors also produced an interesting study of the relationship between fibre type distribution and quality characteristics of bovine muscles. They observed that dark-cutting cattle have a higher percentage of αR fibres in their muscles. However, the relationship between proportion of αR fibres and DFD condition is not absolutely obvious, since the outer part of the ST muscle, which contains less αR fibres than the GM muscle (Hunt and Hedrick, 1977a) shows a higher pH in dark-cutting carcasses (Hunt and Hedrick, 1977b).

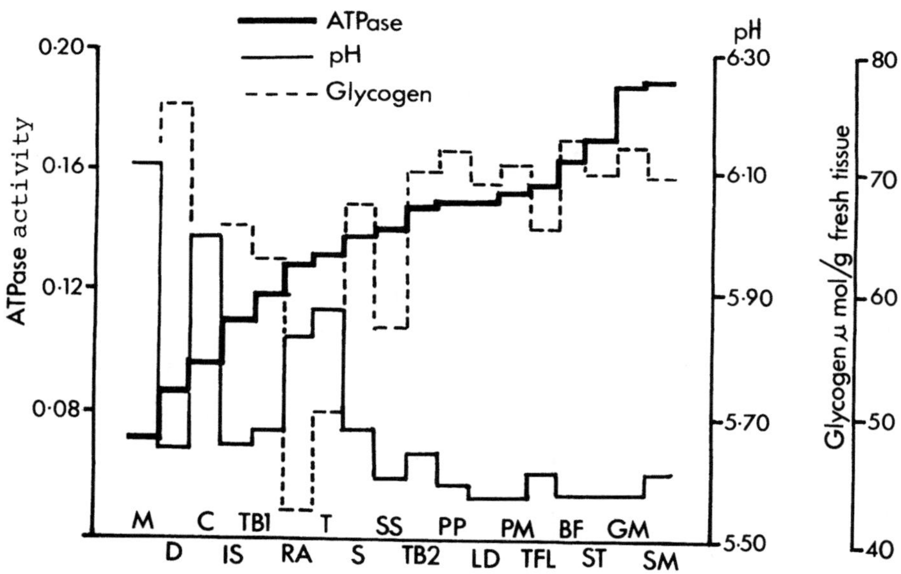

Fig. 5. Myofibrillar adenosine triphosphatase, glycogen (at slaughter) and ultimate pH in eighteen bovine muscles. (Units of ATPase activity are μeq KOH/mg myofibrillar protein/min).

The glycogen concentration in *M. masseter* was 25 $\mu mol.g^{-1}$ and it was not measured in the heart (C).

III - RELATIONSHIPS BETWEEN METABOLIC TYPE, LEVEL OF GLYCOGEN AND GLYCOGEN CONSUMPTION DURING STRESS

3.1. Level of glycogen

The relationship between metabolic type and level of glycogen has been the subject of controversy for some time. Many authors have found higher glycogen levels in 'white' than in 'red' muscles. On the other hand some authors have reported more glycogen in 'red' muscles (Gillespie et al., 1970) or no difference between the two types of muscle (Beecher et al., 1965). This confusion arises from the fact that the various workers did not distinguish between fast-red and slow-red muscles. Peter et al. (1972) showed that in the guinea-pig the highest level of glycogen is found in fast-red muscle and the lowest in slow-red muscle. In well-fed and rested sheep, we observed also a markedly higher level in the fast-red LD and A muscles (90 to 105 $\mu mol.g^{-1}$) than in the fast-white (about 75 $\mu mol.g^{-1}$) or slow-red (about 80 $\mu mol.g^{-1}$) muscles.

In bovine muscle, differences among the sixteen muscles that we studied were not so marked. However there is a trend for a higher glycogen level in faster muscles as illustrated in Figure 5 (except Diaphragm).

3.2. Muscle glycogen consumption during stress as related to metabolic type

It has been known for a long time that 'white' muscle breaks down glycogen and produces more lactate *in vitro* than 'red' muscle (Beatty and Bocek, 1970). Conversely, glycogen synthesis *in vitro* is more active in 'red' than in 'white' muscle (Bocek et al., 1966). However the situation might be different in muscles *in vivo*. Gollnick et al. (1972) showed that glycogen depletion rate may be higher either in α or in β myofibres during exercise in man, depending on the diet ingested before exercise. We were able to compare glycogen decrease during adrenaline infusion or transport stress in fast-white (ST) and slow-red (SS) muscles of sheep (unfortunately not in fast-red muscle). The results are given in Table 1.

TABLE 1

INFLUENCE OF ADRENALINE INFUSION OR TRANSPORT STRESS ON OVINE MUSCLE GLYCOGEN DEPLETION

Muscles	Glycogen $\mu mol.g^{-1}$				
	Control	Adrenaline	ΔA	Transport	ΔT
M. semitendinosus	33.8 ± 1.7	3.8 ± 1.1	30.0	24.4 ± 6.8	9.4
M. supraspinatus	40.7 ± 4.3	7.9 ± 1.0	32.8	19.8 ± 5.8	20.9
M. pectoralis profundus	42.7 ± 5.6	13.3 ± 3.1	29.4	26.5 ± 3.5	16.2

Each experimental group included 5 animals

- Adrenaline was infused for 4 hours at a rate of 30 µg/kg liveweight/h
- Transport stress was produced by transporting animals for 4 hours in a truck.

Lambs were slaughtered immediately after the experimental treatments. Glycogen was measured 20 minutes *post mortem*.

The rather low glycogen levels in control animals are due to the fact that all animals were brought to the slaughterhouse the day before the experiment to be catheterized. They remained there overnight before the experiment, so they experienced some change of environment and some handling stress.

Glycogen decrease during adrenaline infusion was similar in the three muscles studied. During transport stress, glycogen decrease was higher in the slow-red SS than in the fast-white ST; in PP, a muscle which is of intermediate metabolic type (see Figure 1), the decrease was intermediate between those observed in ST and SS muscles. Three different causes could contribute to this finding:

- as pointed out by Lister (1979) for porcine muscle, acidosis provoked by stress could reduce lipolysis and therefore the usual supply of free fatty acids used as fuel by red muscles; consequently red muscles deprived of their 'preferred' substrate could use glycogen more actively.

- in slaughtered sheep, phosphorylase is more activated in red muscles than in white ones, which results in a similar phosphorylase activity in fast-white and slow-red muscles, although total phosphorylase is much more abundant in fast-white muscles (Table 2). These results were obtained in muscles of animals killed at rest, i.e. having experienced only slaughter stress, but the situation could be similar after another type of stress such as transportation.

TABLE 2

PHOSPHORYLASE ACTIVITIES IN SOME OVINE MUSCLES

Muscles	Phosphorylase a + b	Phosphorylase a	a/a + b
M. semitendinosus (fast-white)	69.3	5.8	0.084
M. supraspinatus (slow-red)	34.3	4.2	0.122
M. longissimus dorsi (fast-red)	76.7	7.4	0.096

Phosphorylase activity is expressed as μmol glucose 1-P incorporated in glycogen/mn/g protein at 37°C.

- blood flow is changed by stress to a different extent in white and red muscles (Reis and Wooten, 1970): during excitement in cats, the blood flow is raised selectively in white muscles and does not change in red ones. Obviously, this leads to a better supply of oxygen and nutrients to white muscles, as compared to the supply during rest, but not in red muscles. This could modify the glycogenolysis rate to a different extent in white and red muscles.

Another important point to consider is the amount of glycogen necessary to give the maximal potential pH fall in individual muscles. This amount might vary between muscles, because of variations in buffering capacity; white muscles have a higher buffering capacity than red muscles, so a similar decrease in pH needs more lactate production - and theoretically more glycogen degradation - in the former than in the latter. In practice we found (Gire and Monin, 1979) that in four ovine muscles, differing to some extent in their metabolic type, a similar level of 50 to 60 μmol.g^{-1} glycogen is necessary to obtain the maximal pH fall.

This gives us an explanation of the higher sensitivity of ovine slow-red muscles to transport stress, in terms of increase of ultimate pH. In well-fed rested animals, red-slow and fast-white muscles contain about 70 to 80 μmol.g^{-1} glycogen respectively, and fast-red about 100 μmol.g^{-1} glycogen. So fast-red muscles can 'consume' about 40 μmol.g^{-1} during pre-slaughter stress without noticeable increase in meat ultimate pH, versus only 10 to 20 μmol.g^{-1} in the other muscles. Moreover 'consumption' during stress is greater in slow-red than in fast-white, so the former are more sensitive to the DFD condition than the latter. Even if 'consumption' is high also in fast-red muscles - but we have no result to assess it - these would be protected against DFD condition by their higher glycogen store.

In cattle histochemical data are available. Ashmore and Doerr (1971) reported a faster decrease in the αR myofibres in bovine muscle after adrenaline injection. Lacourt and Tarrant (1980) looked at the selective glycogen depletion induced by stress in myofibres of the different metabolic types. Cattle were stressed by mixing with strange animals for five hours, and samples were taken from the LD muscle using a biopsy technique. They observed that after stress, the glycogen decrease was faster and of greater magnitude in α myofibres, but lasted for a longer time in β myofibres. As pointed out previously, Hunt and Hedrick (1977b) found that muscles from dark-cutting carcasses have a higher proportion of αR fibres than muscle from normal carcasses. They considered that during stress αR myofibres mobilise glycogen more readily than the other types of myofibres. There is an apparent discrepancy between these results and ours obtained on sheep, since we found in the latter that predominantly fast-red muscles are the least prone to DFD condition after preslaughter stress. The explanation could be that in bovine muscle αR fibres have not a higher glycogen content than the other myofibres, conversely to what is observed in ovine muscle: in the outer part of the SM, which was shown by Hunt and Hedrick (1977a) to be rather rich in αR myofibres (32.9 per cent of the total fibres), we found 70 $\mu mol.g^{-1}$ glycogen, versus 71 in PM which according to the same authors is rather poor in αR myofibres (14.9 per cent) of the total fibres). So the 'protective' effect of the very high glycogen level in ovine fast-red muscles probably does not exist in bovine muscles. Clearly more investigation is needed in this field.

IV - GLYCOGEN RESYNTHESIS AFTER STRESS

Using *in vitro* experiments Bocek et al. (1966) showed that in rats the pathway of glucose to glycogen is more active in red muscles than in white ones. This agrees well with the *in vivo* observations of Terjung et al. (1974) in rats. These authors reported that glycogen resynthesis is most active in fast-red muscles and least active in fast-white muscles in fed rats after exhausting exercise. On the other hand Mac Lane and Holloszy (1979) showed that fast muscles can resynthetise glycogen from lactate at a high rate, whereas the rate of synthesis in slow-red muscles is very low. In practice, cattle or sheep encounter very varying conditions before they are slaughtered. In cattle for instance, sometimes stress occurs at a high level between departure from the farm and slaughter (lairage in collective pens with fighting, riding), sometimes not (lairage in individual pens); sometimes they are fed (hay, molasses) or not. Also catecholamine secretion (due to psychic stress) and exercise may induce different balances between lactacidemia and hyperglycemia. It is very difficult to speculate on the relationship between metabolic type and glycogen synthesis rate in such variable conditions.

An experiment was designed to look at the rate of glycogen resynthesis after depletion induced by adrenaline infusion in sheep (see experimental details in the legend of Figure 6). During the entire experiment, the sheep were tied by a belt in order to allow easy blood sampling without having to chase and catch the animals. The animals were accustomed for some days to being tied, but this treatment seemed to remain rather uncomfortable for them during the experiment: probably this situation would compare to that of young bulls put in individual pens for some hours before slaughter without being accustomed to that situation.

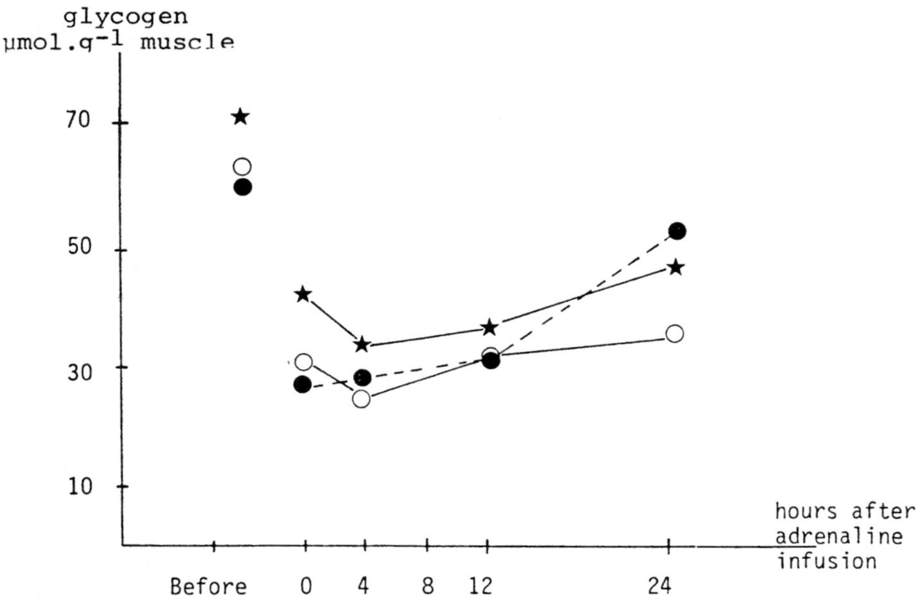

Fig. 6. Resynthesis of glycogen in ovine muscle after depletion provoked by adrenaline infusion.

n = 3 lambs in each group

o *M. semitendinosus* ● *M. supraspinatus* ★ *M. pectoralis profundus*

15 lambs were allotted to five groups of three animals. One group was slaughtered at rest ('before' on the diagram). The other four groups were infused with adrenaline (30 µg/kg liveweight/hour) for four hours and then killed at 0, 4, 12 and 24 hours after the end of the infusion, respectively.

During the experiment, animals were tied by a belt. They were fed hay and water *ad libitum* during the recovery period.

Glycogen was measured 20 minutes after slaughter, and corrected for *post mortem* glycogenolysis using the lactic acid levels in respective muscles (see Gire and Monin, 1979).

Figure 6 shows that resynthesis was much more rapid in the slow-red SS muscle than in the fast-white ST (as for glycogen depletion during stress, the result in PP was very close to that observed in ST). Our results obtained on animals fed during the recovery period agree with those reported in rats by Conlee et al. (1978). They disagree with the histochemical finding of Lacourt and Tarrant (1980) in bovine muscle: these researchers found that glycogen resynthesis is similar in βR myofibres and in α myofibres in bovine LD after stress induced by mixing. But as pointed out above, feeding and conditions during the recovery period are very important and could contribute to the explanation of this discrepancy.

V - EVOLUTION WITH AGE

Monin and Gire (1977) observed that sensitivity to transport stress, in terms of meat ultimate pH, increases with age between 6 to 10 months in lambs. In 6 month old animals, preslaughter transport stress did not induce any significant pH increase; it did in 10 month old lambs. This increase in sensitivity to preslaughter stress was explained partly by a lowered glycogen level and partly by a more active glycogenolysis in muscles of older lambs.

As age increases, a change in metabolic characteristics of muscles is observed. As shown in Figure 7, there is a shift of the metabolic characteristics of muscles to a 'redder' metabolic type. The metabolic (glycolytic and oxidative) activities tend to resemble those of slow-red muscles, although myofibrillar ATPase activity did not change significantly between 2 to 13 months (Talmant et al., 1980). This change could increase the sensitivity of muscles to stress. Moreover there is a decrease of glycogen synthetase activity (Talmant et al., 1980) which could explain the decrease in glycogen content, since Conlee et al. (1978) showed in rat muscles that glycogen content is positively related to glycogen synthetase activity.

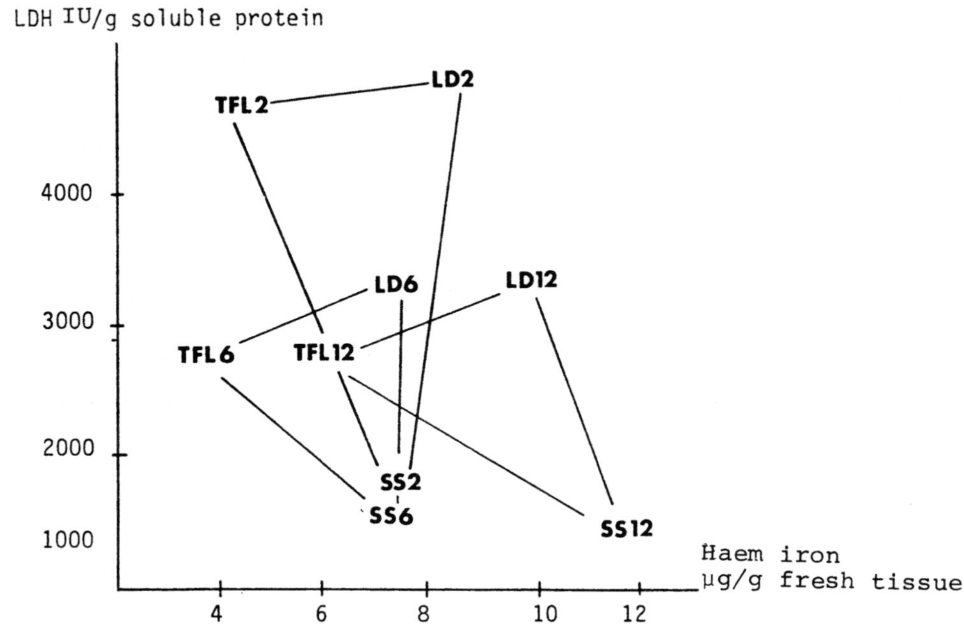

Fig. 7. Evolution of metabolic type with age in 3 ovine muscles.
(Letters indicate muscles, numbers indicate age in months)

CONCLUSION

In sheep, there is an obvious relationship between muscle metabolic type and ultimate pH, in normal as well as in DFD carcasses. Such a relationship is not as clear in bovine muscle, for which really very few results are available from the literature. Further research in this area is therefore necessary.

Except for the studies of Hunt and Hedrick, the results reported here refer mostly to differences between myofibres within the muscle, or between individual muscles within the carcass, with respect to metabolic type and DFD condition. There is a need to establish if the same conclusions are valid in regard to differences between individual animals within a breed or between breeds. There are differences in muscle metabolic characteristics between individual animals within an ovine breed, and these are reflected in the properties of the meat (Valin, personal communication). Valin and his co-workers were able to show that lambs from the Merino d'Arles breed differing in the fibre type distribution in *M. stylohyoïdeus*, differed also in the organoleptic properties of their meat. It seems possible to influence the metabolic characteristics of muscles of live animals in view of the work of Ianuzzo et al., (1977): in the future this could be perhaps one of the most accurate and powerful ways of controlling meat quality.

ACKNOWLEDGEMENTS

We wish to acknowledge A. Lacourt and P.V. Tarrant for communication of their results before publication and Miss Sarah Pengelly for her help in preparing this paper.

REFERENCES

Ashmore, C.R. and Doerr, L., 1971. Comparative aspects of muscle fibre types in different species. Exptl. Neurol., 31, 408-418.

Beatty, C.H. and Bocek, R.M., 1970. Biochemistry of red and white muscle. In Briskey, E.J., Cassens, R.G. and Marsh, B.B. (editors). The Physiology and Biochemistry of Muscle as a Food II University of Wisconsin Press, Madison.

Beecher, G.R., Cassens, R.G., Hoekstra, W.G. and Briskey, E.J., 1965. Red and white fibre content and associated post mortem properties of seven porcine muscles. J. Food Sci. 30, 969-976.

Bocek, R.M., Peterson, R.D. and Beatty, C.H., 1966. Glycogen metabolism in red and white muscle. Am. J. Physiol. 210, 1101-1107.

Briand, M., Talmant, A., Briand, Y., Monin, G. and Durand, R., 1980. Metabolic type of muscles of the sheep: myosin ATPase, glycolytic and mitochondrial enzyme activities (in preparation).

Conlee, R.K., Hickson, R.C., Winder, W.W., Hagberg, J.M. and Holloszy, J.O., 1978. Regulation of glycogen resynthesis in muscle of rats following exercise. Am. J. Physiol., 235, R 145-R 150.

Gillespie, C.A., Simpson, D.R. and Edgerton, V.R., 1970. High glycogen content of red as opposed to white skeletal muscle fibres of guinea pigs. J. Histochem. Cytochem., 18, 552-558.

Gire, P. and Monin, G., 1979. Taux de glycogène musculaire, stress de transport et pH ultime de la viande chez le mouton. Ann. Technol. Agric., 28, 443-444.

Gollnick, P.D., Piehl, K., Saubert, C.W., Armstrong, R.B. and Saltin, B., 1972. Diet, exercise and glycogen changes in human muscle fibres. J. Appl. Physiol., 33, 421-425.

Hunt, M.C. and Hedrick, H.B., 1977a. Profile of fibre types and related properties of five bovine muscles. J. Anim. Sci. 42, 513-517.

Hunt, M.C. and Hedrick, H.B., 1977b. Histochemical and biochemical characteristics of bovine muscles from four quality groups. J. Anim. Sci. 42, 578-581.

Ianuzzo, D., Patel, P., Chen, V., O'Brien, P. and Williams, O., 1977. Thyroidal trophic influence on skeletal muscle myosin. Nature, 270, 74-76.

Lacourt, A. and Tarrant, P.V., 1980. Selective glycogen depletion and recovery in skeletal muscle fibre types of young bulls. EEC Seminar 'The problem of dark-cutting in beef'. Brussels, 7-8 October 1980.

Lister, D., 1979. Some physiological aspects of the stress cycle in relation to muscle function and meat quality. Acta agric. Scand. Supplementum 21, 281-288.

Mac Lane, J.A. and Holloszy, J.O., 1979. Glycogen synthesis from lactate in the three types of skeletal muscle. J. Biol. Chem., 254, 6548-6553.

Monin, G. and Gire, P., 1977. Mobilisation du glycogène musculaire et hépatique au cours du stress de transport chez le Mouton. Influence de l'âge et du mode d'élevage. 23e Réunion Européenne des Chercheurs en Viande, BO, Moscou.

Peter, J.B., Barnard, R.J., Edgerton, V.R., Gillespie, C.A. and Stempel, G.E., 1972. Metabolic profiles of three fibre types of skeletal muscles in guinea pigs and rabbits. Biochemistry, 11, 2627-2633.

Ranvier, P.L., 1874. De quelques faits relatifs à l'histologie et à la physiologie des muscles striés. Arch. Physiol. Norm. Pathol., 6, 1-7.

Reis, D.J. and Wooten, J.F., 1970. The relationship of blood flow to myoglobin, capillary density, and twitch characteristics in red and white skeletal muscle of the cat. J. Physiol., 210, 121-135.

Sornay, J. and Legras, P., 1978. Cartographie du pH dans les carcasses de gros bovins. Ind. Alim. Agric., 4, 392-397.

Suzuki, A., 1971. Histochemical classification of individual skeletal muscle fibres in the sheep. II. On *M. serratus ventralis, M. supraspinatus, M. infraspinatus, M. semimembranosus* and *M. triceps brachii*. Jap. J. Zootech. Sci., 42, 463-473.

Talmant, A., Briand, M., Monin, G. and Durand, R., 1980. Evolution of glycogen level,phosphorylase activity and glycogen synthetase activity in various lamb muscles during growth. 26th European Meeting of Meat Research Workers, A3, Colorado Springs, USA.

Tarrant, P.J.V., 1976. The occurrence of dark-cutting beef. B8. 22nd European Meeting of Meat Research Workers, Malmö, Sweden.

Terjung, R.L., Baldwin, K.M., Winder, W.W. and Holloszy, J.O., 1974. Glycogen repletion in different types of muscles and in liver after exhausting exercise. Am. J. Physiol., 226, 1387-1391.

DISCUSSION

J.J.A. Heffron *(Ireland)*

Biochemically, we recognise three fibre types. There is the fast-twitch glyolytic fibre, the fast-twitch oxidative glycolytic fibre and there is the slow-twitch oxidative fibre. How does your classification relate to this? What I am saying is that the biochemist recognises three fibre-types in muscles, but if you are to believe the histochemist there are several fibre types - more than three!

G. Monin *(France)*

I think the histochemists disagree on this point. I understand that Ashmore, or Peter in the USA, found only three types of myofibres. I think it is possible to find many types of myofibres, but I would prefer to consult a histochemist about it. However, many people can accept three types of fibres.

J.J.A. Heffron

Does your β red fibre correspond to the fast-twitch oxidative glycolytic fibre?

G. Monin

No, α is fast and β is slow.

B.L. Dumont *(France)*

Is there any relationship between buffering capacity of muscles and fibre-types?

G. Monin

I did not state this in my paper, but buffering capacity is higher in white muscles. It is rather strange to find that approximately the same level of glycogen is needed in the different types of muscle to obtain the maximal pH fall. Theoretically, more glycogen is needed in a white muscle to get the same ultimate pH because more lactate is required to produce a comparable effect.

B.L. Dumont

At the moment is there any clear basic explanation of that factor?

G. Monin

I think Dr. Davey proposed an explanation on the basis of carnosine and anserine levels in muscles.

C.L. Davey *(New Zealand)*

Our work showed that the dipeptides, carnosine and anserine have a broad inverse relationship to aerobic activity. I suppose the conclusion we can reach from this is that when there is a high concentration of the dipeptides, the muscle can produce lactic acid and sustain a higher steady state of lactate as it is being transferred to the blood system. This means that a muscle can function, *in vivo* in an anaerobic way for a much longer period.

T.R. Dutson *(USA)*

Do you think that the differences between red and white glycogen levels, found by different researchers, may be due to different methods of extracting the muscle, or for example to differences in freezing techniques. We found quite a lot of difference in the rate of glycogen breakdown in white muscle, as you extract it, versus red muscle. A few minutes delay in freezing may allow enough glycogen breakdown to cause a discrepancy.

G. Monin

Generally I correct muscle glycogen content by taking account of the lactate content. There is, of course, some lactate in the living muscle but I think it is very low - 3 to 5 μmol/g - compared to the level of glycogen. In *M. semitendinosus* we find about 15 μmol lactate/g just after slaughter, but only 6 - 8 μmol/g in *M. supraspinatus*.

<u>J.J.A. Heffron</u>

Do you freeze clamp your tissues when you are taking samples?

<u>G. Monin</u>

No, they are frozen in liquid nitrogen approximately 15 - 20 min after slaughter.

<u>J.J.A. Heffron</u>

This has a bearing on the point made by Dr. Dutson: whether the animal is under anaesthesia or whether you are taking samples from *post mortem* muscle.

<u>G. Monin</u>

I think that freezing with clamps is better of course, but it is not always possible! In any case if you correct for lactate levels due to *post mortem* glycogenolysis you will have a rather good estimate. The difference from the true glycogen level must be only about 5 μmol/g as compared with 70 - 100 μmol/g total.

<u>C.L. Davey</u>

Muscles are the major source of body heat. Large muscles, which have to release this heat through heat transfer fairly efficiently, could well have a different type of muscle fibre deep within the body of the muscle in contrast to the surface tissue. Would you care to comment on this?

<u>G. Monin</u>

This is a very serious problem when working with cattle because the muscles are so large and heterogeneous. My results refer to the outer part of the muscle; it is very difficult and very expensive to get inner samples of 16 muscles in a carcass.

However, the literature shows that muscles are very heterogeneous from this point of view. The problem is to take the measurements of pH and metabolites in the same part. For example *M. triceps brachii* in the shoulder is very heterogeneous: the part *caput longum* and the part *caput laterale* are very difficult to compare.

CONTROL MECHANISMS FOR THE ENZYMES OF GLYCOGEN METABOLISM IN MUSCLE

J.J.A. Heffron
Department of Biochemistry, University College Cork,
Prospect Row, Cork, Ireland.

ABSTRACT

Glycogen metabolism in skeletal muscle is regulated by three inter-connected networks. Firstly, catecholamine hormones cause cyclic-3', 5'-AMP to be elevated in the sarcoplasm; this 'second messenger' binds to the inhibitory sub-unit of protein kinase and releases the catalytic sub-unit. The latter, in the presence of calcium ions, proceeds to phosphorylate phosphorylase kinase b *which in turn converts phosphorylase* b *to* a *by another phosphorylation. Secondly, calcium ions alone, when released from the sarcoplasmic reticulum after neuronal stimulation of the muscle, activate phosphorylase kinase* b *by combining with calmodulin, the* δ *sub-unit of the kinase. Thirdly, insulin regulates glycogen synthesis by a poorly understood mechanism, but probably involving the recently-discovered cAMP-independent glycogen synthase kinases.*

A single, multifunctional protein phosphatase I is responsible for dephosphorylation of phosphorylase a*, phosphorylase kinase* a *and glycogen synthase D. Phosphatase I is itself inhibited by a newly-discovered inhibitory protein, inhibitor I, after it has been phosphorylated by cAMP-dependent protein kinase. However, inhibitor I is inactivated by phosphatase I. A second protein phosphatase, phosphatase II, is involved in regulating the duration of the active state of phosphorylase kinase by removing a phosphoryl group from the* α *sub-unit of the enzyme.*

Glycogen, glucose-6-phosphate and 5'-AMP act as allosteric modulators of glycogen synthase and phosphorylase, respectively.

INTRODUCTION

In the tissues of mammals virtually all of the glycogen is found in the liver and skeletal muscles. In general, the glycogen content of the liver will vary greatly with the diet of the animal while that in skeletal muscle will be less affected. On the other hand, exercise and other activity will quickly deplete the glycogen store of muscle compared with that of liver. Although the liver usually contains some six times the concentration of glycogen in skeletal muscle, the muscles contain the bulk of the total body glycogen owing to their large mass.

Mammalian muscles, however, are not homogeneous for fibre-type. They differ not only in colour but also in their biochemical, physiological and histochemical characteristics (Gauthier, 1970; Peter, 1971). Muscle fibres can be classified into three principal types based on their contraction times (fast-twitch or slow-twitch), their concentration of mitochondria and mitochondrial enzyme activities and their concentration of phosphorylase. This classification overcomes the considerable confusion caused by classification according to coloration, which may or may not vary directly with mitochondrial density. The three fibre types have been termed fast-twitch white, fast-twitch red and slow-twitch red (intermediate). Virtually all muscles are mixed in type but are described according to the predominant fibre-type in each muscle. The most noteworthy exception to this is *M. soleus* which in most species is homogeneously composed of slow-twitch intermediate fibres. For the purposes of this paper the discussion of the control of glycogen-metabolising enzymes is based on studies of enzymes purified from muscles containing the two fast-twitch fibres, but there is good reason to believe that the control mechanisms are qualitatively similar in all fibre types. Since control of the enzymes of the glycolytic pathway is well known and described in most text books of biochemistry, I will concentrate in this review on the recent and exciting developments in the control of the reversible breakdown of glycogen to glucose-1-phosphate (i.e. glycogenolysis and glycogen synthesis).

CATABOLISM OF GLYCOGEN

In skeletal muscle, glycogen is one of the principal sources of energy which powers muscle contraction. When a muscle contracts glycogen is broken down to yield ATP by substrate and oxidative phosphorylation. Glycogen is degraded by phosphorolysis of the 1,4-glucosidic bonds to form glucose-1-phosphate; this is accompanied by cleavage of the 1,6-glucosidic branches by the enzyme, amylo-1,6-glucosidase. The first and principal reaction is catalysed by the enzyme, glycogen phosphorylase a, which cleaves the terminal 1,4-glucosidic bond with inorganic phosphate to produce glucose-1-phosphate and, in the process, shortens the chain by one glucose residue. Phosphorylase a continues to remove glucose residues in this manner until it reaches the fourth residue from a 1,6-branch; then amylo-1,6-glucosidase, acting as a glucosyl transferase, transfers the three end glucose residues to another four-residue branch linking them with a 1,4 bond. The 1,6-glucosidase then removes the single branched residue by simple hydrolysis thus exposing a 1,4-linked chain for continued phosphorolysis by phosphorylase a. In general, the degree of branching in the glycogen molecule is such that 11 - 14 molecules of glucose-1-phosphate are released for every one free glucose produced by the action of 1,6-glucosidase. Although the breakdown of glycogen to glucose-1-phosphate is freely reversible, glycogen synthesis does not take place by simple reversal of breakdown reactions *in vivo*. Formation of glycogen is catalysed by a separate enzyme system known as glycogen synthase. The apparent reason for this separation of glycogen breakdown and synthetic pathways will be dealt with in a later section.

GLYCOGEN SYNTHESIS

Formation of glycogen takes place by addition of single glucosyl residues to the ends of existing glycogen molecules or primers. The starting point for glycogen synthesis is the formation of UDP-glucose in the following reaction catalysed by glucose-1-phosphate uridylyltransferase:

D-glucose-1-phosphate + UTP → UDP-D-glucose + PPi

Under the influence of the enzyme glycogen synthase, UDP-glucose acts as a glucosyl donor to the 4-hydroxyl of the terminal residue of an existing chain:

$$\text{UDP-D-glucose} + (\text{glucose})_n \rightarrow \text{UDP} + (\text{glucose})_{n+1}$$

Branching of the straight chain glucose polymer formed by glycogen synthase is catalysed by another enzyme, 1,4-α-glucan branching enzyme. This enzyme transfers six or seven residue fragments from the main glycogen chain to the 6-hydroxyl of a glucose residue of the same or another chain. In this way, branch points are set up from which further straight chains of glucose residues can be built.

REGULATION OF GLYCOGEN BREAKDOWN

From the foregoing, no indication of the mode of control of glycogen breakdown and synthesis is given but it must be obvious that efficient metabolism requires that synthesis of glycogen is gradually turned off when breakdown is accelerated, and *vice versa*. Absence of control of glycogen metabolism would mean that a major futile cycle would exist resulting in a net hydrolysis of ATP. Many studies over the past twenty years have shown that very fine control of the rates of glycogen synthesis and breakdown is made possible by the existence of two molecular forms, one inactive and the other active, of the two principal enzymes, phosphorylase and glycogen synthase.

Phosphorylase is subject to control by both covalent modification (phosphorylation) and allosteric modulation by certain metabolites. The inactive form of phosphorylase, known as the b form, is a dimer having a sub-unit molecular weight of 98 000 daltons. It is activated by phosphorylation at a specific serine residue at the expense of ATP in a reaction catalysed by the enzyme phosphorylase kinase a, as illustrated in Figure 1. The active phosphorylase a then commences degradation of glycogen to glucose-1-phosphate. It is important to note that phosphorylase a is itself a dimer of the inactive b

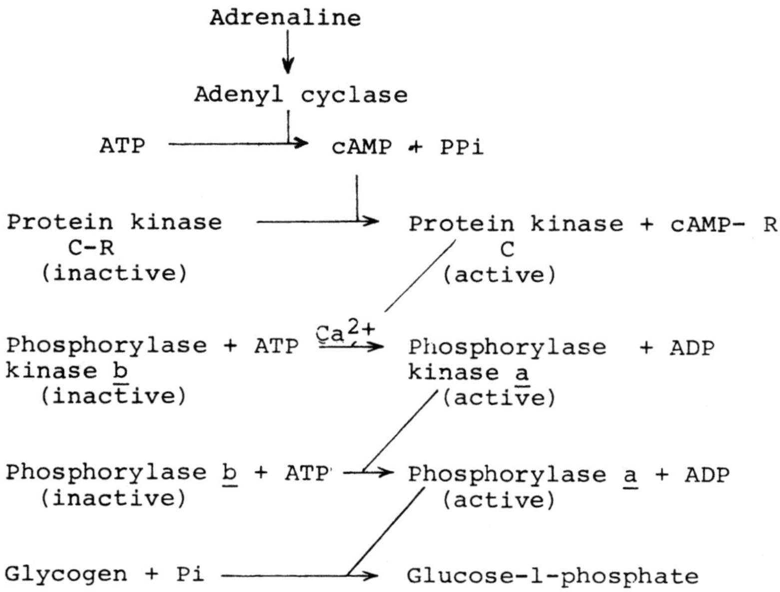

Fig. 1. Outline of the activation of the glycogenolytic cascade by adrenaline and Ca^{2+}. R denotes the inhibitory polypeptide of protein kinase. The amplification produced by adrenaline is several-million-fold. Additional control by protein phosphatases I and II and by the protein, inhibitor I, is described in the text.

form having one phosphorylated serine residue on each sub-unit. However, phosphorylase b is active in the unphosphorylated form when it complexes with 5'-AMP. Since the AMP concentration rises rapidly when there is a high demand for high-energy phosphates, it is probable that its effect on phosphorylase b is of physiological importance in adjusting the level of glycogen breakdown to the demand for ATP. AMP also binds to phosphorylase a which is fully active; here its function seems to be related to making the phosphoenzyme a poor substrate for protein phosphatase I, the enzyme which normally turns off glycogenolysis (McGilvery, 1979).

The stimulus for glycogen breakdown

So far, only the direct control of phosphorylase has been discussed. In normal skeletal muscle, it is known that the hormone adrenaline and Ca^2 both initiate the sequence of events, outlined in Figure 1, leading to the final activation of phosphorylase. During muscular contraction, it is necessary to co-ordinate energy consumption and energy production so as to maintain a metabolic steady state. This is achieved by the Ca^{2+} released from the sarcoplasmic reticulum following surface membrane depolarisation (Carlson and Wilkie, 1974); Ca^{2+} initiates contraction by binding to troponin C and it activates phosphorylase b indirectly by stimulating its kinase, phosphorylase kinase b (Figure 1). When an animal finds itself in an emergency situation which demands immediate, strenuous physical activity (the 3F situations), the adrenal medulla increases its output of adrenaline which, by combination with a specific receptor on the muscle cell membrane, initiates the cascade of events leading to the activation of phosphorylase b (Figure 1). This process also requires Ca^{2+} because phosphorylase kinase is completely dependent on Ca^{2+} (Klee et al., 1980); this point will be dealt with in the next paragraph. It is well known that adrenaline binding to the plasma membrane leads to the activation of adenyl cyclase, production of cyclic-3', 5'-AMP and activation of protein kinase as shown in Figure 1. Cyclic-AMP-dependent activation of the inactive form of protein kinase does not require any phosphorylation but, rather, the nucleotide binds to and removes an inhibitory polypeptide from the kinase. The liberated, active protein kinase (so-called C-form) then phosphorylates phosphorylase kinase b, the next enzyme in the cascade. A minute amount of adrenaline stimulates the initial enzyme, adenyl cyclase; in fact, nanomolar concentrations of the hormone lead to micromolar concentrations of cAMP within the cell (cf. Lehninger, 1975) and an amplification of the rate occurs at each subsequent enzyme-catalysed step (except activation of protein kinase). In muscle, it has been estimated that a given concentration of cAMP initiates the formation of 25 000 times as much glucose-1-phosphate per minute.

Phosphorylase kinase

There have been several important studies of the structure of this enzyme (Cohen, 1979) in the past three years. Its structure, and by implication its control, has turned out to be exceedingly complex. Although it was previously thought that phosphorylase kinase b was composed of equimolar amounts of the three sub-units, α, β, and γ, and that the smallest active species was the dodecamer (Cohen, 1973), it has recently been shown that the enzyme contains an additional, low molecular weight sub-unit (Cohen et al., 1978) and this is identical with the low molecular weight Ca^{2+} binding protein, calmodulin, which is present in many other tissues (Klee et al., 1980). According to Cohen (1979), the γ sub-unit of phosphorylase kinase is the catalytic one while the α and β sub-units are involved in the activation of the catalytic sub-unit after their phosphorylation. The δ sub-unit, calmodulin, is the Ca^{2+} binding one which confers Ca^{2+}-sensitivity on the whole enzyme. A diagrammatic representation of the basic tetramer of phosphorylase kinase is shown in Figure 2.

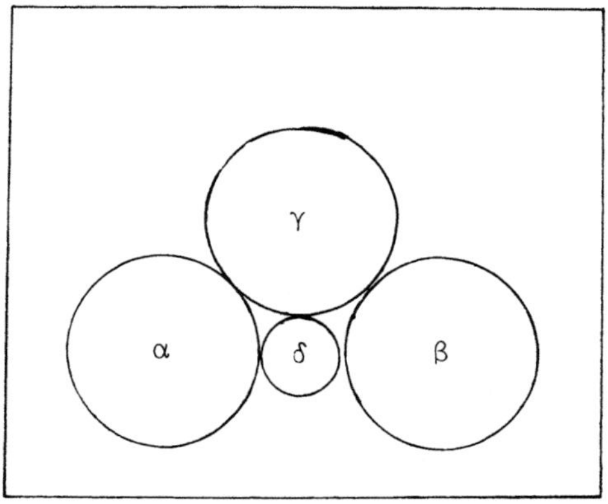

Fig. 2. The basic tetramer of phosphorylase kinase. The α and β sub-units are phosphorylated by cAMP-dependent protein kinase; the rate of phosphorylation of the β sub-unit is several-fold greater than that of the α sub-unit. Only the β sub-unit phosphorylation is necessary for activation of the kinase while phosphorylation of the α sub-unit acts as a control of the rate of dephosphorylation of the β sub-unit. The δ sub-unit, known also as calmodulin, confers sensitivity to Ca^{2+} to the kinase. The functional form of phosphorylase kinase is a complex of four tetramers.

The hormonal control of phosphorylase kinase activity by adrenaline has been very considerably revised by the elegant studies of Cohen and his group (see reviews, Cohen, 1978, 1979) and this will be examined in the rest of the paragraph. cAMP-dependent protein kinase plays two separate roles in regulating the activity of phosphorylase kinase. Firstly, it catalyses phosphorylation of the β sub-unit, and, secondly, it phosphorylates the α sub-unit but at a severalfold slower rate. Phosphorylase kinase, activated by phosphorylation of the β sub-unit only, is only slowly inactivated by protein phosphatase I; but when the α sub-unit is also phosphorylated, the phosphatase rapidly dephosphorylates the β-chain and thus terminates activation of phosphorylase b. Thus, it appears that the slower phosphorylation of the α sub-unit leads to a period of time when there is no competition between cAMP-dependent protein kinase and phosphatase I with one another; this should prolong the active state of phosphorylase kinase and, consequently, that of phosphorylase. Further studies have shown that a separate phosphatase, protein phosphatase II, dephosphorylates the α sub-unit of phosphorylase kinase thus making the a-form of the latter a poorer substrate for phosphatase I. The physiological function of the α-chain phosphorylation therefore appears to be inhibition of the termination signal of hormonal activation of phosphorylase kinase.

Phosphorylation of the β-chain of phosphorylase kinase presumably via a conformational shift, activates the γ sub-unit, a process which also requires Ca^{2+}. But Ca^{2+} alone will also lead to the assumption of the active state by phosphorylase kinase. Thus the effect of adrenaline is to potentiate the activation caused by Ca^{2+}. This activation occurs at similar Ca^{2+} concentrations which initiate muscle contraction (i.e. $\sim 10^{-6}$M). It must be emphasised that the source of this Ca^{2+} is the sarcoplasmic reticulum in fast-twitch fibres though mitochondria may play some role in supplying Ca^{2+} in those fibres having a relatively high mitochondrial density and poorly developed SR (cf. Gronert et al., 1979).

REGULATION OF GLYCOGEN SYNTHESIS

The regulatory enzyme, glycogen synthase, is a tetramer of just one type of sub-unit with a molecular weight of 88 000 (Nimmo et al., 1976). It is active in the dephosphorylated form or I form, and inactive in the phosphorylated D form; this is exactly the reverse of the situation described for phosphorylase. In addition to being covalently modulated by phosphorylation/dephosphorylation reactions, the I form of glycogen synthase is allosterically inhibited by glycogen while the D-form is active in the presence of millimolar concentrations of glucose-6-phosphate. An outline of the mechanism of regulation of glycogen synthase is shown in Figure 3. It is noted that the same cAMP-dependent protein kinase which activates phosphorylase kinase b switches off glycogen synthase. Thus, in principle, this mechanism ensures that glycogen synthesis does not take place simultaneously with glycogen breakdown and *vice versa*. However, the situation is apparently not so simple for Cohen and his colleagues have found that skeletal muscle contains two further kinases, not dependent on cAMP, which specifically phosphorylate glycogen synthase I (Cohen, 1979).

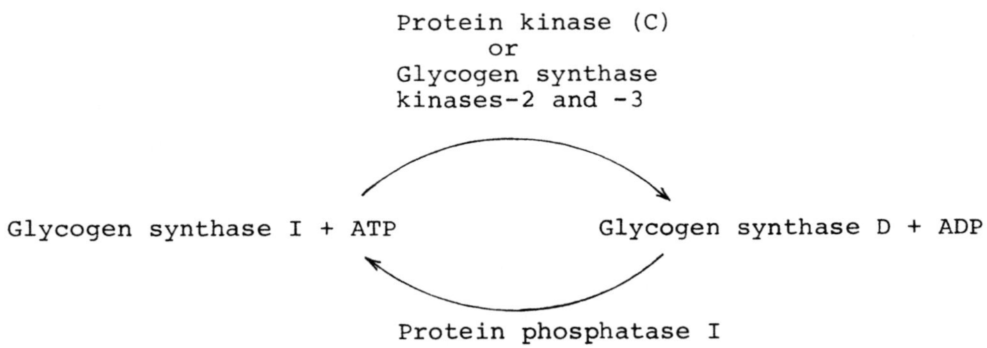

Fig. 3. Outline of the activation and inactivation of glycogen synthase. Synthase D is also activated allosterically by glucose-6-phosphate while synthase I is negatively modulated by glycogen. Additional control of the enzyme is achieved by the action of protein phosphatase I and inhibitor I (see text).

cAMP-independent glycogen synthase kinases

Glycogen synthase kinase-2 and kinase-3 both convert glycogen synthase I into the D-form which is more dependent on glucose-6-phosphate for activity. The kinase-2 phosphorylates the synthase at a different site to kinase-3; in fact, kinase-3 catalyses formation of a glycogen synthase D with a lower activity ratio when assayed in the absence and presence of excess glucose-6-phosphate than is formed by kinase-2. The key point is that the activities of these kinases are independent of cAMP and cGMP.

Insulin and glycogen synthesis

It has been known for quite some time that the hormone insulin stimulates glycogen synthesis and that it does so by activation of glycogen synthase. At one time, it was thought that insulin might act by depressing the synthesis of cAMP or even by increasing cGMP levels in muscle cells. It is, of course, now known that insulin does not affect cAMP levels in muscle under conditions where it stimulates glycogen synthesis (cf. Cohen, 1979). In the normal, fed state, Cohen (1979) has shown that glycogen synthase is highly phosphorylated and that this phosphorylation must be catalysed by either glycogen synthase kinase-2 or -3. The existence of these kinases provide a possible site of action of insulin on glycogen synthase which is completely independent of cAMP and cAMP-dependent protein kinase.

PROTEIN PHOSPHATASE I AND INHIBITOR I

Reference has already been made to protein phosphatase I, the enzyme we now know dephosphorylates phosphorylase *a*, phosphorylase kinase *a* and glycogen synthase D. It was previously thought that separate phosphatases were required in all three processes but the studies of Cohen and colleagues have convincingly shown that phosphatase I is a multifunctional enzyme (Cohen, 1979).

The existence of a heat-stable protein termed inhibitor I (it inhibits phosphatase I) in skeletal muscle was shown by Huang and Glinsmann (1976a,b). However, it only inhibits phosphatase I when it has been phosphorylated by cAMP-dependent protein kinase. Inhibitor-I is an unusual protein of molecular weight 20 000, is very low in aromatic amino acid content but some one-third of its residues are glutamate and proline (Nimmo and Cohen, 1978a). Further, it was found to be phosphorylated at a threonine residue and not serine as in the other phosphoproteins described so far (Cohen, 1979). The inhibitor is phosphorylated by cAMP-dependent protein kinase at a rate similar to the other enzymes involved in glycogen metabolism. Inhibitor I inhibits the dephosphorylation of phosphorylase a, phosphorylase kinase a and glycogen synthase D in an identical manner. Thus, it appears that glycogenolysis is stimulated by (1) activation of phosphorylase kinase and (2) phosphorylation of inhibitor I resulting in inhibition of protein phosphatase I.

This is, however, not the end of the story since Nimmo and Cohen (1978b) made the remarkable discovery that inhibitor I does not inhibit its own dephosphorylation by phosphatase I. These workers also showed that inhibitor I is preferentially dephosphorylated by phosphatase I *in vivo*. It was suggested that this dephosphorylation may be the initial step in the reversal of hormonal stimulation of the glycogenolytic pathway.

FINAL COMMENTS

From the foregoing discussion, it should be clear that the regulation of glycogen breakdown and synthesis is not yet completely understood though it is both an intense and exciting area of current research. Although the actions of adrenaline and Ca^{2+} on glycogen metabolism are now reasonably well documented, the control of glycogen synthesis by insulin still remains fairly obscure. It will be interesting to follow the further studies of the possible interaction of insulin, probably by a new 'second messenger', with the glycogen synthase kinases.

REFERENCES

Carlson, F.D. and Wilkie, D.R., 1974. Muscle Physiology, p. 24. Englewood Cliffs, N.J.: Prentice Hall, Inc.

Cohen, P., 1973. The Subunit Structure of Rabbit-Skeletal-Muscle Phosphorylase Kinase, and the Molecular Basis of Its Activation Reactions. Eur. J. Biochem. 34, 1-14.

Cohen, P., 1978. The Role of Cyclic-AMP-Dependent Protein Kinase in the Regulation of Glycogen Metabolism in Mammalian Skeletal Muscle. Curr. Top. Cell Regul. 14, 117-196.

Cohen, P., 1979. The Hormonal Control of Glycogen Metabolism in Mammalian Muscle by Multivalent Phosphorylation. Biochem. Soc. Trans. 7, 460-480.

Cohen, P., Burchell, A., Foulkes, J.G., Cohen, P.T.W., Vanaman, T.C. and Nairn, A.C., 1978. Identification of the Ca^{2+}-dependent Modulator Protein as the Fourth Subunit of Rabbit Skeletal Muscle Phosphorylase Kinase. FEBS Lett. 92, 287-293.

Gauthier, G., 1970. The Ultrastructure of Three Fibre Types in Mammalian Skeletal Muscle. In: The Physiology and Biochemistry of Muscle as a Food (Eds. Briskey, E.J., Cassens, R.G. and Marsh, B.B.), pp. 103-130. Madison: University of Wisconsin Press.

Gronert, G.A., Heffron, J.J.A. and Taylor, S.R., 1979. Skeletal Muscle Sarcoplasmic Reticulum in Porcine Malignant Hyperthermia. Eur. J. Pharmacol. 58, 179-187.

Huang, F.L. and Glinsmann, W.H., 1976a. A Second Heat-Stable Protein Inhibitor of Phosphorylase Phosphatase from Rabbit Muscle FEBS Lett 62, 326-329.

Huang, F.L. and Glinsmann, W.H., 1976b. Separation and Characterisation of Two Phosphorylase Phosphatase Inhibitors from Rabbit Skeletal Muscle. Eur. J. Biochem. 70, 419-426.

Klee, C.B., Crouch, T.H. and Richmann, P.G., 1980. Calmodulin. Ann. Rev. Biochem. 49, 489-515.

Lehninger, A.L., 1975. Biochemistry, 2nd Ed., p. 814 New York: Worth Publishers, Inc.

McGilvery, R.W., 1979. Biochemistry. A functional approach, 2nd Ed., p 494 Philadelphia: W.B. Saunders Company.

Nimmo, G.A. and Cohen, P., 1978a. The Regulation of Glycogen Metabolism - Purification and Characterisation of Protein Phosphatase Inhibitor-1 from Rabbit Skeletal Muscle. Eur. J. Biochem. 87, 341-351.

Nimmo, G.A. and Cohen, P., 1978b. The Regulation of Glycogen Metabolism: Phosphorylation of Inhibitor-1 from Rabbit skeletal Muscle and its Interaction with Protein Phosphatases-III and -II. Eur. J. Biochem. 87, 353-365.

Nimmo, H.G., Proud, C.G. and Cohen, P., 1976. The Purification and Properties of Rabbit Skeletal Muscle Glycogen Synthase. Eur. J. Biochem. 68, 21-30.

Peter, J.B., 1971. Histochemical, Biochemical and Physiological Studies of Skeletal Muscle and Its Adaptation to Exercise. In: The Contractility of Muscle Cells and Related Processes. (Ed. Podolsky, R.J.), pp. 151-173. Englewood Cliffs, N.J.: Prentice Hall, Inc.

DISCUSSION

P.V. Tarrant *(Ireland)*

First of all I would like to thank Dr. Heffron for a lucid presentation of a difficult subject. My question is in relation to the insulin concentration in plasma. It appears to be a very important factor in glycogen resynthesis. We have measured insulin concentration in bovine plasma and found values close to 20 μU/ml of plasma in animals deficient in muscle glycogen. Can you estimate how much this would have to fall before glycogen synthase would be inactivated?

J.J.A. Heffron *(Ireland)*

I am sorry, I do not know what the dose-response curve is for insulin-mediated dephosphorylation of the enzyme.

T.R. Dutson *(USA)*

Are the sites on calmodulin similar to those for troponin C in that they also bind magnesium? Troponin C has two sites that are obligatory for calcium and two that are obligatory for magnesium, and two that combine either. Is that the same for calmodulin?

J.J.A. Heffron

No, it is not. They are, in fact, all calcium specific sites. Sometimes the protein binds 4 calcium ions per molecule. However, as you decrease the ionic strength, it only binds 3. Therefore, the question of the physiological stochiometry of binding has not been established.

T.R. Dutson

Does its effect decrease as you decrease from 4 to 3?

J.J.A. Heffron

It does, yes. I think it is even effective with 2 calcium ions per molecule. Although the maximum effect apparently is achieved with 4. To my knowledge, very little has been done in detail on this. In their review, Klee et al., (1980) point out that very little has been done on the ionic strength effect which is obviously very important for assessing the detailed physiological results.

G. Eikelenboom *(The Netherlands)*

Can you comment as to the action of sex hormones? One of your slides referred to insulin and other hormones; I was wondering if sex hormones are involved in breakdown of glycogen or have specific effects on the enzyme systems you discussed.

J.J.A. Heffron

I cannot really say. Virtually all this work on the glycogen synthases and kinases, that is the cyclic-AMP-dependent ones (they are normally cyclic-AMP-independent) - has been done by Cohen in Dundee. He works mainly on insulin to my knowledge. Indeed, this work has all been done on rabbit muscle and may not be totally representative of beef or pig muscle, for instance. This has not been examined at all in relation to fibre type: clearly, one must have enormous quantities of muscle to get these proteins.

CHARACTERISTICS OF THE METABOLISM OF CARBOHYDRATE IN RUMINANTS COMPARED WITH OTHER MAMMALS

D.B. Lindsay
Biochemistry Department, ARC Institute of Animal Physiology, Babraham, Cambridge CB2 4AT, UK.

ABSTRACT

Differences in carbohydrate metabolism between ruminants and non-ruminants are almost all quantitative rather than qualitative. The pattern of carbohydrate digestion, i.e. the microbial fermentation of cellulose and starch and the absorption of the digestive products such as glucose, lactate and the short-chain volatile fatty acids, can occur to some extent in most species although the relative importance of these processes differs markedly between ruminants and non-ruminants. Differences in the rate of glucose production and the fractional contribution from gluconeogenesis depend very much on the type of diet as well as on the type of animal. The use of glucose for fatty acid synthesis is also very much diet-dependent and it is probable, although not formally demonstrated, that this is also true for the use of glucose as an energy source. In muscle, there is a quantitative difference in the use of fatty acids and ketones as energy sources between ruminants and other species, but the relative importance of long-chain fatty acids and glucose for the two groups is not well-defined.

INTRODUCTION

Clear evidence that there is a marked difference in the mode of digestion of carbohydrate in ruminants was established nearly 40 years ago by the work of Sir Joseph Barcroft and his colleagues at Cambridge. Since then it has gradually become apparent that there are also differences in the mode of digestion of fats and proteins. As a result, the pattern of metabolism - perhaps even to some degree the mechanism of hormonal control - has undergone some modification, although we have some way to go to understand fully the implication of these changes. In the present context I propose to discuss particularly the metabolism of carbohydrate since this is most likely to be relevant to the theme of this meeting. In parenthesis, I think it likely that changes in carbohydrate metabolism may have been primary in the development of the characteristic pattern of ruminant metabolism.

DIGESTION

The basic advantage gained by ruminants has been a fostering of the capacity to digest cellulose, by encouraging the development of a suitable range of micro-organisms in the gastro-intestinal tract. We have to recognise however that the difference from non-ruminants is quantitative rather than qualitative. Most herbivorous or omnivorous species seem to have some capacity to digest cellulose. Quantitative estimates vary widely, but in sheep and cattle, digestibility seems to be around 60 per cent or more (Armstrong and Beever, 1969; Hoover, 1978), whereas in horses, rabbits, guinea-pigs and pigs, it is nearer to 25 - 40 per cent (Slade and Hintz, 1969).

In all species there is a significant digestion in the hind-gut (large intestine or caecum) and ruminants have no advantage in this respect. Their crucial advantage has been the development of extensive fermentation in the fore-stomach, a development which has probably permitted the growth of a wider range of micro-organisms as well as increasing the total time in which cellulose digestion may occur. The disadvantage resulting from this development has been the fermentation of all dietary carbohydrate, i.e. including starch and soluble sugars. On nearly all diets, at least 80 per cent of starch ingested is digested in the rumen: on certain diets however, particularly those containing ground maize or sorghum, appreciable amounts of starch escape rumen fermentation so that up to 15 - 20 per cent may be digested in the small intestine. In contrast, in non-ruminants, while generally most of the starch is digested in the small intestine, on some diets significant amounts of starch may pass to the large intestine or caecum, to undergo fermentation.

ABSORPTION OF NUTRIENTS

The differing modes of digestion affect the pattern of nutrients absorbed. The products of fermentation are the volatile fatty acids - acetic, propionic, butyric and valeric acids (small amounts of branched-chain acids, isobutyric and isovaleric acids are also produced by microbial fermentation of branched-chain amino acids) - while enzymatic digestion of starch in the small intestine results in formation of maltose and glucose. During absorption, there is some catabolism of the absorbed nutrients by the epithelial cells of the gut. In recent studies in the author's laboratory, Pethick (unpublished) has established that at least 25 per cent of acetate taken up from the rumen in sheep is oxidised. It is also probable that propionate is to some degree oxidised, while butyrate is known to be converted in part to 3-hydroxy butyrate and acetoacetate (Pennington, 1952). A quantitative estimate of nutrients absorbed in sheep receiving their food at 2 h intervals over 24 h, has been made by Pethick. He was able to account for about 63 per cent of the metabolisable energy (ME), almost entirely in the form of volatile fatty acids and ketones. There was no detectable glucose absorption, but lactate appearance might account for 2.5 - 3 per cent of ME. Lactate is also produced by glycolysis of blood-derived glucose, and this estimate is based on the difference in lactate production in fed and fasted animals. It is thus likely to be a maximal estimate, since glycolysis might well be greater in fed than fasted animals. A similar although more approximate estimate has been made for lactating cattle by Baird et al (1975) - about 65 per cent of ME, including about 2.5 per cent from lactate. Symonds and Baird (1975) have also provided some information on the absorption of glucose from the gut in cattle, from the rise in glucose in the mesenteric vein. On this basis, together with my estimate of mesenteric blood flow, I estimate that on hay diets about one per cent of ME might be absorbed as glucose; even when a substantial amount of ground maize is fed, this increases only to about 2.5 per cent. This finding is perhaps difficult to reconcile with the observations discussed earlier, that substantial amounts of starch may escape fermentation on such a diet, and may disappear during passage along the small intestine. It is likely however, that maltase activity in the ruminant small intestine is limited; moreover there is some evidence that glucose absorption occurs by a process that is heavily concentration-dependent, rather than a true active transport, as is known to occur in the rat intestine. Maltose and glucose in the small intestine may therefore undergo fermentation rather than absorption, particularly in the lower part of the small intestine.

The author is not aware of comparable studies in non-ruminants, although there has been much dispute as to the extent to which glucose is absorbed unchanged from the gut. Shoemaker et al. (1963) demonstrated in unanaesthetised dogs that, following an oral dose of 50 g glucose, there was an increase in glucose in portal blood equivalent to 77 per cent of the dose. Appearance of lactate was equivalent to only about 5 per cent of the oral glucose dose. When fructose was given by mouth, there was evidence that nearly half was converted to glucose, but overall carbohydrate recovery was similar to that of glucose.

In contrast to these observations, Shapiro and Shapiro (1979) have claimed that in rats only about 10 - 15 per cent of administered glucose is absorbed unaltered, and as much as 50 per cent may be absorbed as lactic acid, although Windmüller and Spaeth (1980) have recently presented evidence, also in rats, that only a small amount of glucose absorbed is glycolysed during absorption (about 3 per cent).

I have attempted to estimate absorption of products in pigs, using the results of Anderson and Northrop (1973), Anderson (1974) and some unpublished observations made by the author with Anderson. About 50 per cent of the ME may be accounted for by absorbed glucose and only 2 - 3 per cent as lactate. Rérat (1978) has presented figures suggesting that 4 - 6 per cent of starch intake by pigs might be accounted for as lactate - a figure which is quite comparable to our estimate. As he recognised, it is likely to be an over-estimate in that the lactate need not be derived only from dietary carbohydrate. In contrast, it is estimated that about 11 per cent of the ME is absorbed as volatile fatty acids - with acetic and propionic of about equal significance. Thus, in these young growing pigs on a high-starch diet about 65 per cent of the ME is accounted for, a figure very similar to that seen in ruminants, although the proportions of the various constituents are very different. Most of the remaining ME intake may reasonably be attributed to long-chain fatty acids and amino acids.

HEPATIC METABOLISM OF ABSORBED NUTRIENTS

Glucose is known to be required by all animals. Thus in ruminants, where we have seen that there is at best only a trivial amount of glucose absorbed from the gastro-intestinal tract, there must be extensive gluconeogenesis. Some glucose synthesis (about 10 - 15 per cent of the total) occurs in the kidney, at least in sheep (Kaufman and Bergman, 1971, 1974) but the major site is the liver. The relative contribution of various precursors has been assessed by both isotope dilution techniques and measurement of hepatic uptake, in relation to glucose output (Lindsay, 1978). Both techniques have potential limitations, but since there is quite good correspondence between results obtained by the two methods, they are likely to give a reasonably accurate picture. Propionate is undoubtedly the major component, and about 90 per cent is normally extracted by the liver accounting for up to 50 per cent of glucose output. The other glucogenic volatile fatty acids, isobutyrate and valerate, are also substantially extracted by the liver, but since the total amount available is limited, they contribute 5 per cent or less to glucose output. Amino acids, mainly alanine and glutamine, may provide carbon for about 15 - 20 per cent of glucose output. The remainder is derived from lactate and glycerol. Since, as we have seen, little lactate is absorbed from the gut (and the same applies to glycerol) these metabolites are derived from endogenous sources, probably ultimately mainly from glucose. Thus up to a third of the glucose that is synthesised is involved in internal recycling of carbon. In fasting, the major change is that there is a rapid decline in the availability of propionate, and a corresponding rise in the contribution of lactate and glycerol.

In non-ruminants, the immediate effect of a large entry of glucose into the portal circulation is to suppress the post-absorptive production of glucose by the liver. In experiments in man, Felig et al., (1975) observed that following ingestion of an oral glucose load (about 100 g), there was substantial hepatic uptake of glucose, so that only about 15 per cent of the ingested glucose passed the liver to the peripheral circulation. This capacity of the liver to remove a large part of the absorbed glucose load seems to depend in part on an induced insulin secretion; when the experiment was repeated in maturity-onset diabetics, nearly twice as much glucose passed to the peripheral circulation. We cannot, however, suppose that this extensive uptake of dietary glucose is the invariable response in non-ruminants to dietary carbohydrate. While Anderson and the author, in an unpublished study, observed a large uptake of glucose by the liver in young pigs after a carbohydrate meal, in a much larger study (15 pigs) Anderson and Northrop (1974) found that during 4 h following a high carbohydrate meal only 11 per cent of the glucose absorbed was removed directly by the liver. Probably an important factor in the ability of the liver to remove a glucose load is the presence and activity of the enzyme glucokinase, which is characterised by a high K_m; thus at high glucose concentrations it becomes more and more effective in initiating the metabolism of glucose through the formation of glucose-6-phosphate. Hexokinase, which is invariably present in liver, has a low K_m so that it is saturated with respect to glucose below the normal blood-glucose concentration. It is striking that the ruminant liver, which never faces a large glucose load, is characterised by total absence of glucokinase although a low K_m hexokinase is present (Ballard et al., 1969). The enzyme is known to be adaptive (Walker, 1966) although whether dietary factors affect it is uncertain.

Although the output of glucose by the liver of non-ruminants is suppressed following a carbohydrate meal, we should not suppose that gluconeogenesis does not occur. In the pig, for example, the lactate released into the portal vein is extensively removed by the liver - to be used partly no doubt as an oxidative source, but also in the formation of liver glycogen. Moreover, in animals fed once or twice per day, elevated glucose concentration in the portal vein occurs only for 12 - 18 of the 24 h (Anderson, 1974). As soon as this declines the liver begins to put out glucose. Nilsson et al. (1973) showed that in man, in these circumstances, glucose from the liver was about 63 per cent derived from glycogen and the remainder from lactate, glycerol and amino acids. Dr. H.R. Watson (unpublished results) estimated the extent of gluconeogenesis in rats by measuring the incorporation of ^3H (supplied as ^3H_2O in the drinking water) into glucose. This method has some limitations; in particular, it probably over-estimates the rate of gluconeogenesis. Nevertheless, it was striking that even on high-carbohydrate diets (about 50 per cent carbohydrate) about 20 per cent of the glucose appeared to be derived by gluconeogenesis.

RATE OF GLUCOSE SYNTHESIS

Following the original observations of the Barcroft school on the extensive fermentation of dietary carbohydrate in ruminants, a view developed that glucose availability may be much less in ruminants. I suggested however (Lindsay, 1959), on the basis of fairly slender data, that glucose turnover rates were probably not much different in ruminants and non-ruminants. Ballard et al. (1969) had substantially more information available and concluded that the rate of glucose production was approximately proportional to a power ($W^{0.8}$) of body-weight and that ruminants and non-ruminants showed little difference in this respect. There is now sufficient evidence to suggest that this view should be qualified. In all species there seems to be a fall in glucose flux, or turnover, as fasting develops. Choosing an exact time for comparison of fasting in different species is not easy. In small animals, a fast of 24 h must be regarded as substantially more severe than a comparable time for a much larger animal, and in comparing ruminants and non-ruminants, account must be taken of the very different residence time of food in the gastro-intestinal tract. Nevertheless, it seems probable in fasting animals that the view developed by Ballard et al. (1969) is essentially correct. In fed animals, however, we have to take account of the nature of the diet. Belo et al. (1976) have determined rates of glucose production in dogs on different diets. In dogs receiving high-protein or high-fat diets, there was not much difference in the rate of production and it was only about 5 - 30 per cent greater than that observed in fasting. On a high carbohydrate diet (62 per cent carbohydrate) the rate was almost double that observed on other diets or on fasting. Freeman et al. (1970) also observed a rate of glucose production in pigs on a high-carbohydrate diet more than double that observed after about 16 h fasting. Watson, in the study referred to above, found that in rats on a high-carbohydrate diet the rate of glucose production was more than twice as great as that on a high-fat diet. Moreover, these estimates may actually under-estimate the effect of a high-carbohydrate diet. Glucose production rate is determined by isotope dilution techniques. When these are applied to conditions in which there is a large absorption of glucose from the gut, followed by significant uptake by the liver, the circulating glucose no longer constitutes a single uniformly mixed pool.

To meet the requirements of the isotope dilution technique, it is necessary that the ^{14}C-glucose being utilised be of the same specific activity at different sites. When glucose is absorbed from the gut and removed by the liver, this will be at lower specific activity than that utilised at peripheral sites. In effect what is measured lies somewhere between what is being absorbed from the gut, and what is entering the peripheral circulation. This limitation to isotope dilution techniques was noted by Annison and Lindsay (1962) with respect to propionate production in sheep, its relevance to glucose absorption studies was emphasised by Freeman et al., (1970), but it does not generally seem to have been appreciated. It seems therefore highly probable that in non-ruminants on a high-carbohydrate diet, there will be substantially more glucose available than on other diets, or for ruminants on any diet.

UTILISATION OF CARBOHYDRATE

Oxidation

It is to be expected that, in part, dietary carbohydrate will be used as an energy source. In a number of whole-animal studies, in which ^{14}C-glucose has been used as tracer for turn-over studies, the amount oxidised has also been determined by measurement of the $^{14}CO_2$ expired. It is important to recognise that estimates of the proportion of carbon dioxide derived from glucose in such studies have often significant limitations. If one makes a constant infusion of labelled glucose and compares the specific activity of circulating glucose with that of expired air, it is difficult to be sure when the specific activities, particularly that of carbon dioxide, are constant. This is probably because the glucose-carbon, before being oxidised, passes through many pools with very differing turnover rates. If, on the other hand, one makes a single injection of labelled glucose and again follows the specific activity of carbon dioxide and glucose until both are negligible, it may take an unacceptably long time, quite apart from the difficulty of deciding when specific activities really are negligible.

These features apply generally to studies of the oxidation of metabolites, but they seem to be particularly marked with respect to glucose. There is a further difficulty in studies in non-ruminants. As we have discussed, the liver may remove a significant fraction of the glucose absorbed after feeding. This will have a different specific activity from that available to peripheral tissues. Thus, the contribution of the liver to glucose oxidation will be underestimated and if the liver is a significant contributor to overall oxidative metabolism (as it usually is) this will lead to a significant overall underestimation.

This limitation clearly does not apply to ruminants where in most studies it has been estimated that about 10 (4 - 15) per cent of carbon dioxide is derived from glucose, this not being greatly different in fed and fasted animals. In fasted chickens (Annison et al., 1969) the proportional contribution was quite similar (9 per cent) but in fasted dogs (Paul et al., 1975), pigs (Freeman et al., 1970) and rats (Shipley et al., 1970) the estimate was appreciably higher (14 - 20 per cent). Even higher estimates have been obtained in post-absorptive man (Long et al., 1971) and in fed pigs (Freeman et al., 1970) and rats (Shipley et al., 1970) - from 30 - 44 per cent of carbon dioxide from glucose. After allowing for the underestimation, for reasons set out above, it suggests that in the immediate post-prandial period, some 2 - 5 h after a meal, glucose may be the major energy source, in striking contrast to ruminants.

Fat synthesis

Although there is extensive oxidation of carbohydrate in non-ruminants, this is certainly not the fate of all the carbohydrate absorbed. Shipley et al. (1970) in studies in rats with ^{14}C-glucose, attempted to construct a balance-sheet and were able to account for about 90 per cent of the flux in fed and 80 per cent in fasted rats. Of this, about 70 per cent is accounted for through oxidation. It is natural to suppose that a significant fraction is used for fat synthesis. Stetten and Boxer

(1944) from studies with rats on a fat-free diet concluded, from the incorporation of D of deuterated water supplied to the animals, that as much as one-third of the glucose was used for the synthesis of fatty acids. Masoro et al. (1949) drew similar conclusions from studies with ^{14}C-glucose using mice. Masoro has more recently pointed out (Masoro, 1977) that significant rates of incorporation of glucose into fatty acids are found only under the unusual conditions of a totally fat-free diet. In more usual conditions (e.g. with about 60 per cent carbohydrate, 10 per cent fat, in the diet) only about 3 - 4 per cent of glucose flux is converted to fatty acids (Masoro et al., 1957; De Freitas and Depocas, 1965). It has been suggested that as little as 2.5 per cent fat in the diet may result in a significant decrease in lipogenesis (Hill et al., 1958). The only comparable study with larger non-ruminants is that of O'Hea and Leveille (1969). In young pigs, about 12 - 15 kg weight, it may be estimated from their results that about 12 - 13 per cent of glucose flux was recovered in fatty-acids - almost entirely in adipose tissue. The diet used in these studies contained about 70 per cent carbohydrate, and perhaps more significant, only about 3 per cent fat.

Most studies in ruminants have been made with tissues *in vitro*. The author however, has made experiments in mature sheep, in which ^{14}C-glucose was infused and incorporation into tissues estimated (Beneke and Lindsay, 1967; Lindsay, 1970). Rather less than one per cent of glucose flux was used for fatty acid synthesis, this being almost entirely in adipose tissue; although about 5 per cent of the flux was incorporated in the glycerol of the triacylglycerols of adipose tissues. From the results of Prior (1978) in which ^{14}C-lactate was infused into sheep, it may be calculated that about 6 per cent of the lactate flux was converted into depot fat. It was implied, although not explicitly stated that this was recovered in the depot fatty acids, and recovery in glycerol was not stated. It is difficult to understand how lactate can be much more effective than glucose *in vivo* since the two are so rapidly interconvertible. In contrast to glucose, acetate is more readily used as a source of depot fatty-acids in sheep. Beneke and Lindsay (1967) recovered about 5 per cent of acetate flux in depot-acids in mature sheep at maintenance level of feeding. Prior recovered about 5 - 13 per cent, depending on dietary intake, in younger animals, and Ingle et al. (1972) recovered between 6 - 9 per cent also in young animals. A rough calculation suggests that this means that about 1 - 3 per cent of ME is used for lipogenesis in ruminants. This is probably only about half the value for the pig (on a low fat diet), but perhaps not so different from non-ruminants on more usual diets. The striking difference, however, is that the carbon source for this is almost entirely acetate for ruminants, whereas it is glucose for non-ruminants. The most usual reason advanced for this limited use of glucose in ruminants stems from the finding (Hanson and Ballard, 1967) that the activities of ATP citrate lyase and malic (carboxylating) dehydrogenase activity in ruminant liver and adipose tissue are negligible compared with the activities in corresponding tissues of many non-ruminants. Lipogenesis from glucose carbon requires formation of acetyl CoA from pyruvate in mitochondria, transfer back to the cytosol as citrate, and cleavage (via ATP citrate lyase) to acetyl CoA and oxaloacetate. The latter is returned to the mitochondria via malate, the malic enzyme providing at the same time $NADPH_2$, which is specifically required for fatty acid synthesis. In contrast in synthesis from acetate, acetyl CoA can be formed directly in the cytosol. The necessary $NADPH_2$ is partly formed from glucose oxidation, by the pentose phosphate reactions, and in part from acetate, since cytosolic isocitric dehydrogenase is present in ruminant adipose tissue at enhanced activity (Ingle et al., 1972). This biochemical explanation (limiting activity of ATP citrate lyase) is further supported by the findings of Hardwick (1966). He found that, while the enzyme was absent from ruminant mammary tissue (where it is known that fatty acid synthesis from glucose is very small), it was present in nervous tissue, where it is required for the synthesis of acetyl choline. It has also been shown (Ballard et al., 1972) that prolonged infusion of glucose into sheep both increases citrate lyase and stimulates incorporation of glucose into fatty acids *in vitro*.

Finally, in foetal lambs, where glucose is virtually the only available source for lipogenesis, citrate lyase activity (in the liver) is significant (Muramatsu et al., 1970). (In the foetus, in contrast to the adult ruminant, the liver is probably the major site for fatty acid synthesis).

There is thus a plausible case for activity of citrate lyase being the factor involved in the limited use of glucose for fatty-acid synthesis. At the same time, it has to be recognised that enzyme activities may reflect, rather than determine, a pathway. It is still possible that low hexokinase activity, limiting uptake in adipose tissue, or low pyruvate dehydrogenase activity, limiting availability of acetyl CoA, may be the determining factors, although there is no direct evidence for either of these possibilities.

METABOLISM IN MUSCLE

Until about twenty years ago, it was generally held that glucose was the important energy source for muscle. However, Andres et al. (1956) found in studies of forearm muscle in men in the post-absorptive state, i.e. fasted overnight, that there was substantial lactate production by muscle, even in the face of a marked consumption of oxygen. Glucose uptake, corrected for lactate output, could account for at most 7 per cent of the oxygen consumption. This is supported by the observations of Ruderman et al. (1971) that in the isolated rat hindquarter, perfused with ^{14}C-glucose, only 1 - 3 per cent of oxygen consumed appeared to be derived from oxidation of glucose. With the recognition of free (non-esterified) fatty acids (FFA) as a major vehicle for the transport of lipid in blood, it seemed likely that this might be a major energy-source for skeletal muscle. In initial studies (Baltzan et al., 1962) no significant A-V difference was observed across human muscle. Later, Friedberg et al. (1960) demonstrated a consistent uptake of ^{14}C-FFA. In general, there is an output of FFA from adipose sites in close connection with muscle, and this may mask the uptake, until this is shown by isotopic studies. By using this technique it has been shown that FFA uptake is generally sufficient (if oxidised) to account for most of the oxygen consumed by muscle. Studies of $^{14}CO_2$ output across muscle however, generally suggest a much lower amount of oxidation of FFA. It is argued (e.g. Zierler, 1976) that FFA taken up by muscle is first incorporated into lipid, and that fatty acid derived intracellularly is the direct source of most muscle carbon dioxide. Other sources of energy for muscle include 3-hydroxybutyrate (Ruderman et al., 1971) which might account for up to 15 per cent of oxidation; and acetate (Karlsson et al., 1975). This latter substrate is likely to be significant only following alcohol ingestion in man. The role of glucose is not very clear, although Ruderman et al. (1979) have suggested that it might account for up to 17 per cent of oxygen consumption on the basis of studies with 1-^{14}C-lactate. This is presumably used as a marker for intracellular pyruvate, and suggests that the authors supposed that muscle glycogen was a more immediate source for oxidation.

With this background, we may turn to examine energy sources in ruminant muscle. Studies of the uptake of metabolites across the sheep hind-limb and their role as fuels have been made by Jarrett et al. (1976), Domanski et al. (1974) and Lindsay and Setchell (1976); and across the hind-limb of steers by Bell et al. (1974, 1975) Bell and Thompson (1979). There is much variation in the estimates of the contribution of particular metabolites. Probably this in large part reflects differing techniques as well as different conditions, especially in relation to feeding. Nevertheless, some generalisations seem permissible. In normally fed animals, where there is little variation in blood-ketone concentrations, the uptake of ketones could account for 9 - 12 per cent of oxygen consumption. Acetate uptake varies greatly with concentration, but in animals fed at two hourly intervals, when the arterial concentration is fairly constant, at about 1 - 1.2mM, about 35 - 40 per cent of oxygen consumption may be accounted for, assuming acetate taken up is oxidised. In experiments with ^{14}C-labelled ketones or acetate, direct estimates of the degree of oxidation were about 65 - 80 per cent of these values. Since the latter are probably under-estimates (because of hold-up of isotope in metabolic pools) it is probable that most of the metabolites taken up are indeed oxidised. Thus nearly half the energy needs of ruminant muscle are derived from ketones and acetate. In non-ruminants (pig and neonatal lamb) in contrast, these metabolites will account for only about 10 per cent of oxygen consumption.

The remaining sources of energy must be FFA and glucose. From the estimate of true uptake of FFA by the steer hind-limb (Bell and Thompson, 1979) one may calculate that almost 50 per cent of oxygen consumption could be derived from FFA, yet measurements of $^{14}CO_2$ output indicated that only 2 per cent of oxidation was derived from FFA oxidation. This could be explained as already discussed, by supposing that FFA pass through an intramuscular lipid pool before oxidation. The results of Bell and Thompson (1979) however, point rather to a slow exchange of metabolic carbon dioxide with a slowly turning-over pool of carbon dioxide. Pethick and Lindsay (unpublished) have studied FFA in pregnant sheep. We find there is a linear relation between FFA concentration and uptake (expressed as a maximum contribution to oxidation). If this relation holds also in non-pregnant, fed animals, it suggests that uptake of FFA would account for only 15 - 20 per cent of oxidation. Moreover, in contrast to other workers, we find little evidence of an intramuscular lipid pool - estimates of FFA oxidation from $^{14}CO_2$ output suggest at least 65 per cent of FFA is promptly oxidised.

Finally, we may consider the role of carbohydrate. Varied results are reported for glucose uptake and lactate output. We find, however, that glucose uptake is greatest in fed, non-pregnant, non-lactating sheep, and in these conditions there is no consistent lactate output. The amount taken up, if oxidised, could account for 30 - 40 per cent of oxygen consumption. This agrees with the evidence detailed above, that other metabolites account for 65 per cent of oxygen consumption, although it is excessively large if FFA provide half the energy required. When we used ^{14}C-glucose however, variable results were obtained, but on average only 6 per cent of carbon dioxide appeared to be derived from glucose. This could be explained if the major fate of glucose taken up was formation of muscle glycogen, which would then be the direct source of carbohydrate oxidised. Earlier experiments, however, (Annison et al., 1963) produced little labelling of muscle glycogen following infusion of ^{14}C-glucose, suggesting that the turnover was only 1 - 2 per cent per day. Glucose uptake of neonatal lamb muscle was larger than that of adult sheep, but there was also substantial lactate production. Net carbohydrate uptake was still sufficient to account for about 35 per cent of oxygen consumption. In preliminary studies of pigs, using the same technique, glucose uptake was even larger, and there was also an uptake of lactate. Total carbohydrate uptake was sufficient to account for nearly 95 per cent of oxygen consumption.

We are left with a rather unsatisfactory conclusion. The metabolism of pig muscle may be dominated by carbohydrate to a greater degree than in sheep and cattle. Nevertheless, the oxidation of carbohydrate in ruminant muscle may be at least as important as in that of men and rats. Before accepting this, we need to identify metabolic pools in muscle, which have a long turnover time, and through which glucose apparently must pass.

REFERENCES

Anderson, D.M., 1974. The effect of feeding on the concentration of glucose and insulin in the portal and atrial plasma of pigs. J. Agric. Sci. 82, 29-36.

Anderson, D.M. and Northrop, A.J., 1973. The diurnal variation in volatile fatty acids concentration in portal and atrial plasma in pigs. Proc. Nutr. Soc. 32, 37A.

Anderson, D.M. and Northrop, A.J., 1974. The absorption of glucose from the gut and the amount removed by the liver in young pigs. Proc. Nutr. Soc. 33, 91A.

Andres, R., Cader, G. and Zerler, K.L., 1956. The quantitatively minor role of carbohydrate in oxidative metabolism by skeletal muscle in intact man in the basal state. Measurements of oxygen and glucose uptake and carbon dioxide and lactate production in the forearm. J. Clin. Invest. 35, 671-682.

Annison, E.F. and Lindsay, D.B., 1962. The measurement of entry rates of propionate and butyrate in sheep. Biochem. J. 85, 474-479.

Annison, E.F., Lindsay, D.B. and White, R.R., 1963. Metabolic interrelations of glucose and lactate in sheep. Biochem. J. 88, 243-248.

Annison, E.F., Shrimpton, D.H. and West, C.E., 1969. Glucose and fatty acid metabolism in chickens in relation to overall energy expenditure. In: Energy metabolism of farm animals. Ed. Blaxter, K.L., Kielasowski, J. and Thorbeck, G. pp. 339-347. Oriel Press, Newcastle.

Armstrong, D.G. and Beever, D.E., 1969. Post-abomasal digestion of carbohydrate in the adult ruminant. Proc. Nutr. Soc. 28, 121-131.

Baird, G.D., Symonds, H.W. and Ash, R., 1975. Some observations on metabolite production and utilization *in vivo* by the gut and liver of adult dairy cows. J. Agric. Sci. Camb. 85, 281-296.

Ballard, F.J., Filsell, O.H. and Jarrett, I.G., 1972. Effects of carbohydrate availability on lipogenesis in sheep. Biochem. J. 126, 193-200.

Ballard, F.J., Hanson, R.W. and Kronfeld, D.S., 1969. Gluconeogenesis and lipogenesis in tissue from ruminant and nonruminant animals. Fedn. Proc. Fedn. Am. Socs. Exp. Biol. 28, 218-230.

Baltzan, M.A., Andres, R., Cader, G. and Zierler, K.L., 1962. Heterogeneity of forearm metabolism with special reference to the free fatty acids. J. Clin. Invest. 41, 116-125.

Bell, A.W., Gardner, J.W. and Thompson, G.E., 1974. The effects of acute cold exposure and feeding on volatile fatty acid metabolism in the hind leg of the young ox. Br. J. Nutr. 32, 471-477.

Bell, A.W., Gardner, J.W., Manson, W. and Thompson, G.E., 1975. Acute cold exposure and the metabolism of blood glucose, lactate and pyruvate and plasma amino acids in the hind leg of the fed and fasted young ox. Br. J. Nutr. 33, 207-217.

Bell, A.W. and Thompson, G.E., 1979. Free fatty acid oxidation in bovine muscle *in vivo*: effects of cold exposure and feeding. Am. J. Physiol. 237(4), E309-315.

Belo, P.S., Romsos, D.R. and Leveille, G.A., 1976. Influence of diet on glucose tolerance, on the rate of glucose utilization and on gluconeogenic enzyme activities in the dog. J. Nutr. 106, 1465-1474.

Beneke, H.G. and Lindsay, D.B., 1967. Fatty acid synthesis in sheep. Proc. Aust. Biochem. Soc. 1, 28.

De Freitas, A.S.W. and Depocas, F., 1965. Fatty acid and glyceride glycerol synthesis from glucose during high rates of glucose uptake in the intact rat. Can. J. Biochem. 43, 437-450.

Domanski, A., Lindsay, D.B. and Setchell, B.P., 1974. Blood flow and substrate uptake and oxidation in the hind limb muscles of sheep. J. Physiol. 242, 28-29P.

Felig, P., Wahren, J. and Hendler, R., 1975. Influence of oral glucose ingestion on splanchnic glucose and gluconeogenesis substrate metabolism in man. Diabetes 24, 468-475.

Freeman, C.P., Noakes, D.E. and Annison, E.F., 1970. The metabolism of glucose, acetate, palmitate, stearate and oelate in pigs. Br. J. Nutr. 24, 705-716.

Freidberg, F.J., Klein, R.F., Trout, D.L., Bogdonoff, M.D. and Estes, E.H. Jr., 1960. The characteristics of the peripheral transport of ^{14}C-labelled palmitic acid. J. Clin. Invest. 39, 1511-1515.

Hanson, R.W. and Ballard, F.J., 1967. The relative significance of acetate and glucose as precursors for lipid synthesis in liver and adipose tissue from ruminants. Biochem. J., 105, 529-536.

Hardwick, D.C., 1966. The fate of acetyl groups derived from glucose in the isolated perfused goat udder. Biochem. J. 99, 228-231.

Hill, R., Linazasoro, J.M., Chevallier, F. and Chaikoff, I.L., 1958. Regulation of hepatic lipogenesis: the influence of dietary fats. J. Biol. Chem. 233, 305-310.

Hoover, W.H., 1978. Digestion and absorption in the hind gut of ruminants J. Anim. Sci. 46, 1789-1798.

Ingle, D.L., Bauman, D.E. and Garrigus, U.S., 1972. Lipogenesis in the ruminant: *in vivo* site of fatty acid synthesis in sheep. J. Nutr. 102, 617-624.

Jarrett, I.G., Filsell, O.H. and Ballard, F.J., 1976. Utilization of oxidizable substrates by the sheep hind limb: effects of starvation and exercise. Metabolism 25, 523-531.

Karlsson, N., Fellenius, E. and Kiessling, K.H., 1975. The metabolism of acetate in the perfused hind-quarter of the rat. Acta Physiol. Scand. 93, 391-400.

Kaufman, C.F. and Bergman, E.N., 1971. Renal glucose, free fatty acid and ketone body metabolism in the unanaesthetised sheep. Am. J. Physiol. 221, 967-972.

Kaufman, C.F. and Bergman, E.N., 1974. Renal ketone body metabolism and gluconeogenesis in normal and hypoglycaemic sheep. Am. J. Physiol. 226, 827-832.

Lindsay, D.B., 1959. Significance of carbohydrate in ruminant metabolism. Vet. Rev. Annot. 5, 103-128.

Lindsay, D.B., 1970. In: Physiology of digestion and metabolism in ruminants. Ed. A.T. Phillipson and others pp. 438-451. Oriel Press, Newcastle.

Lindsay, D.B., 1978. Gluconeogenesis in ruminants. Trans. Biochem. Soc. 6, 1152-1156.

Lindsay, D.B. and Setchell, B.P., 1976. The oxidation of glucose, ketone bodies and acetate by the brain of normal and ketonaemic sheep. J. Physiol. 259, 801-823.

Long, C.L., Spencer, J.L., Kinney, J.M. and Geiger, J.R., 1971. Carbohydrate metabolism in normal man and effect of glucose infusion. J. App. Physiol. 31, 102-109.

Masoro, E.J., 1977. Lipids and lipid metabolism. Ann. Rev. Physiol. 39, 301-321.

Masoro, E.J., Asuncion, C.L., Brown, R.K. and Rapport, D., 1957. Lipogenesis from carbohydrate in the negative caloric balance state induced by exposure to cold. Am. J. Physiol. 190, 177-179.

Masoro, E.J., Chaikoff, I.L. and Dauben, W.G., 1949. Lipogenesis from glucose in the normal and liverless animal as studied with C^{14}-labelled glucose. J. Biol. Chem. 179, 1117-1125.

Muramatsu, M., Ambo, K. and Tsuda, T., 1970. ATP citrate lyase activity in the liver of newborn lambs. J. Biochem. (Tokyo) 67, 727-729.

Nilsson, L.H.son, Furst, P. and Hultman, E., 1973. Carbohydrate metabolism of the liver in normal man under varying dietary conditions. Scand. J. Clin. Lab. Invest. 32, 331-337.

O'Hea, E.K. and Leveille, G.A., 1969. Significance of adipose tissue and liver as sites of fatty acid synthesis in the pig and the efficiency of utilization of various substrates for lipogenesis. J. Nutr. 99, 338-344.

Paul, P., Donohue, M. and Holmes, W.L., 1975. Glucose metabolism in thyroid-ectomised and normal dogs during rest and acute cold exposure. J. Appl. Physiol. 38, 236-240.

Pennington, R.J., 1952. The metabolism of short-chain fatty acids in the sheep. 1. Fatty acid utilization and ketone body production by rumen epithelium and other tissues. Biochem. J. 51, 251-258.

Prior, R.L., 1978. Effect of level of feed intake on lactate and acetate metabolism and lipogenesis *in vivo* in sheep. J. Nutr. 108, 926-935.

Rérat, A., 1978. Digestion and absorption of carbohydrates and nitrogenous matters in the hindgut of the omnivorous nonruminant animal. J. Anim. Sci. 46, 1808-1837.

Ruderman, N.B., Goodman, M.N., Conover, C.A. and Berger, M., 1979. Substrate utilization in perfused skeletal muscle. Diabetes 28, Suppl. 1., 13-17.

Ruderman, N.B., Houghton, C.R.S. and Hems, R., 1971. Evaluation of the isolated perfused rat hindquarter for the study of muscle metabolism. Biochem. J. 124, 639-651.

Shapiro, A. and Shapiro, B., 1979. Role of the liver in intestinal glucose absorption. Biochem. Biophys. Acta. 586, 123-127.

Shipley, R.A., Chudzick, E.B. and Gibbons, A.P., 1970. Rate of disposal of glucose carbon to carbon dioxide, fat, protein and glycogen in the diabetic rat. Am. J. Physiol. 219, 364-373.

Shoemaker, W.C., Yanof, H.M., Turk, L.N. and Wilson, T.H., 1963. Glucose and fructose absorption in the unanaesthetized dog. Gastroenterol, 44, 654-663.

Slade, L.M. and Hintz, H.F., 1969. Comparison of digestion in horses, ponies, rabbits and guinea pigs. J. Anim. Sci. 28, 842-843.

Stetten de Witt Jr. and Boxer, G.E., 1944. Studies in carbohydrate metabolism. 1. The rate of turnover of liver and carcass glycogen studied with the aid of deuterium. J. Biol. Chem. 155, 231-236.

Symonds, H.W. and Baird, G.D., 1975. Evidence for the absorption of reducing sugar from the small intestine of the dairy cow. Brit. Vet. J. 131, 17-22.

Walker, D.G., 1966. The nature and function of hexokinases in animal tissues. In: Essays in Biochemistry 2 pp. 33-67. Campbell, P.N. and Greville, G.D. eds. Academic Press, London and New York.

Windmüller, H.G. and Spaeth, A., 1980. Respiratory fuels and nitrogen metabolism *in vivo* in small intestine of fed rats. J. Biol. Chem. 255, 107-112.

Zierler, K.L., 1976. Fatty acids as substrates for heart and skeletal muscle. Circ. Res. 38, 459-463.

DISCUSSION

P.V. Tarrant *(Ireland)*

I would like to ask Dr. Lindsay if the observations he made on muscle carbohydrate metabolism referred to resting animals, and how would they change in the event of heavy exercise or exertion?

D.B. Lindsay *(UK)*

I have not made any studies under the conditions you describe. The animals were conscious and standing quietly. I think standing is important. If one supports an animal on a sling, so that the muscles of the hind legs are not doing any work, particularly if one anaesthetises the animal, then the whole metabolic rate drops very substantially. I think it drops more in terms of oxidative metabolism than in terms of glycolytic, but I do not have any good evidence for that. In the studies that have been made in Australia on exercising sheep - and there are also some being made in cattle at present - the indication is that the ability to use acetate and hydroxybutyrate does not increase with an increased demand for oxygen. There is some indication that, in this case, carbohydrate is used substantially more, but we have no direct information about this. I should add that the same thing happens if you cold-stress the animals; it does not matter if it is a particular limb or the animal as a whole, if it is sufficient to produce shivering the carbohydrate consumption goes up very substantially. Again, I do not have much evidence of whether there is a direct oxidation of glucose which is rather puzzling. Definitive experiments have not been done on that.

J.J.A. Heffron *(Ireland)*

You said that, in man, free fatty acids were a source of energy in muscle. Is that under resting conditions?

D.B. Lindsay

That is what is suggested. I think that most of the

people who have done these studies have, in fact, chosen conditions which emphasise this. There was a classical view that muscle relied on carbohydrate as an energy source but it was changed about 20 years ago. It was changed because the studies were made in the post-absorptive state. To my knowledge there have been no satisfactory studies in man within 2 - 3 h after a meal, during peak carbohydrate availability. That may be one of the reasons why we have got this emphasis on free fatty acids as the energy source in man.

J.J.A. Heffron

It is not my area but I believe a Swedish group have shown that carbohydrate is involved under active conditions and that it also depends on the particular fibre type of the muscle.

D.B. Lindsay

It is a little more complicated than that. The effectiveness of training of the distance athelete is believed to depend very much on the ability of his muscles to use fatty acids. If he is not very well trained then, certainly, he uses a lot of carbohydrate.

P.V. Tarrant

I would like to add a comment to Dr. Heffron's remarks. Some cattle are well-exercised, where they are reared under extensive conditions; others in intensive systems get very little exercise. I am sure this may have an important bearing on the incidence of dark-cutting beef in extensive and intensive beef production systems. In the intensive system, where animals are housed and perhaps individually tied, their muscles may have a reduced capacity for oxidative metabolism of free fatty acids. In the extensive system the muscles may be well adapted to exercise and consequently have a high oxidative capacity. Take Lawrie's classical studies in Australia for example, which showed that it was practically impossible to produce dark-cutting beef by exercising cattle. Presumably this was because they were very well adapted animals; would you agree?

D.B. Lindsay

I think that sounds quite reasonable.

P.V. Tarrant

A further question concerning results on a poster by McVeigh and Tarrant. We have studied hay-fed heifers, probably similar to some of the hay-fed animals which you showed us during your talk. We induced a glycogen-depleted condition and measured the time it took to return to the normal muscle glycogen concentration, and this was in excess of 10 days. Have you any suggestions as to the factors responsible for this very slow rate of glycogen repletion in hay-fed heifers? If you compare this rate with that reported for other species, there is an enormous difference. Is it simply a factor of diet or is there something peculiar to the ruminant which leads to a very slow rate of glucose assimilation by the muscles?

D.B. Lindsay

I cannot answer your question with certainty. However, there are one or two points: you say that, with hay-fed animals, there was a long recovery period. Have you any evidence that it is much shorter when the animals are given concentrate?

P.V. Tarrant

It comes down to about 7 days with 7 kg of barley per day, which is a fairly substantial supplement.

D.B. Lindsay

There are supposed to be well-marked differences in insulin concentration in the two circumstances. The other point is that I have noticed that the ruminant muscle seems to be rather sluggish to respond to insulin treatment. When as much as 100 mU/min of insulin are supplied locally to the muscle, it is very hard to see any significant increase of glucose uptake. It is striking in contrast to the rat, for example, and, I would guess, to the dog. There are one or two factors which might affect that. One of them is that fatty acids, and acetate in particular, are said to minimise the effect of insulin; I do not know how important that is. The other possibility is that insulin receptors are not present in the ruminant muscle to the same degree as in other species, there is some evidence of marked differences in sensitivity. It may be that this is an important factor in recovery of glycogen. On the other hand, there is evidence that there may be markedly rapid resynthesis of glycogen in some of the studies that have been made.

P.V. Tarrant

In concentrate-fed young bulls, we have observed a pretty substantial recovery of muscle glycogen in 3 days. It is reported in the literature that, with some laboratory animals, recovery takes hours rather than days. Of course the experimental conditions are very different. In man, under optimal conditions, 24 h is adequate for supercompensation of muscle glycogen.

It does appear that a rather lengthy period is required for glycogen repletion in cattle, whether one looks at concentrate-fed young bulls, where we observe about 72 h in the best of circumstances, to about 7 days, using a concentrate supplement for heifers, or up to 2 weeks where the animals are fed a maintenance diet of hay *ad libitum*.

D.B. Lindsay

Another point is, how long are the effects of catecholamines persisting, they are notorious for their effects of antagonising, not only the actions of insulin, but of antagonising secretion of insulin as well. You could keep getting maintained sympathetic discharge; it is not until that stops that you start getting normal insulin secretion and normal sensitivity.

SESSION III

ANIMAL BEHAVIOUR AND THE ENVIRONMENT

Chairman: L. Schön

ENVIRONMENTAL AND BEHAVIOURAL INFLUENCES ON THE SUPPLY OF ENERGY FOR MUSCLE DURING LIFE AND CONSEQUENCES *POST MORTEM*

D. Lister and G.S.G. Spencer
ARC Meat Research Institute, Langford, Bristol, BS18 7DY, UK.

ABSTRACT

The paper attempts to account for the production of dark-cutting meat in terms of the fundamental mechanism controlling the supply of energy to working muscle. The conclusion is reached that excessive use of glycogen in stressed animals is attributable to inadequate aerobic metabolism and to stimulation of anaerobiosis under the influence of the β-adrenergic mechanism. The consequent reduction of FFA supply for energy purposes contributes to an increased reliance on carbohydrate stores and ultimately to limited acidification in muscle post mortem.

INTRODUCTION

The metabolic regulation of energy production and utilisation, whether by cell, tissue or whole organism, is of fundamental importance to all creatures. Not only does it dictate an animal's ability to be physically and metabolically active for short or long periods, but it also determines the potential to survive unfavourable environments and even to grow. Control is exercised and modulated by a combination of nervous, hormonal and enzymic activity which allows energy expenditure of varying degrees and, if necessary, permits later recovery if the demand for energy temporarily exceeds current production. The system of operation is analogous to that in banking through current and deposit accounts. The biological 'cash' is largely ATP; deposits are in the form of glycogen, adipose tissue and, occasionally, protein. All the metabolic problems which relate to meat quality, like those in the financing of our own lives, stem from deficit or overdraft financing. Success or failure in supporting energy metabolism, like banking, depends on how the various assets are used. The size of any deficit at the time an animal dies is indicated by the final level of acidity which develops in muscle *post mortem*. The purpose of this paper is to suggest some possible physiological and biochemical mechanisms which lead to a loss of energy substrate in muscle during life and hence modify the development of muscle acidity *post mortem*.

Whatever combinations of energy substrates, glucose, glycogen or fatty acids (FFA) are used to support respiration, glycogen predominates overwhelmingly *post mortem*. The key issue in relation to dark-cutting muscle is, therefore, how muscle glycogen may be drawn upon, prior to an animal's death.

Sufficient depletion of glycogen to produce dark-cutting meat is difficult to induce experimentally, for neither fasting, exercise nor a combination of the two will readily precipitate it (Howard and Lawrie, 1956; Lawrie, 1958; 1966). Behavioural reactions will initiate it and dark-cutting beef often results when strange young bulls are mixed, even for a short period, prior to slaughter (Duchesne, 1978).

In the fed monogastric animal the main fuel for oxidation is glucose. During starvation the concentration of fatty acids in the plasma rises and their utilisation is increased. *In vitro* evidence suggests that the increasing availability of fatty acids for oxidation leads to inhibition of glycolysis and glucose utilisation in muscle. There is no doubt that this occurs, for even in prolonged starvation the circulating glucose level falls by only 20 - 25 per cent. A constant supply of glucose can, thus, be maintained to satisfy the continual requirement for glucose by the brain and nervous tissue. Starvation is unlikely, therefore, to lead to substantial glycogen depletion in muscle.

Exercise is also a possible cause of glycogen depletion. It is seen as a common, temporary occurrence in experimental animals and man during short periods of heavy exercise (Havel, 1970; Issekutz, 1970; Pernow and Saltin, 1971). As the work intensity by muscle increases, the respiratory quotient (RQ) approaches 1.0 which indicates an increase in the rate of glucose and/or glycogen utilisation. At even higher work-loads the supply of fuel and oxygen is likely to be limited by the supply of blood to tissues, and anaerobic glycolysis of muscle glycogen must provide energy for a short period of time. When the supply of glycogen falls, if adequate oxygen levels are restored a low level of activity can be maintained for a further short time by the oxidation of plasma glucose. Ultimately, however, this too falls and physical exhaustion results.

The 'playful' bulls whose carcasses develop the dark-cutting condition do not appear, however, to indulge in physically exhausting antics prior to slaughter. Such activity as they take is nevertheless sufficient to reduce glycogen levels in muscle and probably liver. This is difficult to explain for although the body's limited stores of carbohydrate will, as we have seen, in emergency sustain metabolic activity through anaerobic glycolysis for a few minutes, they are rarely required to be the sole energy source. At relatively moderate levels of activity fatty acids will provide the major substrate. At such levels of demand the large stores of depot fat from which FFA are mobilised are virtually inexhaustible. In the dark-cutting syndrome, where muscular activity is not necessarily predisposing, it seems more likely, therefore, that the cause is the premature enlistment of anaerobic glycolysis for energy provision rather than excessive energy demand. The important physiological question is, therefore, - how can this occur?

EXPERIMENTAL INVESTIGATION OF SUBSTRATE UTILISATION

There have been few experimental studies of metabolic stimulation in farm animals. Amongst the most comprehensive are those of the condition known as 'porcine malignant hyperthermia' (MH) (Hall et al.,1980). This reaction, which is similar in many ways to those observed as responses to stress (Lister et al., 1976), can be readily induced in susceptible pigs by the anaesthetic drugs halothane and suxamethonium, although all the potent inhalational agents can trigger the syndrome. The main responses during the development of the reaction are summarised in Table 1. Of these, the increase in oxygen consumption and carbon dioxide production (RQ > 1), the developing lactic acidosis, tendency for hyperglycaemia and unchanged or decreasing plasma FFA concentration are of note and all point to the syndrome's similarity to exhaustive physical exercise (Pernow and Saltin, 1971). The features which are, perhaps, surprising are the inconsistency of the hyperglycaemia and the FFA response. Both are stimulated by adrenergic and catecholaminergic mechanisms which are of demonstrable consequence in the aetiology of MH (Hall et al., 1980). The hyperglycaemia results mainly from glucose production by the liver and is derived from glycogenolysis and gluconeogenesis from lactate, alanine and glycerol. Terminally, hepatic glycogen is depleted.

Lipolysis, as indicated by a rising glycerol concentration in plasma, is stimulated by catecholamines during MH, but plasma

TABLE 1

MAIN METABOLIC, HORMONAL AND ELECTROLYTE CHANGES DURING PORCINE MH.

Metabolic	Hormonal	Plasma electrolytes
↑ O_2 consumption } RQ 1.0	↑↑↑ plasma noradrenaline	↑↑ inorganic phosphate
↑↑ CO_2 production } RQ 1.0	↑↑ plasma adrenaline	↑ potassium
↓↓ arterial pH	↑↑ plasma glucagon	↔ magnesium
↑↑ arterial pCO_2	↑ plasma cortisol	↔ calcium
↑↑ blood lactate	↔ plasma insulin	↓ sodium
↑ blood pyruvate		↓ chloride
↑↑ blood glucose		
↑ plasma glycerol		
↔ or ↓ plasma FFA		

The increase or decrease in plasma electrolyte values are relative to the observed haemoconcentration.

FFA values, if anything, decline. It is thought (Hall et al., 1980) that this is explained by the re-esterification of FFA.

These observations suggest new possible causes for the failure of energy substrate provision during stress which lead to the production of dark-cutting meat. We have, therefore, conducted experiments in sheep and cattle to explore some of the possibilities, in particular, the suggestion that the failure of FFA supply may be a major cause of muscle glycogen depletion in stressed animals.

In the first experiments (Lister and Spencer, 1980 - in preparation) adult ewes were infused for 8 h prior to slaughter with α- or β-adrenergic agonists. Half of each treatment group were given the potent anti-lipolytic drug MPCA (methyl pyrazole carboxylic acid: Upjohn Co.). Blood parameters were measured throughout the infusions and at the end the sheep were slaughtered for analyses of muscle and liver glycogen and assessment of meat quality. Some of the results are given in Tables 2 and 3.

α-stimulation with phenylephrine had minimal effect on blood constituents or appearance of the meat. On the other hand, administration of isoprenaline stimulated both glycolysis and lipolysis, giving rise to an elevation in the plasma concentrations of lactate, FFA, glycerol and glucose. Prolonged infusion with isoprenaline caused a decrease in muscle glycogen at slaughter, but a net increase in liver glycogen content, the latter presumably as a result of increased gluconeogenesis from lactate and glycerol. Under these conditions the decrease in muscle glycogen was not sufficient to cause dark-cutting, being comparable with the concentration following α-stimulation plus MPCA.

Blockade of isoprenaline-stimulated lipolysis, by simultaneous administration of MPCA, produced the expected decrease in plasma FFA and glycerol concentrations, and also reduced the rise in lactate and glucose. Under these conditions, with less

TABLE 2

CHANGES (%) IN PLASMA CONSTITUENTS AFTER 8 h INFUSION WITH SYMPATHOMIMETICS (SHEEP)

Treatment	Glucose	FFA	Glycerol	Lactate
α - stimulation	-5	+5	+10	0
α - stimulation + MPCA	-10	-10	-10	-30
β - stimulation	+85	+100	+110	+280
β - stimulation + MPCA	+10	+15	+20	+120

α - stimulation - phenylephrine (0.5 μg/kg/min)

β - stimulation - isoprenaline (0.1 μg/kg/min)

MPCA - 30 mg methyl pyrazole carboxylic acid 2 hourly

TABLE 3

GLYCOGEN CONCENTRATION IN MUSCLE[+] AND LIVER, AND MUSCLE[+] QUALITY AFTER 8 h INFUSION WITH SYMPATHOMIMETICS (SHEEP)

Treatment	Liver glycogen (mg/g)	Muscle glycogen (mg/g) *post mortem*		Muscle pH	Muscle Quality[++]
		0 h	24 h	at 48 h	
Control (saline)	3.8	10.4	2.7	6.03	35
α - stimulation	1.6	14.4	2.2	5.91	37
α - stimulation + MPCA	1.3	6.3	1.2	5.97	29
β - stimulation	46.1	5.5	1.5	6.07	26
β - stimulation + MPCA	20.5	1.2	0.6	6.51	20[+++]

α - stimulation - phenylephrine (0.5 μg/kg/min)

β' - stimulation - isoprenaline (0.1 μg/kg/min)

MPCA - 30 mg methyl pyrazole carboxylic acid 2 hourly

\+ *M. longissimus dorsi*
++ Measured by Fibre Optic Probe (see Macdougall and Jones, 1980)
+++ All carcasses dark-cutting

energy available from fat and less gluconeogenic precursors, muscle glycogen was severely depleted and dark-cutting resulted in all the carcasses, even though there was still appreciable liver glycogen present.

Although these effects were produced by infusions under experimental conditions, additional evidence of the importance of fat mobilisation in preventing dark-cutting, under practical conditions of animal husbandry and slaughter, has been obtained using cattle. In two separate experiments (each using 12 bulls, but under slightly differing experimental conditions) depletion of muscle glycogen was enhanced by the administration of an anti-lipolytic agent, in these cases, nicotinic acid.

The basic design of the experiments was that 12 bulls, from the same farm, were selected from three or more previously unfamiliar groups. Six of the animals were treated with nicotinic acid (through an indwelling jugular vein catheter) and 6 were similarly treated with saline. The bulls were then mixed together in a single pen for eight hours. The appropriate treatments were repeated at 2 h intervals, when blood samples were also taken. The total dose of nicotinic acid administered was 90 g per animal. After 8 h the bulls were slaughtered. Some of the results are given in Table 4.

In these experiments, the animals used and the handling treatments employed were such that all animals risked becoming dark-cutting. The results showed this to be the case. Nevertheless, the reduction of lipolysis, plasma FFA and glycerol with intravenous nicotinic acid (results not shown) dramatically exaggerated the effects of behavioural activities in the bulls and caused the induction of very high ultimate pH in muscle.

All the results taken together confirm the proposition (Lister, 1979) that excessive glycogen usage by muscle and production of high pH meat are the usual consequences of profound muscular stimulation when the availability and utilisation of other energy substrates, notably FFA, are reduced. The

TABLE 4

EFFECTS OF NICOTINIC ACID^{+}, ADMINISTERED BEFORE SLAUGHTER, ON SOME MUSCLE^{++} AND LIVER MEASUREMENTS IN FIFTEEN MONTH OLD FRIESIAN BULLS

	Experiment 1		Experiment 2		Significance of Pooled data
	Control	Treated	Control	Treated	(Treated vs control)
Liver glycogen (mg/g)	2.4	0.2	13.1	0.1	NS
Muscle glycogen (mg/g) (at death)	0.9	0.2	0.5	0.3	*
Muscle pH (48 h *post mortem*)	6.42	6.92	6.40	6.90	***
Muscle quality^{+++}	25	20	27	21	*

+ Nicotinic acid, 20 g intravenously at 2 h intervals over 8 h

++ *M. longissimus dorsi*

+++ Fibre Optic Probe (MacDougall and Jones, 1980)

* $P < 0.05$

*** $P < 0.001$

NS Not statistically significant

indications are that β-adrenergic stimulation is important in perpetuating the development of the syndrome through stimulation of anaerobic glycolysis. But a contribution from the sympathetic nervous system in initiating the reaction and adrenal medullary involvement cannot be ruled out. It is clear, however, that β-adrenergic stimulation alone, unless severe and likely to lead to a sizeable lactacidosis and suppression of FFA concentrations in the blood, may not be accompanied by the development of the classical dark condition in muscle. This possibly explains why adrenaline treatment of cattle (Hedrick et al., 1959) does not, in our experience, consistently induce dark-cutting carcasses. Why some breeds of cattle, like certain breeds of pig, should be more susceptible to these metabolic problems than others, is still not clear.

Paper read by Dr. D.B. McDougall in Dr. D. Lister's absence.

REFERENCES

Duchesne, H.E., 1978. The aetiology of dark-cutting beef - a study on the management and behavioural factors that affect meat quality in entire male cattle. Ph.D thesis, University of Bristol.

Hall, G.M., Lucke, J.N. and Lister, D., 1980. Malignant Hyperthermia - Pearls out of swine? Br. J. Anaesth. 52, 165-171.

Havel, R.J., 1970. Lipid as an energy source. In: The Physiology & Biochemistry of Muscle as a Food II (Eds) Briskey, E.J., Cassens, R.G. and Marsh, B.B., University of Wisconsin Press, Madison pp 609-621.

Hedrick, H.B., Boillet, J.B., Brady, H.E. and Naumann, H.D., 1959. Etiology of dark-cutting beef. Univ. Missouri Coll. Agr. Res. Bull., No. 717.

Howard, A. and Lawrie, R.A., 1956. Special report of the Food Investigation Board. HMSO London No. 63.

Issekutz, B. Jr., 1970. Interrelationships of Free Fatty Acids, Lactic Acid and Glucose in Muscle Metabolism. In: The Physiology & Biochemistry of Muscle as a Food II (Eds) Briskey, E.J., Cassens, R.G. and Marsh, B.B., University of Wisconsin Press, Madison pp 623-643.

Lawrie, R.A., 1958. Physiological stress in relation to dark-cutting beef. J. Sci. Fd.Agric. 9, 721-727.

Lawrie, R.A., 1966. Metabolic stresses which affect muscle. In: The Physiology and Biochemistry of Muscle as a Food (Eds) Briskey, E.J., Cassens, R.G. and Trautman, J.C., University of Wisconsin Press.

Lister, D., 1979. Some physiological aspects of the stress cycle in relation to muscle function and meat quality. Acta. agric. Scand. Suppl. 21, 281-288.

Lister, D., Lucke, J.N. and Hall, G.M., 1976. Pale, soft, exudative (PSE) meat, stress susceptibility and MHS in pigs - endocrinological and general physiological aspects. In: Production Diseases in Farm Animals. Pudoc. Wageningen, pp 144-150.

MacDougall, D.B. and Jones, S.J., 1980. Translucency and colour defects of dark-cutting meat and their detection. In: Proc. EEC Seminar - The problem of dark-cutting in beef - Brussels.

Pernow, B. and Saltin, B., 1971. Muscle metabolism during exercise. Plenum Press, New York and London.

BEHAVIOUR OF DOMESTIC CATTLE UNDER MODERN MANAGEMENT TECHNIQUES

Marie-France Bouissou
INRA Station de Physiologie de la Reproduction
37380 Nouzilly, France.

ABSTRACT

For domestic animals, modern management techniques lead to a very different way of life compared to the natural one.

Generally, animals adapt without major problems. However, several precise studies have shown that certain problems arise which are associated with social relationships. Reduction of available space per animal, crowding, competition induced by localisation of food resources, introduction of unfamiliar animals into established groups, mixing of groups and other disturbances lead to an increase in intraspecific aggressiveness and to exacerbation of dominance relationships. As a result production is reduced (i.e. reduction in growth rates, decrease in milk yield etc) as some animals are subjected to a social stress.

On the other hand, animals can also be stressed by various environmental situations and inappropriate handling techniques.

The study of the behaviour of domestic animals is an essential prerequisite to the development of rational management techniques which take into account the demands of the various species and which allow a reduction in stress.

INTRODUCTION

During the past thirty years, the intensification of animal production systems has resulted in the development of industry-like structures in agriculture from both technical and economic points of view. In order to improve the efficiency of animal husbandry, large production units have been created and the various treatments mechanised. The animals' way of living thus differs more and more from their natural way of life.

The changes in the way of life of animals induced by man bring about 'uncomfortable' situations which may be stressful under certain circumstances. Dark-cutting in beef is caused by exposure to pre-slaughter stress; cattle are obviously subjected to numerous stressors at this particular time.

Until recently, research has been particularly devoted to problems concerning animal nutrition, reproduction and pathology; the behaviour of animals in relation to changes in the environment have been little investigated. However, it is only through a thorough knowledge of the mechanisms of animal behaviour, and the psychological requirements and limits of adaptation of the various species, that efficient management techniques can be developed which will acnieve optimum production objectives and at the same time take account of animal welfare.

In this paper, we shall review some aspects of cattle behaviour under modern management systems together with their consequences in various respects. This could help us to understand which situations should be avoided and which management techniques might be improved in order, in particular, to reduce pre-slaughter stress.

SOCIAL BEHAVIOUR

Domestic mammals are generally kept in groups. In natural conditions, the group is the result of an equilibrium between opposing tendencies e.g. cohesion and dispersion. Thus, conflicts resulting from competitions for food, reproduction, occupation of a favourable site, etc., lead to aggressive manifestations which tend to disperse the individuals.

The intensity of these phenomena (cohesion and dispersion) varies according to whether the animals live in natural or semi-natural conditions or are confined in a restricted area.

In the first case, the conflicts are rare since competition is reduced or even non-existent (especially for food), whereas in the second situation, competition for limited sources of food in a small area is strong. Increase in population density brings about a constant violation of the space between individuals. In such conditions aggressiveness is increased whereas the mechanisms ensuring group cohesiveness decrease and even disappear. The attention paid to these two types of phenomena has been unequal: the majority of studies have been devoted to problems concerning aggressiveness and its unfavourable consequences, as well as to events related to dominance.

Dominance relationships in cattle

In wild species it is often difficult or even impossible to show a hierarchical organisation between females within family groups, while the existence of a dominant animal in domestic cattle herds is now well established (for review see Hafez and Bouissou, 1975; Syme and Syme, 1979). The existence of this hierarchy can easily be observed because of events such as butts, threats and priorities at feeding or more simply because of withdrawals or displacement of one animal by another.

Hierarchical relationships involve aggressive events in most cases, but it is important not to confound aggressiveness and social rank order, the dominant animal being rarely the most aggressive one. For a given pair of animals, the aggressive interactions are unidirectional i.e. always directed from A towards B, and it is always B which runs away. In short, A dominates B. Thus, the criterion used to determine dominance-subordination relationships is the direction of the agonistic interactions. The simple observation of a group of animals allows the determination of its structure. However, when animals with low aggressiveness are together for rather a long time, the manifestation of dominance-subordination relationships is often discreet and may rarely occur. In such a case it is difficult to determine all the relationships between animals. The confrontation of two animals in a food competition test clearly reveals these dominance relationships: in all cases, the dominant animal eats during almost all the test and the aggressive interactions occurring during the test are always identical to those observed within the undisturbed group (Bouissou, 1970a).

All groups exhibit a hierarchical organisation which may be of the linear type, with an absolute dominant animal and an 'omega' animal dominated by all the others; on the other hand, the organisation may be more complex, involving a variable number of triangular relationships such as A dominates B, B dominates C and C dominates A (Figure 1).

The study of dominance-subordination relationships gives rise to several problems: how do these relationships become established and what are the factors responsible for the social rank of an animal? How are these relationships maintained and what are the consequences of hierarchy?

Establishment of dominance-subordination relationships and rank factors

Grouping of adult unfamiliar animals or the introduction of new individuals into a group are seldom encountered in natural conditions, but occur frequently with domestic animals. In such conditions, important aggressive reactions often occur.

The establishment of hierarchical relationships takes place very rapidly and mostly through the recognition of physical attributes, postures or other signals made at a distance. The social experience of the animals increases the speed at which these relationships become established and

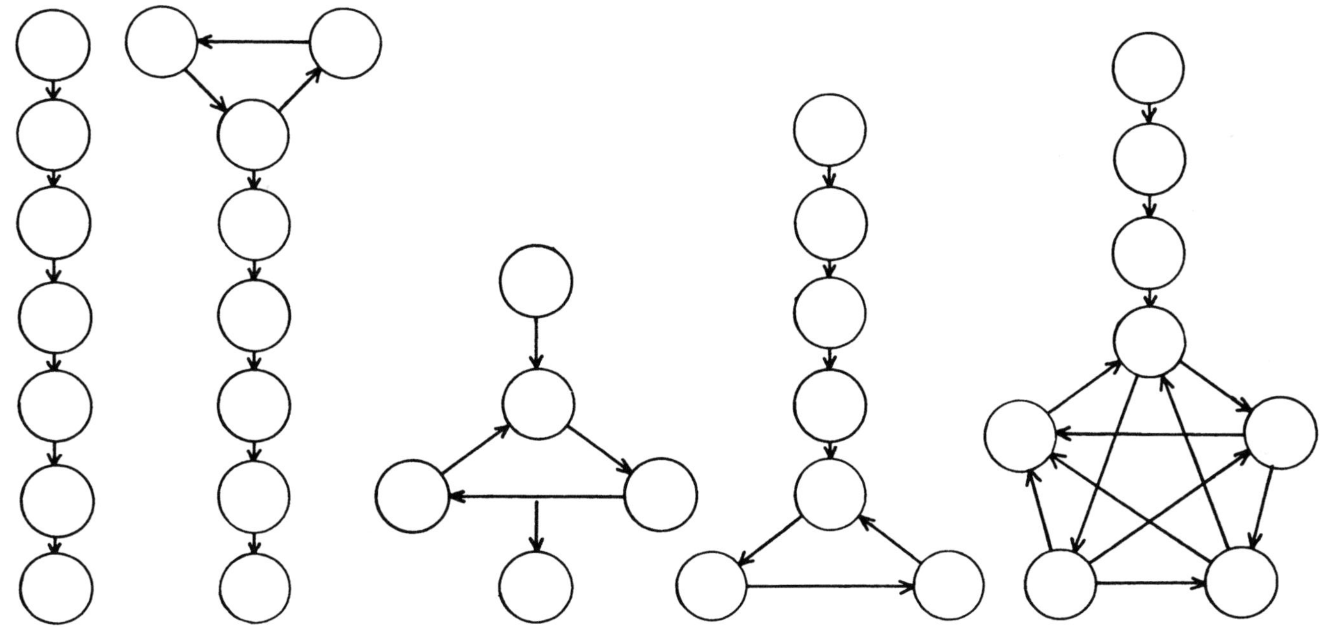

Fig. 1. Different hierarchies observed in groups of heifers.
The animals are represented by circles. The direction of the arrows indicates the direction of dominance and if there is no other indication an animal dominates all those located below it on the graph.

reduces the necessity of a real challenge. Thus, a study of the formation of 25 experimental groups of 4 heifers has shown that about 70 per cent of the relationships were established 10 min after the animals were put together, and almost all of them 1 h after. Suprisingly, the establishment of these relationships mostly takes place without any fighting (65 per cent of the cases) and sometimes even without any aggressive interaction. In almost half the cases, the relationships are immediately unidirectional. Comparison of results obtained with animals meeting strangers for the first time or, conversely, having acquired a social experience during previous meetings, clearly shows the important role played by the latter factor: 'experienced' animals determine their relationships much more rapidly than the 'inexperienced' ones (66 per cent within 10 min versus 13 per cent) and more frequently without fighting (65 per cent versus 40 per cent). The relationships are more frequently immediately unidirectional (48 per cent versus 17 per cent) and less subject to further modifications (14 per cent versus 42 per cent) (Bouissou, 1974a, 1974b, 1975) (Figure 2).

It has also been shown that neither sight nor smell deprivation prevents the formation of hierarchical relationships (Mansard and Bouissou, 1980).

Knowledge of the criteria by which one animal accepts the superiority of another, even in the absence of any contact, is very important in understanding dominance phenomena. In the determination of social rank, many authors consider that weight, size, age and seniority in the group and presence of horns play a part. However, only a few accurate studies have been made and almost all the observations have been made on adult animals with unknown 'past experience'.

It seems that some physical factors such as weight and the presence of horns are important as they favour a high social rank order (Bouissou, 1972), and this is also the case for age and seniority in the group (but weight, age and seniority in the group are often correlated). However, the most important factor

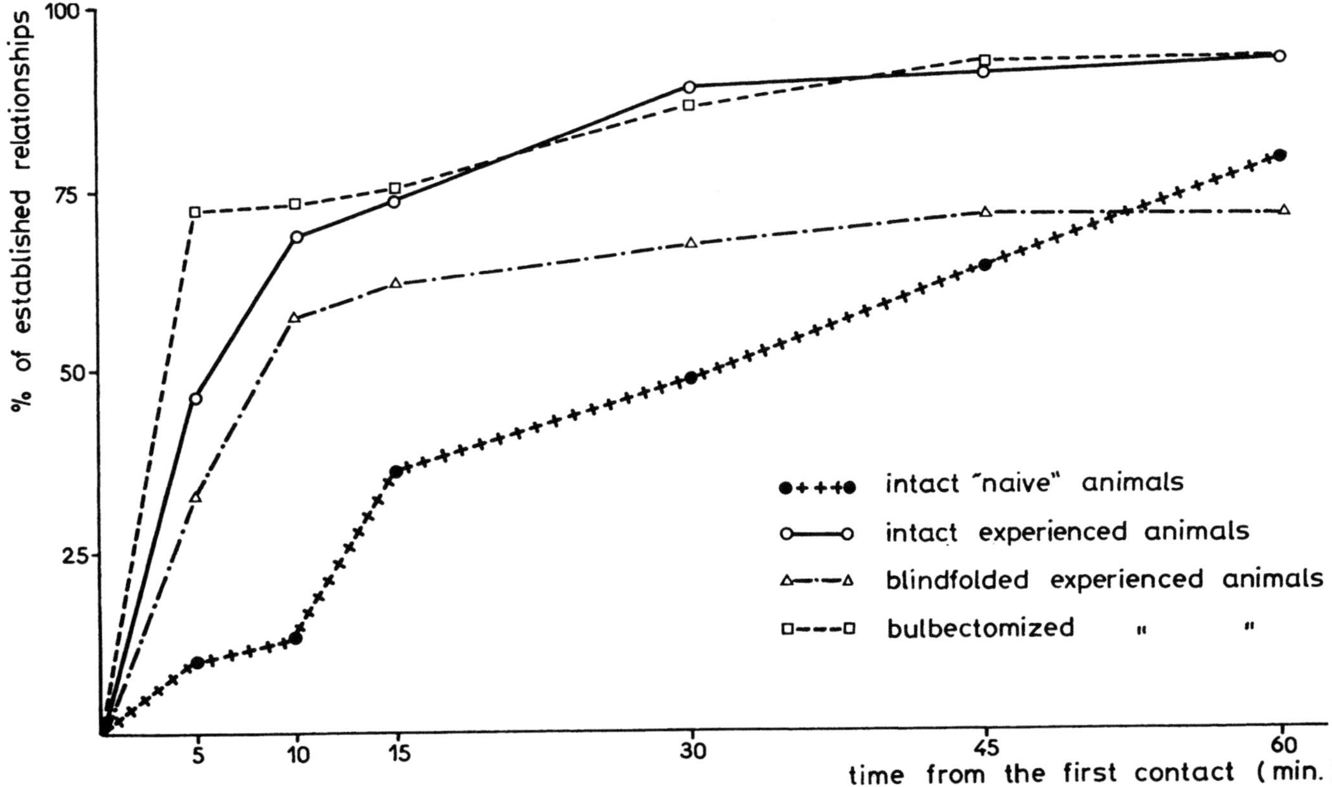

Fig. 2. Establishment of dominance-submissive relationships in cows.

seems to be the experience acquired by the animal; for each individual the relative importance of the other factors seems to depend on this experience.

Consequently, the study of the development of social relationships during ontogeny appears to be essential for a better understanding of these phenomena. The results obtained by various authors are, again, contradictory. Some have found a hierarchy between calves a few weeks old (Stephens, 1974), whereas others have not been able to show it before the age of one year (Schake and Riggs, 1970). This is due in particular to management techniques used. It seems that animals reared in groups of young of the same sex, without any contact with adults, exhibit dominance relationships very late, around puberty (Bouissou, 1977). Conversely, when the same animals are mixed with young of the same age, from foreign groups, they are able to establish dominance relationships before 6 months (Bouissou and Andrieu, 1977). For calves reared in groups by their dam these relationships are established after 2 - 3 months and sometimes even after the first weeks of life (Bouissou, unpublished data). The appearance of hierarchical relationships in the young therefore depends on the social context in which the animals live.

Stability of hierarchical relationships and mechanisms of their maintenance

The dominance-subordination relationships established between 2 animals are very stable, most of them persisting for several years. Although it is very rare, some relationships may be reversed. Such modifications usually occur abruptly without fighting and they are difficult to explain. Established relationships normally remain stable, even after a period of separation of 45 days, during which the animals are either isolated or placed in other groups and subjected to various experiences.

After the establishment of the social rank order, the hierarchical relationships are generally maintained by simple postures or by the spontaneous withdrawal of the subordinate animal.

It therefore seems justified to impute an important role to sight whilst physical contact seems to be of secondary importance. However, the deprivation of sight from all members of a group of cows does not lead to any modification of their social relationships. On the other hand, although physical contact is not necessary, it has to be possible, since its total suppression hinders the manifestation of hierarchical relationships (Bouissou, 1971).

Individual recognition also plays an important role in the maintenance of social relationships.

The social group

Spontaneous associations between some individuals when eating or resting, accompanied by a decrease in aggressiveness among these animals, are often observed in cattle herds. A certain number of observations show that the presence of a kind of familiarity between animals at a given moment of their existence may lead to subsequent preferential relationships (Ewbank, 1967; Zimmermann-Müller and Zeeb, 1971). When the animals are reared together from birth, preferential relationships between them are observed; these result in lower aggressiveness, a larger proportion of some types of positive interactions and a spatial association of the animals when they eat or are at rest in the stable or on pasture, whatever their activity. In addition there is a mutual tolerance in the case of competition. This behaviour can be observed for at least 1 year after regrouping these animals with strangers. A special period of sensitivity for the creation of this type of relationship seems to exist before 6 months of age (Bouissou and Hövels, 1976a; Bouissou and Andrieu, 1978).

These phenomena partly explain the stability of family groups and the apparent absence of a hierarchical structure in the social organisation of females of many wild ungulates.

CONSEQUENCES OF MODERN MANAGEMENT TECHNIQUES AND POSSIBLE REMEDIAL MEASURES

Modern management of domestic animals has led to important improvements, especially with respect to returns and labour-saving, but it has also given rise to various problems.

It has been suggested that the housing conditions of animals are adapted to man rather than to animals (Ross, 1960).

The surface available per animal tends to decrease: 6 to 10 m^2/cow. Now, each animal possesses an 'individual distance' beyond which the presence of a congener constitutes an aggression; this distance varies according to species and within one and the same species according to individuals, to their social 'role', to their physiological state and so on.

When the area is reduced, the animals cannot avoid each other and the individual distances are constantly violated, leading to a considerable increase in the number of aggressive interactions; inversely, on pasture this number is extremely low (Bouissou and Signoret, 1971) (Table 1).

TABLE 1

FREQUENCY OF AGONISTIC INTERACTIONS IN A GROUP OF 10 COWS ACCORDING TO THE SURFACE AREA AVAILABLE

	Free stable		Pasture
Total surface area	60 m^2	120 m^2	5.5 ha
Surface area/animal	6 m^2	12 m^2	5 500 m^2
Number of agonistic interactions (butts and threats)/hour	22.6	9.0	2.2

Feed is often supplied partly in the form of a rapidly consumed concentrate and it is offered to the animal on a given area for a given period. This situation, which normally does not exist for herbivorous animals, leads to considerable competition and also favours aggressive reactions. In addition, if the number of animals exceeds the number of places available at the feeding trough, some, and always the same ones, consume their food later. They consequently eat the foodstuffs left after the first animals have made their choice.

The housing conditions, especially feeding devices, milking parlours, waiting areas, etc. may also be at the origin of conflict situations, or be detrimental to the welfare of animals obliged to be in close body-to-body contact. The very design of the buildings, entries, boxes and so on, may also play a part.

Manipulation of the animals may result in stress. Wittlestone et al. (1969) showed that the leukocyte count in milk, a measure of stress, increases when cows are chased by a herdsman or by a dog. One of the major causes of stress during handling is when people handle animals in a rough manner, yelling at or hitting them when they refuse to move.

Change in the physical environment brings about fright reactions, be it change of room, a sudden change in illumination, violent noise, and so on, or even a simple disturbance of habits (change of side in the milk parlour, for example). Milk production can then be reduced by 20 per cent (Kilgour, 1969). Excessive temperature and humidity, an excess or absence of sensory stimulations from the environment also have detrimental effects on the physiology and on the behaviour of animals, with subsequent repercussions on their production.

Various disturbances (moving of the animals, restraining for treatment purposes, etc.) or human interventions considered as 'neutral' (cleaning and any work in the stable) lead to a considerable increase in all social and especially aggressive interactions during the following hour (Bouissou, 1976) (Figure 3).

The different species of domestic mammals belong to families which live naturally in groups. These groups are either mixed (cattle), or composed of females only, the males being

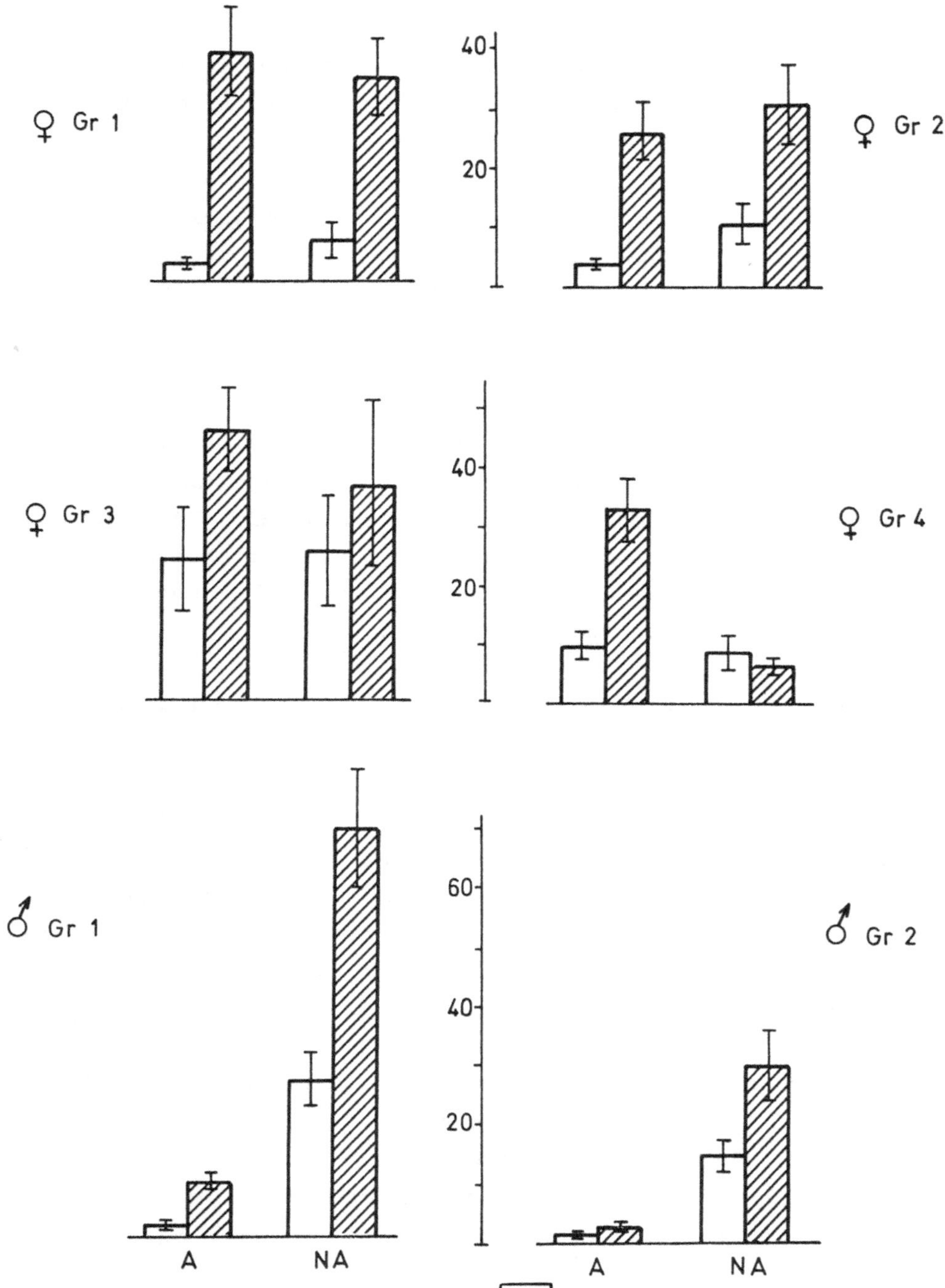

A Agonistic interactions
NA Non agonistic interactions

Before disturbance
After disturbance

Fig. 3. Mean number of social interactions in groups or four animals during the hour preceding and following a disturbance.

isolated or associated in more fluctuating structures (pigs, sheep, goats) or they have harems.

The herds constituted by modern management techniques are substantially different from those of the corresponding or similar wild species. The sexes are separated and in some cases never meet (artificial insemination). In cattle, the young are mostly separated from their dams at birth and reared in unisex groups of animals of the same age without any contact with adults. The groups are frequently changed, for example, according to milk production. Especially when in market channels, livestock are continuously being mixed with strange animals.

One of the most striking consequences of this modern management is increased aggressiveness among animals; it may be caused by a great number of factors concerned with physical environment, some of which have already been mentioned above. The disturbance of social relationships by the introduction of foreign animals to the herd or any changes in the latter represent a very important factor.

The increase of aggressiveness due to the concentration of many animals and body-to-body contact with animals of higher rank (e.g. at the point of milking) bring about a true social stress which leads in particular to an increase in the weight of the adrenal glands of dominated animals (Bouissou, unpublished)

The tremendous amount of agonistic interactions occurring when the animals first meet can create a large amount of stress which appears to be more severe than moderate feed or water deprivations. It has been shown that cattle become stressed if they are sorted and regrouped more than once during a 48 h period. Results from a study by Grandin (1978) indicated that mixing strange steers was the major cause of dark cutters.

The effects on production are obvious. A 5 per cent lowering of milk production is observed when a foreign cow is introduced into a group (Schein et al., 1955) or when the animals are transferred to another group (Arave et al., 1973). When a temporarily isolated animal is introduced into the herd, after calving, for instance, a fall in milk production that may reach 20 per cent and continue for several months can be observed. The effect is more marked when one animal is introduced alone than when several animals are introduced together. High yielding cows are more affected than others (Porzig, 1977)(Figure 4).

The social hierarchy itself has unfavourable consequences on the dominated animals whose eating or resting times are sometimes greatly reduced. It has also been observed that the dominant animals profit from priorities in the choice of best place for eating or resting; even when they are no longer hungry they may temporarily prevent access to feed for the dominated animals.

Another factor, little studied up till now, is that of group size. It is most likely that aggressiveness is more marked in a big group. It has not yet been established what the maximum number of individuals is that cattle, for instance, are able to recognise. It is possible that in a very large group all animals do not know (or do not recognise) each other, resulting in unfavourable social tensions.

The Beef recording association 1968 (in Kiley-Worthington, 1977) showed that young bulls kept in groups of 18 exhibited a higher production than those kept in groups of 28. Some reports on herds of 200 - 350 individuals indicate that the production of the animals is lower than in small herds. Fertility problems occur in such large herds and may lead to a 10 per cent decrease in conception rate, a large proportion of short cycles, and of 2 year old non-cycling cows. Additionally, milk production may be reduced by 5 per cent or more (Albright, 1971).

Conversely, for an animal living naturally in a group, its separation from this group may constitute a true stress and reduce its performance. Thus, a decrease in the growth rate was observed in calves (Coffey, unpublished, in Kiley-Worthington, 1977) and a rise in the milk level of leukocytes in isolated

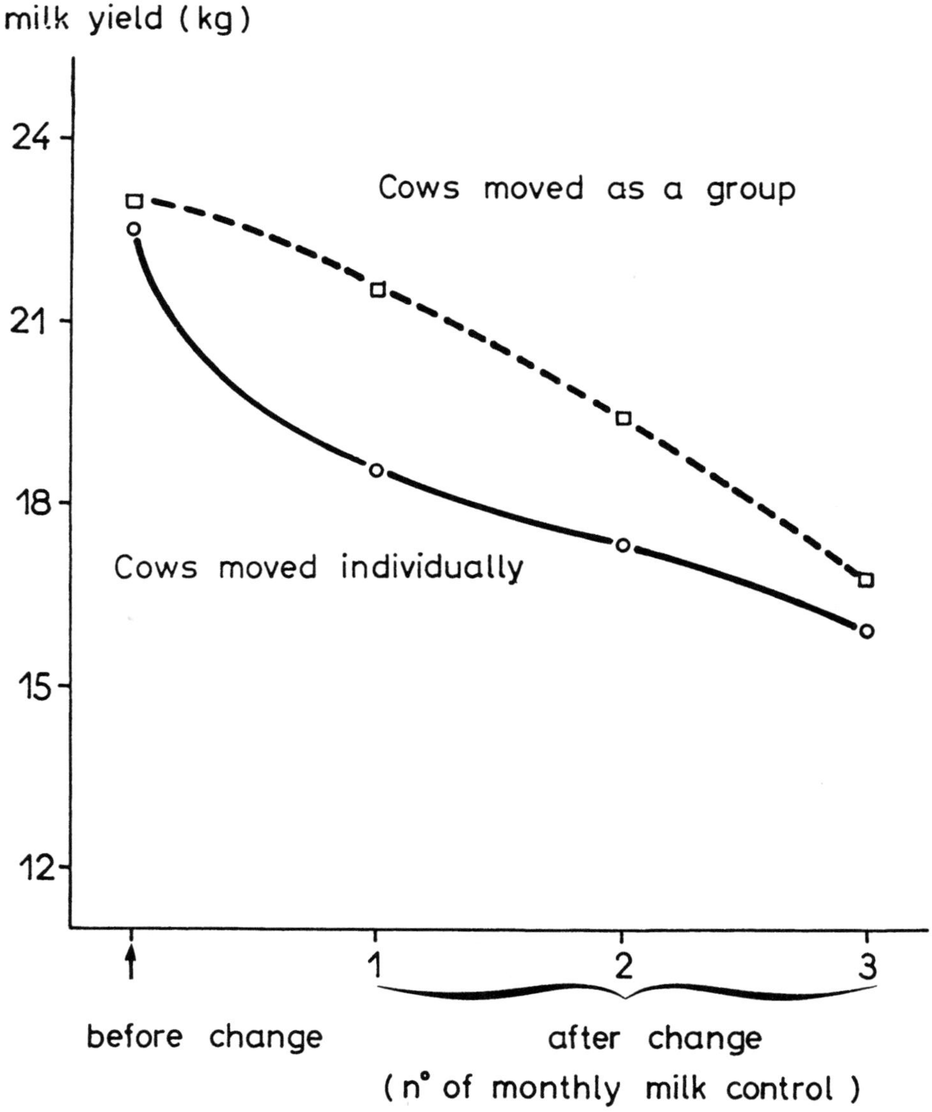

Fig. 4. Effect of transfer of dairy cows from reproduction stable into production stable (Porzig, 1977)

cows (Arave, 1974). Isolated individuals may become stressed and agitated; they may injure themselves attempting to rejoin their herdmates and they may become aggressive towards handlers.

Isolation has a depressive effect on growth rate in sheep (Scheibe, personal communication) and the mortality rate is higher Weaning, separation from the mother, as well as events occurring when the young are transferred to the fattening house, for example also represent stress factors giving rise to important problems.

Can solutions be found for these problems?

Economic conditions are such that only optimum performance of the animal is able to ensure the maximum efficiency of the farm. In the USA bruising and carcass damage are a major source of financial loss for the cattle industry ($22 million annually; Grandin, 1980). In order to obtain optimum performance it is necessary to develop methods aimed at decreasing aggressiveness and reducing stress of the animals. Some of the methods suggested at the present time are not always fully efficient, although they lead to a marked improvement. The most visible consequences may disappear (lesions after dehorning, for example) but the basic causes of the problems still persist. In other cases empirical solutions have been adopted as a consequence of anthropomorphic considerations.

In the light of the research results obtained on cattle behaviour various possibilities may be considered. Let us give some examples:

a. The first one concerns a change in physical environment which interferes with the consequences of the dominance relationships in the case of competition. It was shown that in the absence of any possibility of physical contact during food-competition tests, the manifestations of dominance are ignored by subordinates (Bouissou, 1971). In such conditions the dominated animal continues to eat during the same time as the dominant one. A progressive reduction of the separation between the animals has permitted us to show the existence of what may be called the 'notion of protection' in cattle. Protection of the head is essential and may be reduced almost to a symbolic state (Bouissou, 1970b) (Figure 5). This finding may be compared with the almost 2 h increase in resting time/animal kept in cubicles as compared to the loose-housing system. This 'notion of protection' is most likely important in some other situations, especially in the milking parlour, and must be taken into consideration when designing or changing the different types of equipment for cattle.

b. The existence of preferential relationships between animals of the same rearing group, resulting in lowered aggressiveness and a trend towards remaining together, is of considerable importance in practice. In a herd composed of 4 rearing groups we did not notice any significant difference between the length of eating time of the dominant animals and the dominated ones when competition is weak. The animals of the same group generally remain together at the same feeding rack and are not aggressive towards each other and this regulatory mechanism still exists when competition is strong. The results of competitive tests between 4 animals of the same rearing group or of different groups show that the eating time of the animals is always longer when they are together with familiar animals and this is even more marked for those who are low in the social rank order. This tolerance between animals of the same rearing group does not exist when the animals have been put together at the age of 6 months (Bouissou and Hövels, 1976b; Bouissou and Andrieu, 1978) (Figures 6 and 7).

Maintenance of animals within the same group from early days until slaughter would reduce aggressiveness and probably social stress, and would partly eliminate the unfavourable effect of competitive situations. This may be possible for fattening groups. If the improvements obtained using this type of management are confirmed and if they appear to be sufficient to justify the acceptance of other necessary constraints, the procedure could be extended to other situations.

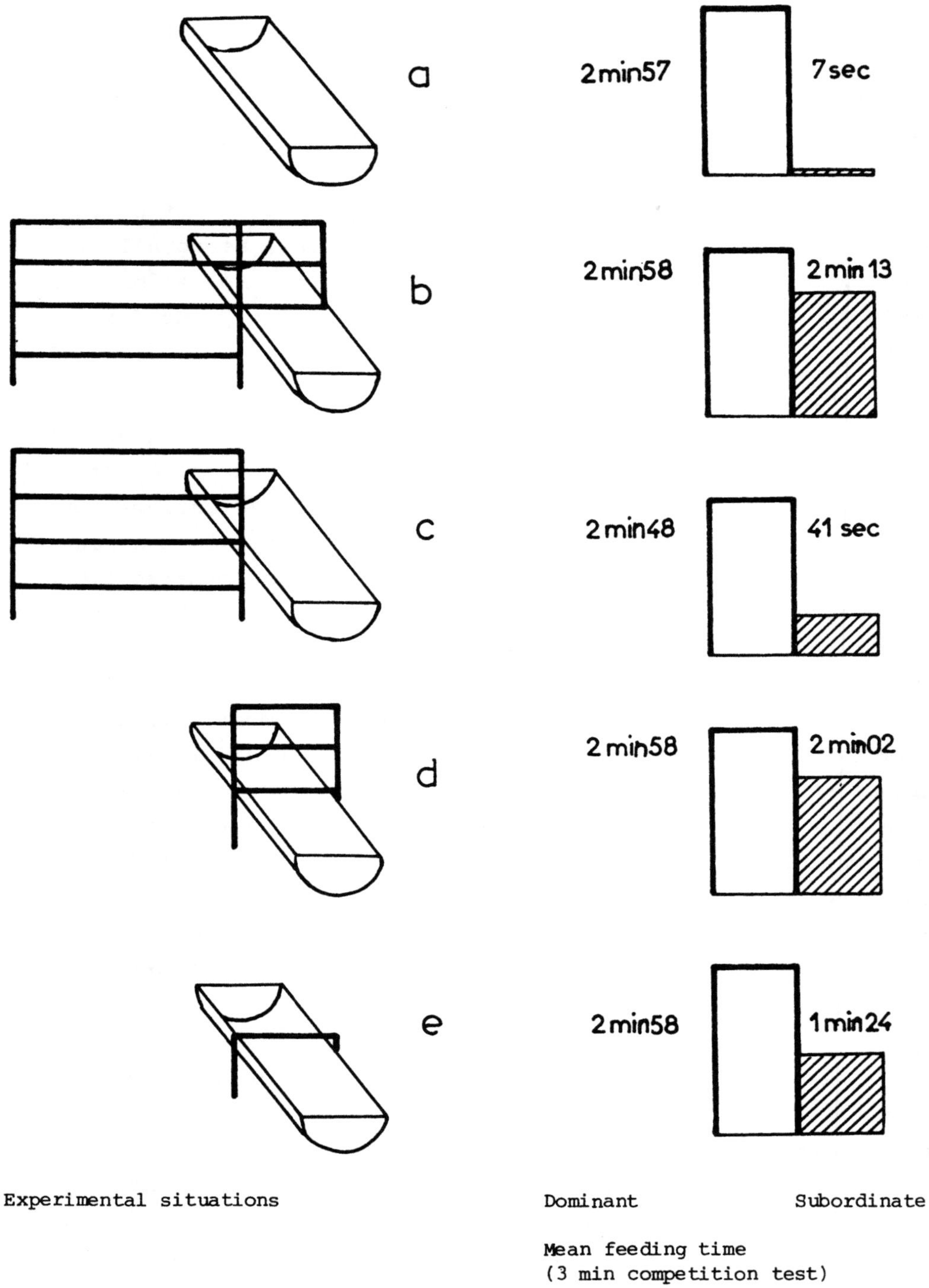
a
2 min57
7 sec
b
2 min58
2 min 13
c
2 min48
41 sec
d
2 min58
2 min02
e
2 min58
1 min24
Experimental situations
Dominant
Subordinate
Mean feeding time
(3 min competition test)

Fig. 5.

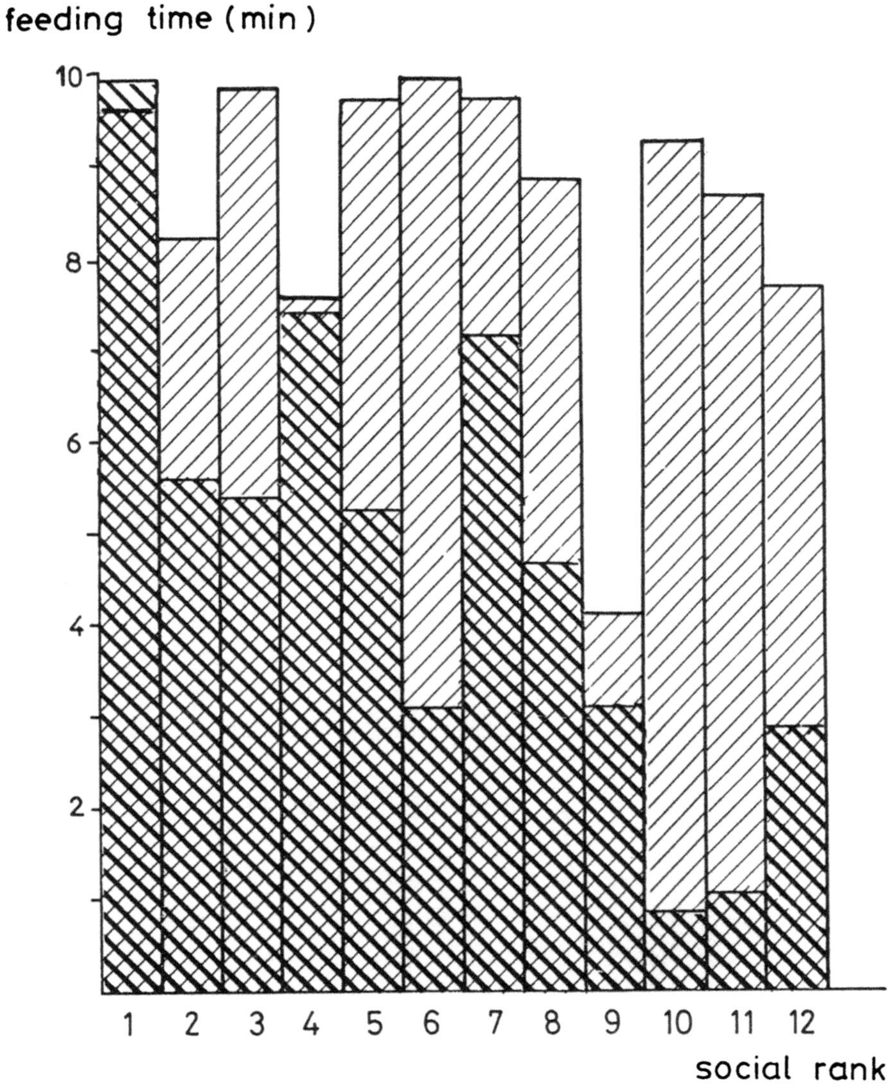

Mean feeding time when tested with animals

- of their own rearing group
- of different rearing groups

Fig. 6. Mean feeding time during 10 min food competition tests involving animals of the same or different rearing groups

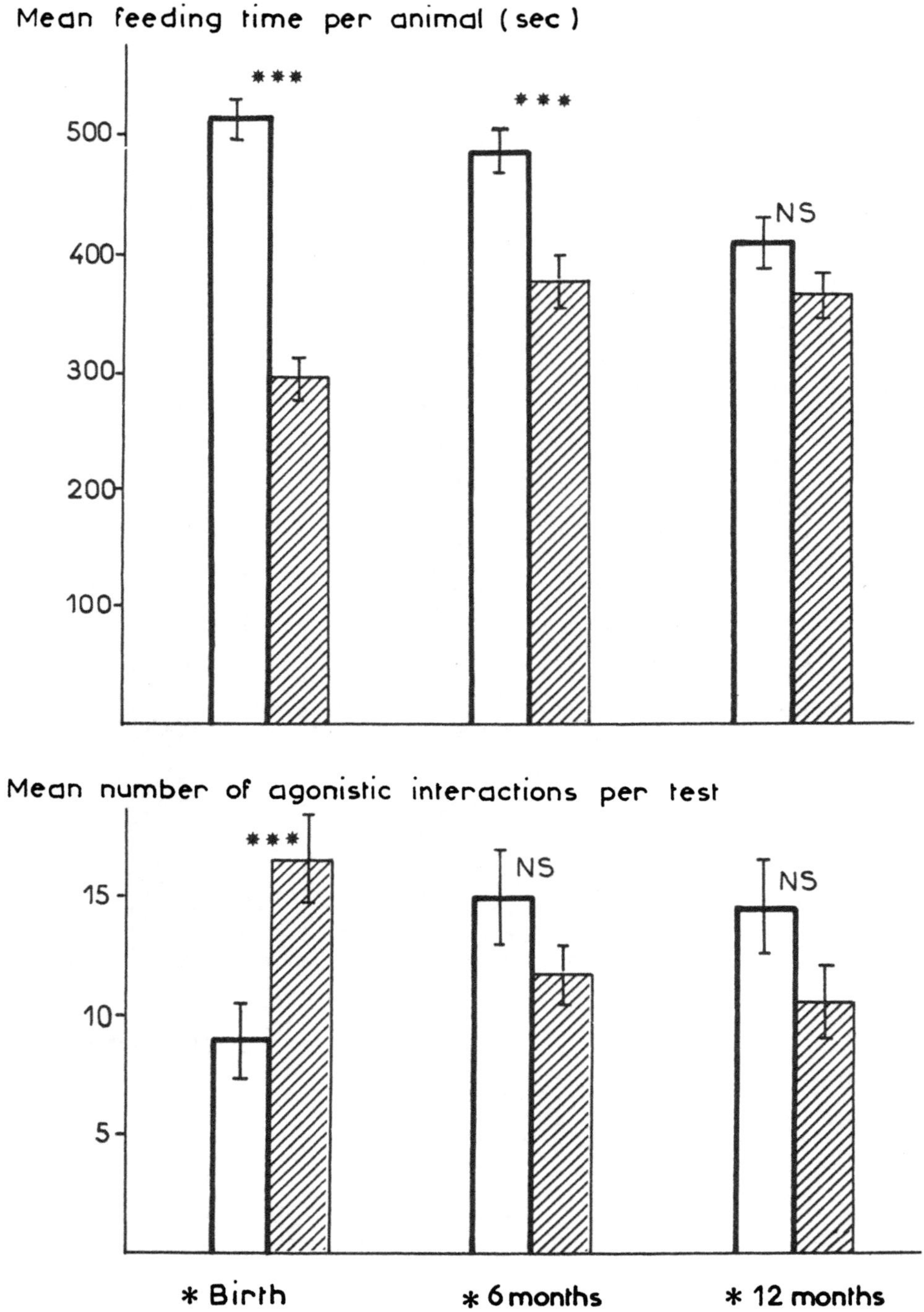

*animals grouped at birth, at 6 or at 12 months

Intra Inter *** P < 0.001

Fig. 7. Food competition tests (10 min) between 4 (or 3) animals of the same (intra) or different (inter) groups.

It has been suggested that one might mix animals on the farm at least a week prior to slaughter; this allows them to establish a social order and to settle down before going to slaughter. This has been shown to reduce the incidence of dark-cutting (Moreton and Hardy, 1977).

c. With respect to handling, Grandin (1978, 1980) using results of cattle behaviour studies and of sensory physiology (especially visual perception) has designed optimal facilities which incorporate features to minimise stress on the animals and maximise the efficiency of movements from holding pen to slaughter

CONCLUSION

For a long time, research on the behaviour of domestic animals was not considered as a priority as it did not compare favourably with what could be expected from research in other fields.

However, animal husbandry has reached a stage where certain aspects previously regarded as secondary are gaining interest. Behavioural problems belong to this group. Success or failure depends on some percentage points earned or lost with respect to feed conversion ratio, age at slaughter etc. Because of the quantity of money invested, it is difficult to modify equipment during use and it is necessary to pre-adapt new methods which take account of animal behaviour. Furthermore, on the basis of a thorough knowledge of the mechanisms involved, some aspects of behaviour can certainly be changed to advantage and behavioural possibilities put to beneficial use.

With respect to the problem of dark-cutting, results of behavioural studies in cattle should lead to an improvement in pre-slaughter techniques so that stress may be considerably reduced.

REFERENCES

Albright, J., 1971. Big herds are O.K. but are best worked in groups. The New Zealand Farmer, 92: 39-41.

Arave, C.W., Albright, J.L. and Sinclair C.L., 1974. Behavior, milk yield, and leucocytes of dairy cows in reduced space and isolation. J. Dairy Sci., 57: 1497-1501.

Arave, C.W., Albright, J.L., Yungblut, D.H. and Malven, P.V., 1973. Social status and physiological traits as affected by group interchanges. J. Dairy Sci., 56: 667 (abstract).

Bouissou, M.F., 1970a. Technique de mise en évidence des relations hiérarchiques dans un groupe de bovins domestiques. Rev. Comp. Anim., 4: 66-69.

Bouissou, M.F., 1970b. Rôle du contact physique dans la manifestation des relations hierarchiques chez les bovins. Conséquences pratiques. Ann. Zootech. 19: 279-285.

Bouissou, M.F., 1971. Effet de l'absence d'information optiques et de contact physique sur la manifestation des relations hiérarchiques chez les bovins domestiques. Ann. Biol. anim. Bioch. Biophys. 11: 191-198.

Bouissou, M.F., 1972. Influence of body weight and presence of horns on social rank in domestic cattle. Anim. Behav. 20: 474-477.

Bouissou, M.F., 1974a. Etablissement des relations de dominance-soumission chez les bovins domestiques. I. Nature et évolution des interactions sociales. Ann. Biol. anim. Bioch. Biophys. 14: 383-410.

Bouissou, M.F., 1974b. Etablissement des relations de dominance-soumission chez les bovins domestiques. II. Rapidité et mode d'établissement. Ann. Biol. anim. Bioch. Biophys. 14: 757-768.

Bouissou, M.F., 1975. Etablissement des relations de dominance-soumission chez les bovins domestiques. III. Rôle de l'expérience sociale. Z. Tierpsychol. 38: 419-435.

Bouissou, M.F., 1976. Effet de différentes perturbations sur le nombre d'interactions sociales echangées au sein de groupes de bovins. Biol. Comp. 1: 193-198.

Bouissou, M.F., 1977. Etude du développement des relations de dominance-subordination chez les jeunes bovins à l'aide d'épreuves de compétition alimentaire. Biol. Comp. 2: 213-221.

Bouissou, M.F. and Andrieu, S., 1977. Etablissement des relations de dominance-subordination chez les bovins domestiques. IV. Etablissement chez les jeunes. Biol. Comp. 2: 97-107.

Bouissou, M.F. and Andrieu, S., 1978. Etablissement des relations préférentielles chez les bovins domestiques. Behaviour LXIV: 148-157.

Bouissou, M.F. and Hovels, J., 1976a. Effet d'un contact précoce sur quelques aspects du comportement social des bovins domestiques. Biol. Comp. 1: 17-36.

Bouissou, M.F. and Hovels, J., 1976b. Effet des conditions d'élevage sur le comportement de génisses dans une situation de compétition alimentaire. Ann. Zootech. 25: 213-219.

Bouissou, M.F. and Signoret, J.P., 1971. Cattle behaviour under modern management techniques. Farm Building Ass. J. 15: 25-28.

Ewbank, R., 1967. Behaviour of twin cattle. J. Dairy Sci. 50: 1510-1512.

Grandin, T., 1978. Transportation from the animal's point of view. ASAE Technical Paper No. 78.6013, 16 pp.

Grandin, T., 1980. Observations of cattle behavior applied to the design of cattle-handling facilities. Appl. Anim. Ethol. 6: 19-31.

Hafez, E.S.E. and Bouissou, M.F., 1975. The behaviour of cattle. In: Hafez, E.S.E. The behaviour of domestic animals, Baillière Tindall, London, 203-245.

Kiley-Worthington, M., 1977. Behavioural problems in farm animals. Oriel Press, Stockfield, London.

Kilgour, R., 1969. Social behaviour in the dairy herd. N.Z. Dept. Agric. Ruakara, Pub 459.

Mansard, C. and Bouissou, M.F., 1980. Effects of olfactory bulbs removal on the establishment of dominance-submission relationships in domestic cattle. Biol. Comp. 5: 169.

Moreton, H. and Hardy, R., 1977. Calm induced before slaughter. Farmer's Weekly, June 17, p. 91.

Porzig, R., 1977. Untersuchungen zur Gruppen - und Einzeltierumstellung von Milchkuhen in industriemassig produzierenden Laufstallanlagen. Montash. Veterinarm. 32: 7-11.

Ross, O., 1960. Swine housing. Agric. Engin. 41: 584-585.

Schake, L.M. and Riggs, J.K., 1970. Activities of beef calves reared in confinement. J. Anim. Sci. 31: 414-416.

Schein, M.W., Hyde, C.E. and Fohrman, M.H., 1955. The effect of psychological disturbances on milk production of dairy cattle. Proc. Ass. South. Agric. Wkrs. 52nd Convention, 79-80.

Stephens, D.B., 1974. Studies on the effect of social environment on the behaviour and growth rate of artificially reared British Friesian male calves. Anim. Prod. 18: 23- 34.

Syme, G.J. and Syme, L.A., 1979. Social structure in farm animals. Elsevier Scientific Publ. Comp. 200 pp.

Whittlestone, W.G., Kilgour, R., de Langen, H. and Duirs, G., 1969. Behavioral stress and the cell count of bovine milk. J. Milk Food. Tech. 33: 217-220.

Zimmermann-Muller, M. and Zeeb, K., 1971. Sozialstruktur und Aktivitat bei Milchkuhen. Der Tierzuchter 9: 251-253.

DISCUSSION

E. Kallweit *(FRG)*

I would like to comment on the ranking within the herd. A colleague of mine, Dr. Unshelm, has investigated the levels of adrenaline and cortisol in tied bulls which were afterwards put together in a group. Factors which may influence the ranking in the group, such as having horns, age or weight, etc. were kept as constant as possible, but there seems to be a predisposition in the animals themselves, even before they are put into a group. He found that the animals with the highest concentrations of adrenaline and cortisol, before they came into the group, were very high in ranking after mixing. After some time in the group, this balance changed completely, so that animals with high ranks may have low concentrations of cortisol and adrenaline, which is the reverse of the earlier situation.

Mme M.F. Bouissou *(France)*

I agree with you. I have mentioned some physical factors which are thought to be important. I agree that if all factors are kept constant there is, nevertheless, a hierarchy. There is a hypothesis that the temperament or emotional status of the animals may play a part. I do not think that physical factors are very important except in the case of huge differences. When we raise animals together from birth, keeping all factors as constant as possible, a social rank emerges.

B.L. Dumont *(France)*

Do we know the exact physiological stimuli that are involved in agonistic interactions between animals? Is it through sight, hearing or touch?

Mme M.F. Bouissou

There are several which provoke aggression. Many interactions are made from a distance. They are provoked by the sight of another animal. I do not think that auditory stimuli are very important, but smell and sight are. However, I have done an experiment in which the sight of the cows was suppressed by fitting them with blindfolds and they could establish relationships as well as normal cows. If you blindfold an established herd, the relationships are maintained. If you suppress smell by removing the olfactory bulbs it does not matter. Animals rely on many sources of information. If one is missing, another can take its place. For the establishment of social ranks there can be fights - very important fights. However, in a number of cases, mainly when the animals have experience, the social rank is established from a distance; that is, only after threats and without any physical contact. Therefore, it seems that sight is very important, but if you suppress it another sensory mechanism takes its place.

J. Wismer-Pedersen *(Denmark)*

I think there might be some genetic background for the ability to dominate.

Mme M.F. Bouissou

I do not have any results on that subject. I do not think that much work has been done on it. With breed differences it is a matter not only of temperament but of size, shape of horns and many other things. However, in the same breed, the only way to study this is to study the social rank of the animals and to compare them with their mothers and, for example, if they had the same father. It is difficult to determine whether it is only genetic or a question of learning the social relationship from the mother. We would need to have calves which were born of dominant mothers, fostered to dominant or subordinate mothers to give us any idea of this. Learning is very important in the development of social relationships. There are huge differences in the development of social relationships if calves are reared by their mothers or with other calves. I have studied groups of Friesian cows and their calves and there was not a good relationship between the rank of the mother and the rank of the daughter. However, I do not think there has been much work on this topic.

G. Eikelenboom *(The Netherlands)*

Is there a relationship with physical traits in the hierarchy?

Mme M.F. Bouissou

Some authors have said that strength, weight, presence of horns, and so on, have importance. However, all their studies were made on herds whose past history was unknown. Because I think previous experience is so important, it is impossible to discriminate.

D.E. Hood *(Ireland)*

I would like to ask Mme Bouissou to comment on her results in relation to pre-slaughter management problems as opposed to those of animal husbandry.

Mme M.F. Bouissou

I suppose that mixing of the animals is a very important problem. I cannot say what the exact pre-slaughter conditions are, but I suppose the animals are mixed frequently. I refer only to social relationships and not to procedures for handling, transport and so on. I think that mixing strange animals can induce aggressiveness and this is detrimental and can be stressful. Even when they do not fight, and the establishment of the social hierarchy appears to be very quiet to the observer, I feel that the dominated animals could be stressed.

C.L. Davey *(New Zealand)*

It was a most excellent paper and I enjoyed it very much. It does not necessarily relate to the DFD condition which we are specifically talking about here, but I should imagine it has great significance to the problem of bruising of animals which is a great source of commercial down-grading. I can understand that it also relates to the better management of animals to slaughter.

However, to return to the DFD condition, it seems possible that the behavioural developments within animals, when changed from their accustomed herding, does not necessarily relate to the DFD condition. It is interesting that the range-fed animals of the southern hemisphere demonstrate the same incidence of the DFD condition as the animals in the northern hemisphere which are husbanded in quite a different way. It also seems surprising that the aggressive characteristics of a group of animals which are brought together for a brief period of time can, in fact, create the DFD condition. If one relates specifically to the amount of physical activity the animal has undergone, the amount of glycogen available which would have to be burnt up, would be far more than the animal could ever utilise by way of chemical activity. So there are some surprising contradictions here. Mr. Chairman, this is more in the way of a comment, but it is interesting that the incidence of the DFD condition with animals in the southern hemisphere, which are managed and husbanded in quite a different way from those in the northern hemisphere, is nevertheless the same.

T.R. Dutson *(USA)*

I have a question about aggressiveness of bulls versus heifers. Is there more actual contact in establishing the social relationships with intact males as opposed to heifers and cows?

Mme M.F. Bouissou

As far as I know, and contrary to popular belief, among cattle females are more aggressive than males. Although, as I said, my work was with females, I had the opportunity to observe two small groups of bulls. In these groups the animals were very quiet but there was a high level of homosexual activity. It appeared that a sexual motivation was more important to them than an aggressive one. I made comparisons mixing four strange bulls, or four strange cows, all in oestrus or all not in oestrus. Even in oestrus, the females were very aggressive, with a great amount of sexual behaviour too; the aggressiveness was higher than with groups of males. From studies in Australia, by Dr. Edey and Dr. Hinch, it appears that groups of bulls are not a problem until they are 15 months of age. Below that age, steers and bulls did not differ. They became more aggressive after 15 months of age.

ANIMAL WELFARE IN RELATION TO TRANSPORT, LAIRAGE AND SLAUGHTER IN CATTLE (A REVIEW)

J.G. Van Logtestijn and A.M.C.S. Romme

Department of the Science of Food of Animal Origin,
Faculty of Veterinary Medicine, Biltstraat 172,
3572 BP Utrecht, The Netherlands.

ABSTRACT

This paper reviews the welfare of slaughter cattle in relation to transport, lairage and slaughter. It considers how to define the welfare of cattle and how to establish the principles of proper treatment. Recommendations on the alleviation of suffering are made.

INTRODUCTION

Much literature is available about transport, lairage and slaughter of cattle. Most of this literature is devoted to technical and economic aspects of slaughtering, and also to the influence of transport and lairage conditions on meat quality of beef cattle after slaughter.

As far as animal welfare is concerned two streams of literature can be distinguished:

- one is concerned with the influence of animal welfare on quantitative and qualitative aspects of the meat (Blount, 1968). The various studies in this subject are primarily of economic interest and suggestions for improvement have in general a symptomatic nature.

- the second one deals with the welfare of the slaughter animals. This literature is in general produced by people who are interested in animal protection (Carson, 1972; Ewbank, 1973; Godlovitch et al., 1971; Melrose et al., 1979; Singer, 1975a,b). Their proposals for improvement have a more causal nature. They try to minimise animal stress while economy is of secondary significance.

During the last decades the concern of the meat industry - and not least the consumer - has grown for animal welfare aspects of meat producing animals during the fattening period and during transport to the slaughterhouse. This growing concern for animal welfare is related to developments in and around modern husbandry, such as:

- larger scale of production - less concern of the owner for the animals, for which he is responsible;
- increased stress susceptibility of the animals by breeding and selection, by modern housing and management, and lack of exercise;
- the growing awareness that these problems have much to do with animal welfare;

- the growing concern (and complaints) of the consumer on the welfare of the meat producing animals (Carson, 1972; Godlovitch et al., 1971). The increase of often negative publicity from the so-called 'bioindustry', and the occurrence of vegetarianism, are symptoms of this.

It may seem hypocritical to discuss 'welfare' aspects of animals, which are destined to be slaughtered, only because man prefers to eat meat. Apart from the answer to this specific and legitimate question we are obliged to do everything to prevent unnecessary and avoidable harm and cruelty to domestic animals, especially in the last period of their lives.

The purpose of this paper is to give a comprehensive review of the welfare of slaughter cattle in relation to transport, lairage and stunning.

WELFARE OF SLAUGHTER CATTLE

It is very difficult or perhaps impossible to give a good definition of 'welfare of slaughter cattle'. An anthropomorphic approach is often followed in discussions on animal rights and animal welfare. We are inclined to place man in the situation of the animals when we attempt to judge their welfare status. Most people would agree that anthropomorphism cannot be our sole guide in fixing a standard of welfare for slaughter cattle. Nevertheless, we do need a certain definition. But how do we define the welfare of these animals and how do we establish the principles of proper treatment?

Historical sources may throw some light on this problem. Religion can also give some indication. The Bible, for instance, does not recognise animal rights, but it strongly advocates respect for animal life.

A good definition of animal welfare seems to be: life in reasonable harmony with the environment, as judged by physiological and ethological points of view. The big problem remains of course: what is 'reasonable'? It has been suggested that a so-called 'ethogram' (behaviour inventory) of the meat producing species will provide the key to better methods of handling, thus reducing stress and fulfilling the requirements of humane handling (Kilgour, 1978).

The behaviour of animals is governed by a number of standards. For the different bio-regulation systems these are concentrated in the nervous system. We do not know so much about these regulation systems in cattle. The standards are partly genetically and partly ontogenetically defined during the first period of life and are settled during later periods of life through learning processes (Brown, 1975; Wiepkema, 1980). According to modern ethologists animal welfare exists only if the animal can establish a good co-ordination between his own standards and the internal or external environment (Wiepkema, 1980).

In relation to animal welfare a major basis for attacking animal production systems is deviations from the genetic and ontogenetic standards. Symptoms of such deviations for instance are continuously repeated, apparently senseless movements. Another deviation is the reduced ability to 'learn' in a simple environment and aberrant standards developed during the learning process.

During transport and lairage slaughter animals are subjected to psychological and physical stress due to treatment which they have usually never experienced before in their lives. Generally speaking it is necessary to avoid any adverse stress during transport and handling of beef cattle, which elicits an abnormal physiological or behavioural response (Hails, 1978).

The famous 'Brambell Report' (1965) mentioned five freedoms of movement. They can be seen as minimal requirements: freedom to lie down, to stand, to stretch the legs, to turn around and to scratch, to lick or do whatever is typical for a particular species. (The Brambell Report did not specifically mention animal welfare in relation to transport and slaughtering). These five freedoms are generally accepted by ethologists as a minimum-packet for the judgement of different situations in animal husbandry.

Several people are in favour of a more fundamental approach rather than observing symptomatic responses resulting, for example, from transport and handling problems (Schulze et al., 1972). If an animal is in a stressful situation, it shows symptoms of discomfort, such as characteristic behavioural or physiological changes (Jedlička et al., 1980; Perry, 1973). Various parameters have been suggested for the measurement of stress in animals e.g. levels of blood glucose, serum enzymes, thyroid hormone, plasma or urine corticosteroids or catecholamines, somatic cell count in milk, pulse rate, blood pressure and respiration frequency.

Westervelt et al. (1976) tried to define a multifactorial terminal stress index to assess the amount of stress from reactions of slaughter animals. To our knowledge, however, studies on this subject have not yet resulted in a physiological parameter which can be used to evaluate objectively the effects of production methods, from the point of view of animal welfare. Although there is an urgent need for such objective criteria, it is doubtful if a single parameter will be found. All EEC countries have their own and in general comparable legislation on animal protection (Allsup, 1977). They make liable to punishment anyone who shows cruelty to animals, or submits them to 'unnecessary' suffering (Drawer and Ennulat, 1977; Ray and Scott, 1973; Tegge, 1976). The European Convention for the protection of animals during international transport (1974) gives some general legislation, on which more detailed regulations for transport are based. Recommendation 641 makes the provision that animals should live in conditions that respect their physiological needs and are as close as possible to natural conditions.

WELFARE AND TRANSPORT

Although there is an extensive literature on the transport of pigs much less has been published and less work has been done on the transport of cattle. The main reason is that in general cattle are regarded as being more resistant to transport stress than pigs. Yet the problem of dark-cutting beef which is associated with stress prior to slaughter, is of considerable concern to the meat industry. Meat from bulls, reared in an 'oversimplified' environment is especially prone to this problem.

Several factors are involved in the damage to cattle which may occur during and after transport:

- neglect by the seller, by the driver and/or the owner of the animals. More direct financial interest would probably result in less losses!
- environmental stressors related to feeding regimen prior to transport or to the transport conditions.
- temperature, humidity and air movement, (climate).
- a disproportionate physical and/or psychological load on the animals relative to their resistance (adaptability).

In the literature we may find quite a number of recommendations for improvement (Dow, 1976; Leach et al., 1977; Taylor, 1978; Pohlcristoph, 1977; Ramsay et al., 1976; Schlicht et al., 1980). Long and tiresome transport should be prevented (Puolanne, 1980). Stress can be markedly decreased by sending the animals directly to slaughterhouses and not via markets or auctions. In Europe the distance between the farm and slaughter plant varies from less than ten to hundreds of kilometers. In general, transport takes place by road, sometimes by rail. It seems that loading and unloading are the major critical points and it does not make much difference if the transport duration-distance varies within a certain limit. In order to reduce stress the animals should be treated gently and with a full knowledge of the possible risks involved (Tegge, 1976). Animals from different sexes, groups or farms should not be mixed (Augustini and Fischer, 1979; Augustini et al., 1979; Wythes and Horder, 1979; Yeh et al., 1978). Clean water should be available for stock at all times and animals should be fed normally before despatch to markets.(Anon, 1971). Special attention has to be given to the problem of transport and slaughtering of low quality, weak animals. It is not known to what extent neuroleptics and other drugs are used in practice as a preventice measure against transport problems. But it is necessary to issue as soon as possible a complete prohibition of pharmaceuticals in the EEC, unless the usefulness and residue aspects have been objectively established (Volker et al., 1974). The use of pharmaceuticals may cause residue problems and may result in a negative image for the product in the eyes of the consumer. Moreover it is preferable to find a causal and not a symptomatic solution to these problems!

WELFARE AND LAIRAGE

There is not much literature available on the relation between welfare and lairage. Most of it is dedicated to the technical construction of stables, the optimum rest-period after transport and the administration of feed and water (Grandin, 1980a,b,c,d). An important question is to establish if a rest period after transport is necessary. Many would recommend a period of rest after transport and before slaughter whilst others cast doubt on the usefulness or advisability of resting and would prefer that animals are slaughtered immediately on arrival at the slaughterhouse. A strong plea has been made for a good delivery system which makes it possible to slaughter the animals directly on arrival. In practice however, a rest period is unavoidable or even necessary because of practical difficulties (e.g. delivery time too late for slaughtering on the same day, inadequacy of delivery or slaughtering systems etc.). It might also be necessary however, in order to avoid meat quality problems which may be expected if animals are very tired or over stressed at slaughter. In relation to 'animal welfare' it is doubtful, given the type of lairage available in our slaughterhouses, if animals are able to recover from the stress of transport and unloading. Moreover, the less social experience the animals have, the more disorder and aggression will arise (Metz, 1980; Schein and Fohrman, 1955). It is probably very difficult in practice to create suitable conditions in the lairages for such a period.

Many countries have legislation which enforces a rest period for all animals or at least for tired and apparently stressed animals. The rest period varies from 3 - 4 h after short journeys up to 72 h. During the rest period animals should be fed up to 8 h before slaughter and water should be available at all times (Anon, 1971).

The lairages must be adequate in construction and size, they must be cool, they must have adequate ventilation and provision must be made for feeding and watering of the animals. The floors must be designed to prevent the risk of slipping or falling. Large farm animals, and particularly bulls, should be tethered during their stay in lairage and mixing of groups should be avoided.

WELFARE AND SLAUGHTER

The stunning operation is a particularly important consideration in the humane treatment of cattle in slaughterhouses. Slaughtering of animals in the sight of other animals must be prevented.

Stunning before slaughter became compulsory in most Western European countries some 60 - 70 years ago. Since that time several methods have been used and these are more or less prescribed in detail by national regulations.

Since November 18, 1974 there has been a Directive in the EEC on 'Stunning of animals before slaughter' (74-577-EEC). In principle slaughter animals are allowed to be stunned by a special mechanical apparatus (as allowed in the different member states) by electricity or by gas (not in use for cattle). It is prescribed that unconsciousness is induced that will last at least until unconsciousness by bleeding occurs. In any case, 'unnecessary' pain has to be avoided. Ineffective stunning must of course be very painful and paralysis may occur without loss of consciousness (Croft, 1952; Hoenderken, 1978). Special attention has to be given to the stunning procedure and it should only be applied by skilled people.

It must be emphasised that 'stunning' means the immediate disappearance of cerebral activity or consciousness. 'Immediate' means within 1 s maximum.

For stunning of cattle, in general only mechanical stunning methods with free-bullet firearms or captive bolt stunners are used and legally acceptable in most countries (Gross, 1976; Lambooy and Spanjaard, 1980a). If applied properly, this method guarantees an immediate unconsciousness (Freesemann, 1975; Gross, 1976; Lambooy and Spanjaard, 1980b; Mickwitz and Leach, 1977).

However, captive bolt pistols are sometimes ineffective and in addition they are noisy, the blanks are not cheap, and they cause brain haemorrhages making the brains unacceptable for consumption. Research on electrical stunning methods for cattle has been investigated before (Hickman, 1954) and is now again receiving attention (Lambooy and Spanjaard, 1980a). In calves with body weights of approximately 200 kg the general epileptic insult showed a relatively short duration compared with pigs, and clonic spasms occur 10 s after stunning (Lambooy and Spanjaard, 1980a). These are major drawbacks to the practical application of this method to calves.

Although electrical stunning is the method of choice for stunning pigs (Hoenderken, 1978; Mickwitz and Leach, 1977; Roos and Koopmans, 1934; Tervoert, 1950; Warrington, 1974) up till now it has not worked so well for cattle. Although it has been used for some time in some slaughterhouses, it is not in general use as a routine method. Good results have nevertheless been obtained for electrical stunning and in principle it is a good method since it is not painful (Leach et al., 1980); sufficiently high current can induce immediate unconsciousness.

Concussion stunning is employed in the USA and in some European countries on cattle. At present non-penetrating mushroomheaded bolts are in use, which derive their power from a cartridge of appropriate charge or from compressed air. In the Netherlands the use of this concussion stunning method is forbidden. This seems to be justified, since heavy haemorrhages of the nose may occur, and the brains are sometimes destroyed by bone fragments; but in particular, stunning is often ineffective (Lambooy et al., 1980; Mickwitz and Leach, 1977; Nilsson and Nordström, 1977; Ommaya and Gennarelli, 1974; Parkinson, 1977).

Special attention should be paid to the ritual slaughtering by Jews and Muslims. Sometimes electric stunning or percussion stunning is allowed by Muslim or Jewish leaders for use before throat cutting. But in most cases the animals are bled directly, without stunning.

The World Federation for the Protection of Animals and many other organisations and people have argued against these ritual methods for many years, holding that they are cruel. This is a very complicated problem and cannot be discussed in detail here. Ritual slaughter is however still allowed - under very strict conditions - in most European countries. It snould be noted that, if the treatment of the animals is gentle and careful enough and if bleeding is performed properly, the animals are generally unconscious within 10 - 12 s (Gross, 1976; Hoenderken, 1978; Levinger, 1979).

REFERENCES

Allsup, T., 1977. Domestic animal transport regulations. Royal Soc. Health J. 97, 232-236

Anon, 1971. Welfare of animals slaughtered for meat. World Fed. for Protection of Animals, Rept. no. 7, Zurich.

Augustini, Chr. and Fischer, K., 1979. Untersuchungen zum Problem des dunklen, leimigen Rindfleisches ('dark-cutting beef'). Fleischwirtsch. 59, 1871-1873

Augustini, Chr., Fischer, K., and Schön, L., 1979. Zum Vorkommen von dark-cutting beef unter Praxisbedingungen. Fleischwirtsch. 59, 342-344.

Blount, W.P., 1968. Intensive Livestock Farming. Heinemann Medic. Books Ltd. London.

Brambell Report, 1965. Command Paper no. 2836. HM Stat. Office, London.

Brown, J.L., 1975. The evolution of behaviour. Norton, New York.

Carson, G., 1972. Man, beasts and gods. A history of cruelty and kindness to animals. Scribner's Sons, New York.

Convention 1974. The European Convention for the Protection of Animals during international transport. Council of Europe. HM Stationery Office, London, UK.

Croft, P.G., 1952. The effect of electrical stimulation of the brain on the perception of pain. J. Mental Sci. 42, 421-426.

Dow, J.K.D., 1976. A survey of the transport and marketing conditions of slaughter cattle, sheep and pigs in the United Kingdom. Anim. Health Trust, Portland Place, London.

Drawer, K. and Ennulat, J., 1977. Tierschutzpraxis. Gustav Fischer Verlag, Stuttgart.

Ewbank, R., 1973. The trouble with being a farm animal. New Scientist 172-173.

Freesemann, L., 1975. Elektroencephalographische und elektrokardiographische Untersuchungen zur Bolzenschussbetaubung beim Schaf. Thesis, Hanover.

Godlovitch, S., Godlovitch, R. and Harris, J., 1971. Animals, men and morals. Gollancz Ltd., London.

Grandin, T., 1980a. Bruises and carcass damage. Int. J. Stud. Anim. Prob. 1, 121-137.

Grandin, T., 1980b. The effect of stress on livestock and meat quality prior to and during slaughter. Int. J. Stud. Anim. Prob. (in press).

Grandin, T., 1980c. Designs and specifications for livestock handling equipment in slaughter plants. Int. J. Stud. Anim. Prob. 1, 178-200.

Grandin, T., 1980d. Livestock behaviour as related to handling facilities design. Int. J. Stud. Anim. Prob. 1, 33-52.

Gross, R., 1976. Elektroencephalographische und Elektrokardiographische Verlaufsuntersuchungen nach Bolzenschussbetäubung und nach Töten durch Enthauten in den Form des Rituellen Schlachtens. Thesis, Hanover.

Hails, M.R., 1978. Transport stress in animals: a review. Anim. Reg. Stud. 1, 289-343.

Hickman, J., 1954. The electrical stunning of animals prior to slaughter. The Vet. Rec. 35, 498-501.

Hoenderken, R., 1978. Electrical stunning of slaughter pigs. Thesis, Utrecht.

Jedlička, J., Moito, J., Vančišin, J., Kmetová, E. and Palenik, S., 1980. Untersuchung der Stresseinwirkung vor der Schlachtung mit Hilfe biochemischer Kriterien und deren Einfluss auf die Fleischqualitat der Bullen und Kühe. Fleischwirtsch. 60 (8), 1532-1534.

Kilgour, R., 1978. The humane handling of stock for slaughter with particular reference to procedures in New Zealand. Anim. Reg. Stud. 1, 235-246.

Lambooy, E. and Spanjaard, W., 1980a. Electrical stunning of veal calves. Meat Science (in press).

Lambooy, E. and Spanjaard, W., 1980b. Stunning of veal calves by means of a captive bolt method. The Vet. Rec. (in press).

Lambooy, E., Spanjaard, W. and Eikelenboom, G., 1980. Concussion stunning of veal calves. Fleischwirtsch. (in press).

Leach, T.M., Warrington, R. and Wotton, S.B., 1980. Use of a conditioned stimulus to study whether the initiation of electrical pre-slaughter stunning is painful. Meat Science 4, 203-208.

Leach, T.M., Akers, M.J., Warrington, R., Warriss, P., Moreton, H., Wilkins, L. and Wotton, S., 1977-79. Identification of causes of stress during rearing, transporting and lairing of meat animals. Meat. Res. Inst. Bienn. Rpt.

Levinger, 1979. Jewish method of slaughtering animals for food and its influence on blood supply to the brain and on the normal functioning of the nervous system. Anim. Reg. Stud. 2, 111-126.

Melrose, D.R., Meadows, F.R. and Hughes, R.B., 1979. The humane treatment of food animals in transit. Proc. Symp. Univ. Fed. Anim. Welfare, July, 1979.

Metz, J.H.M., 1980. Sociaal gedrag van runderen: betekenis voor de practijk. Bedrijfsontwikkeling 11, 674-681.

von Mickwitz, G. and Leach, T.M., 1977. Review of pre-slaughter stunning in the EEC. Commission of the European Communities Inform. on Agriculture 30.

Nilsson, B. and Nördstrom, C.H., 1977. Rate of cerebral energy consumption in concussive head injury in the rat. J. Neurosurg. 47, 274-281.

Ommaya, A.K. and Gennarelli, T.A., 1974. Cerebral concussion and traumatic unconsciousness. Brain, 97, 643-654.

Parkinson, D., 1977. Concussion. Mayo Clin. Proc. 52, 492-496.

Perry, G., 1973. Can the physiologist measure stress? New Scientist 175-177.

Pohlchristoph, H., 1977. Transportschaden bei Schlachttieren Massnahmen zu ihrer Verhutung. SVZ Schlachten u. Vermarkten 77, 147-151.

Puolanne, E. and Aalto, H., 1980. Factors bearing on the formation of DFD meat. Proc. 26 Eur. Meet. Meat Res. Work., paper C7, Colorado Springs.

Ramsay, W.R., Meischke, H.R.C. and Anderson, B., 1976. The effect of tipping of horns and interruption of journey on bruising in cattle. Austr. Vet. J. 52, 285-286.

Ray, Ph. M. and Scott, W.M., 1973. Animal Health and the EEC. Animal Welfare in the EEC. Br. vet. J. 129, 194-201.

Roos, J. and Koopmans, S., 1934. Studies on so-called electrical stunning of animals. The Vet. J. 90, 232-245.

Schein, M. and Fohrman, M.H., 1955. Social dominance relationships in a herd of dairy cattle. Br. J. Anim. Behav. 3, 45-55.

Schlicht, H., Suhr, E. and Rappsilber, E., 1980. Zur Rationalisierung des Schlachttiertransportes. Fleisch 34, 109-111, 129-131.

Schulze, H., Fischer, A. and Palitzsch, A., 1972. Fleischtechnologische, ernährungswirtschaftliche und lebensmittelrechtliche Konsequenzen des Tierschutzes bei der Tierischen Produktion. Schl. u. Viehh. Zeit. 72, 116-121.

Singer, P., 1975a. Animal Liberation. The New York Review.

Singer, P., 1975b. A new ethics for our treatment of animals. The New York Review.

Taylor, G.B., 1978. Welfare aspects of animal transportation. In: The Ethology and ethics of farm animal production, D.W. Folsch, Brinkhauser Verlag, Basle pp. 92-95.

Tegge, G. 1976. Tierschutz und Transport von Tieren. Fortschr. der Vet. Med. 25, 121-126.

Tervoert, F., 1950. Bijdrage tot het electrisch bedwelmen van schlachtdieren. Vlaams Diergeneesk. Tijdschr. 19, 106-118.

Volker, H., Holzel, W. and Gratsch, U., 1974. Indikation von Psychofarmaka bei Tiertransporten. Mhft. Vet. Med. 29, 177-181.

Warrington, R., 1974. Electrical stunning: a review of the literature. The Vet. Bull. 44, 617-635.

Westervelt, R.G., Kinsman, D.M., Prince, R.P. and Giger, W., 1976. Physiological stress measurement during slaughter in calves and lambs. J. Anim. Sci. 42, 831-837.

Wiepkema, P.R., 1980. Wat doet een etholog in de landbouw. Bedrijfsontwikkeling 11, 666-669.

Wythes, J.R. and Horder, J.C., 1979. Bruising and muscle pH with mixing groups of cattle pre-transport. Vet. Rec. 104, 71-73.

Yeh, E., Anderson, B., Jones, P.N. and Shaw, F.D., 1978. Bruising in cattle transported over long distances. Vet. Rec. 103, 117-119.

DISCUSSION

D.E. Hood *(Ireland)*

Could you be a little more specific about the recommendations you would make concerning resting of animals before slaughter? Are you satisfied that the distribution system, or the collection system, for transfer to the slaughterhouse is effective?

G. van Logtestijn *(The Netherlands)*

It would be most profitable to organise transport so that there is a good guarantee that the animals would be slaughtered within half an hour after delivery. In some countries this is possible. In my own country, for instance, the transfer distances are generally not longer than 50 km, with a maximum of 200 km. The problem is that even if you give animals a certain amount of resting time you cannot be sure that they are actually resting. This is especially true for stress-susceptible animals which may be impossible to rest. In my opinion the situation in cattle is different to that in pigs. As we know, with pigs a period of about 2 h rest is optimal, resulting in a smaller amount of high pH and DFD meat. With cattle, I have studied the literature and have done an experiment with 800 bulls in two groups. Our experience was that, after 24 h, the situation in meat from bulls was not improved. Therefore, I would advise that the animals should be slaughtered immediately, without rest. If they are to have rest they need at least 48 h. You must, however, guarantee a favourable environment. Ideally conditions at the slaughterhouse should be comparable with those on the farm; Mme Boussiou also said this. However, in practice, this is very difficult.

R. Moss *(UK)*

What you are saying is that immediate slaughter is something to be aimed at. Surely, that presupposes superb conditions in transport?

G. van Logtestijn

As I said, in The Netherlands we can do this, but I realise that in many countries, and many regions of Europe, it is very difficult to organise good delivery and slaughtering schemes.

E. Kallweit *(FRG)*

I would like to know what are the objections to the concussion method of stunning. Our experiences with pigs are quite positive.

G. van Logtestijn

In the Institute of Animal Husbandry in Zeist, cattle were stunned by this method and the electroencephalograph was recorded. In many cases it showed paralysis of the animals. They appeared to be stunned, but were not, the brain activity was almost normal. One of the major requirements for stunning is unconsciousness - not paralysis. That is my main objection to concussion.

B.L. Dumont *(France)*

What is your opinion on the factors during transport, lairage and just before slaughtering which can affect the integrity of the intestinal wall to prevent invasion of the carcass by bacteria.

G. van Logtestijn

From the literature we have learned that in some extreme cases of stress it is possible for bacteria to invade the muscles from the intestines. However, there is disagreement on this point. We have made some relevant investigations in pigs. In some cases bacteria may be found in the meat, but there are so many possibilities for infection during slaughter and subsequently that I do not know if our results are valid. Also, with salmonellosis research, you may find Salmonella on the surface of the carcass in many cases; they are also in the intestines and in many glands, but you never find them in the meat. We have also done this experiment with *E. coli*; sometimes you find them, sometimes not, but it is difficult to say whether the meat is infected due to stress or otherwise.

C.L. Davey *(New Zealand)*

Adding to what you have said, our most recent knowledge would suggest that there is a continual movement of gut flora from the gut into the mesentery. This triggers the immunological responses of the animal, resulting in the bacteria being killed anyway; for 24 h at least, the carcass with the gut in will remain sterile.

SESSION IV

GENETIC INFLUENCES ON MEAT QUALITY

Chairman: A. Romita

HEREDITARY ASPECTS OF SUSCEPTIBILITY TO STRESS IN MEAT ANIMALS

G. Eikelenboom
Research Institute for Animal Husbandry 'Schoonoord',
Zeist, The Netherlands.

ABSTRACT

During the past few decades much research has been devoted to the problem of susceptibility to stress and abnormal meat quality, particularly PSE and DFD, in certain meaty pigs. Since the introduction of the halothane test as a method of diagnosing this abnormality in the live pig, much more is known about the genetic predisposition, mode of inheritance and its relationship with production traits.

The purpose of this paper is to summarise briefly some of the experimental results obtained in this field in our laboratory and an attempt will be made to draw a parallel between the situation in pigs and similar problems which may exist in certain types of cattle.

In our preliminary experiments with the halothane test (Eikelenboom and Minkema, 1974) we established a relationship between the reaction to the test and various *post mortem* meat quality traits. Meat quality in reactors was inferior to that in non-reactors.

In later studies involving a large number of Dutch Landrace pigs both at our own experimental farm (Van Eldik, 1975) and at national testing stations (Eikelenboom et al., 1978, 1980a), the following differences in production characteristics were found between the halothane phenotypes:

- A slower growth rate was found in reactors owing to their lower feed intake under *ad lib.* conditions. No significant differences were found, however, under restricted feeding conditions.
- Death losses due to stress were consistently higher in reacting pigs than in non-reacting pigs. Table 1 summarises the losses found in the testing station studies. Losses during the fattening period in (individually housed) boars and gilts as well as those recorded during the transport of the gilts to the slaughterhouse, were approximately ten times higher in reactors than in non-reactors.

TABLE 1

DEATH LOSSES RECORDED IN REACTING AND NON-REACTING DUTCH LANDRACE PIGS DURING FATTENING AND DURING TRANSPORT TO THE SLAUGHTERHOUSE

Experiment	Halothane phenotype	Fattening period n	Fattening period % losses	Transport n	Transport % losses	Total losses %
Eikelenboom et al.(1978)	+	364	1.92	179	3.35	5.27
	-	1 266	0.24	611	0.32	0.56
Eikelenboom et al.(1980a)	+	389	2.57	177	5.65	8.22
	-	1 166	0.26	541	0.55	0.81

- Meat quality was inferior in reactors as evidenced by their lower pH_1 and higher muscle temperature and *rigor* values at 45 min *post mortem* and lower quality score and higher transmission percentage observed at 24 h *post mortem*.
- Carcass quality. A lower backfat thickness and carcass length and a higher dressing-, ham-, shoulder- and total meat percentage was found in reactors. This increased meat percentage was not only due to a decreased fat percentage, but also to an increased fat-to-bone ratio. The higher muscling score found in reactors also suggests that muscle hypertrophy is one of their most specific characteristics.

In a separate experiment we have investigated the inheritance of susceptibility to halothane (Minkema et al., 1977). A total of 53 matings were made between, and among, reacting and non-reacting pigs. Nine matings made between reactors resulted solely in reacting offspring, while in the remainder of the matings the whole litter was either complete or partially halothane-negative. The latter matings were used to test the hypothesis that the trait had a single recessive inheritance. In 20 out of 23 of these matings the segregation ratios between reactors and non-reactors found in the litters did not differ statistically from those which would be expected, if a single recessive gene was involved. Therefore, we consider the trait to be inherited as a single recessive gene with complete penetrance. Similar conclusions have been reached by others using different methods (Ollivier et al., 1975; Smith and Bampton, 1977).

Data from our testing-station studies were used to estimate differences in production traits between the three halothane genotypes (Eikelenboom et al., 1980b). It was shown for many traits, in particular carcass quality that the carrier (heterozygote; halothane-negative phenotype) had an intermediate position between the reactor and the non-carrier (homozygote; halothane-negative phenotype). There was also a similar tendency for meat quality score, although both halothane-negative genotypes had markedly higher scores than the reactors. Because of the low incidence of death losses due to stress among the halothane-negative phenotypes, it was not possible to make reliable estimates for the three genotypes with regard to their susceptibility to stress.

Now, keeping in mind the subject of this seminar, let us return to the situation in beef.

In contrast with DFD in pigs, 'dark-cutting' is the most frequently occurring quality deviation in beef and is of much concern to the meat industry. However, beef exhibiting PSE-like characteristics such as pale colour, low water-binding-capacity and high transmission value, has been reported (Fischer et al., 1977; Hunt and Hedrick, 1977). It is interesting to note that *post mortem* electrical stimulation as a means of improving tenderness, which is the subject of my current research, seems to promote such characteristics.

'Dark-cutting' is particularly a problem in beef bulls, cows and heifers being much less affected. The condition is generally associated with stress and excitement prior to slaughter. It is doubtful that within breed and sex the meaty-type animal is more prone to the condition, although in my opinion such a relationship might also be questioned for pigs.

In double-muscled cattle the situation is perhaps even more comparable to the one described before for pigs, since this type of cattle seems to be more susceptible to conditions of stress. During thermal stress conditions they produce more heat and during muscular exercise they are more easily exhausted, showing a more severe metabolic acidosis than normal cattle (Holmes et al., 1972, 1973; Halipré, 1973). It was also observed that the more tender meat from double-muscled cattle is also paler in colour (Boccard and Monin, 1973).

Apart from muscle-fibre hyperplasia, there appeared to be also an increased muscle-fibre diameter in double-muscled animals. This increased diameter coincided with the occurrence of a more anaerobic type of fibre, which was associated with susceptibility to stress and pale meat (Ashmore and Robinson, 1969; Holmes and Ashmore, 1972).

At the recent EEC-seminar on 'Muscle hypertrophy in cattle' held in Toulouse (France) it was generally accepted that muscle hypertrophy in cattle is also inherited as a recessive gene although its expressivity seems to vary. Unfortunately a clear marker gene, such as the halothane gene in pigs, is lacking at the moment in this species.

It is clear that much research still needs to be done on the qualitative and quantitative aspects of beef production. There is no doubt that the knowledge on this subject which has been obtained in recent years in pigs, will contribute to our understanding in cattle.

REFERENCES

Ashmore, C.R. and Robinson, D.W., 1969. Hereditary muscular hypertrophy in the bovine. I. Histological and biochemical characterization. Proc. Soc. exp. Biol. Med. 132, 548.

Boccard, R. and Monin, G., 1973 cited by Menissier, F., 1980. General survey about the incidence of double muscling on cattle performances. Proc. EEC Seminar 'Muscle Hypertrophy in cattle', June 10-12, 1980, Toulouse (France).

Eikelenboom, G. and Minkema, D., 1974. Prediction of pale, soft, exudative muscle with a non-lethal test for the halothane-induced porcine malignant hyperthermia syndrome. Neth. J. Vet. Sci., 99, 421.

Eikelenboom, G., Minkema, D., Van Eldik, P. and Sybesma, W., 1978. Production characteristics of Dutch Landrace and Dutch Yorkshire pigs as related to their susceptibility for the halothane-induced Malignant Hyperthermia Syndrome. Livest. Prod. Sci. 5, 277.

Eikelenboom, G., Minkema, D., Van Eldik, P. and Sybesma, W., 1980a. Results of halothane-testing in offspring of Dutch Landrace A.I. boars of different halothane phenotypes. Livest. Prod. Sci. 7, 283.

Eikelenboom, G., Minkema, D., Van Eldik, P. and Sybesma, W., 1980b. Performance of Dutch Landrace pigs with different genotypes for the halothane-induced malignant hyperthermia syndrome. Livest. Prod. Sci. 7, 317.

Fischer, Chr., Scheper, J. and Hamm, R., 1977. Über das auftreten von wäszrigem blassen Rindfleisch. Fleischwirtsch. 57, 1826.

Halipré, A., 1973. Etude du caractère culard. Sensibilité des bovins culards au stress thermique. Ann. Génét. Sél. anim., 5, 441.

Holmes, J.H.G. and Ashmore, C.R., 1972. A histochemical study of development of muscle fiber type and size in normal and double muscled cattle. Growth 36, 351.

Holmes, J.H.G., Ashmore, C.R. and Robinson, D.W., 1973. Effect of stress on cattle with hereditary muscular hypertrophy. J. Anim. Sci., 31, 776.

Holmes, J.H.G., Robinson, D.W. and Ashmore, C.R., 1972. Blood lactic acid and behaviour in cattle with hereditary muscular hypertrophy, J. Anim. Sci., 35, 1011.

Hunt, M.C. and Hedrick, H.B., 1977. Chemical, physical and sensory characteristics of bovine muscle from four quality groups. J. Food Sci., 42, 716.

Minkema, D., Eikelenboom, G. and Van Eldik, P., 1977. Inheritance of MHS-susceptibility in pigs. In: Proc. 3rd Int. Conf. Production Diseases in Farm Animals, Wageningen, 1976. P.203. PUDOC, Wageningen, The Netherlands.

Ollivier, L., Sellier, P. and Monin, G., 1975. Déterminisme génétique du syndrome d'hyperthermie maligne chez le porc de Piétrain. Ann. Génét. Sél. Anim., 7(2), 159.

Smith, C. and Bampton, P.R., 1977. Inheritance of reaction to halothane anaesthesia in pigs. Genet. Res. Camb., 29, 287.

Van Eldik, P., 1975. Het verband tussen halothane-gevoeligheid en produktiekenmerken bij varkens, in afhankelijkheid van het voerniveau. Res. Institute for Animal Husbandry 'Schoonoord', The Netherlands. Res. Rep. C-265.

DISCUSSION

G. Monin *(France)*

I do not agree with the comparisons between stress susceptible pigs and double muscled cattle with respect to colour of meat. The pale meat in double muscled cattle is due to a lower pigment, but this is not so in pigs. It is the same with respect to tenderness. There is no difference in collagen content between muscular pigs and normal pigs, while double muscled cattle have lower collagen content than normal cattle.

G. Eikelenboom *(The Netherlands)*

I have not done any research on this topic. In Holland there are hardly any double muscled beef cattle so my information is based on the literature, but I think you are right. However, there are some studies on susceptibility to stress which indicate that double muscled cattle are more prone to stress. It has also been suggested that problems occur regarding reproduction with stress susceptible pigs. I am not saying that the condition is essentially the same in the two species. I just wanted to point out that there are some striking similarities - another is the inheritance of the trait.

M. Casteels *(Belgium)*

In your Table 1 you gave the losses in connection with the halothane-positive reactors. Am I correct in thinking it was 10 per cent, and was it with the Dutch Landrace breed?

G. Eikelenboom

These were the recorded losses, yes: during the fattening period and during transport to the slaughterhouse. There were two testing stations involved and these were in the study. One of them had slightly higher losses than the other. Actually, it was approximately 8 per cent. They were very carefully treated. I think these losses, due to stress, are overlooked by many people and they are often not recognised as such.

P.V. Tarrant *(Ireland)*

Dr. Eikelenboom, would you agree that the breed effect in relation to DFD beef is probably there but is much less prominent than in the case of stress susceptibility in pigs?

G. Eikelenboom

Yes, I discussed it with various participants yesterday. I think there may be two types of DFD in pigs. There is one type which is a stage further than PSE. If the animal had been slaughtered at an earlier time, it would probably have been PSE. There is another type which may occur in more resistant types of animals. We did a breed comparison, which included Yorkshire Large White pigs. This was a study made by Walstra. He had some 15 meat quality parameters. If you look at these data, and at ultimate pH in particular, which is a good indicator of DFD, there were quite a few animals among the Yorkshire which had to be qualified as DFD. Yet it has always been considered a resistant breed. These were samples taken from a large number of breeders and also a testing station, and the results showed that the incidence of halothane reactors was very low. However, I agree with what Dr. Monin said; it is less related to halothane susceptibility than is PSE.

P.V. Tarrant

Yes, I would agree that DFD can be induced by illtreatment or exhaustion in any animal if the treatment is sufficiently severe. But, obviously, stress-susceptible animals would show the condition at an earlier stage. Am I right in saying that Dr. Sornay, in his survey of about 5 years ago, found a tendency among French cattle towards a higher incidence of DFD in the dairy breeds than in the beef breeds?

M.J. Sornay *(France)*

Yes, I can confirm that. At the moment, we find more susceptibility among American Holstein Friesians than in Charolais, Limousin or Maine Anjou breeds. But these are just observations and not statistical information. However, I was interested in Dr. Puolanne's results which seem to lead in the same direction.

DOUBLE-MUSCLING AND SENSITIVITY TO STRESS

G. Monin
Station de Recherches sur la Viande, INRA, Theix,
63110 Beaumont,
France

ABSTRACT

Double-muscled (DM) cattle are reputed to be more sensitive to stress than normal animals. Sensitivity to stress has many implications with respect to breeding qualities (viability of calves, adaptation to management conditions) and meat quality. Such sensitivity to stress has often been associated with meat qualities defined as pale-soft-exudative (PSE) or dark-firm-dry (DFD) pork and DFD (i.e. dark-cutting) beef (Lawrie, 1966; Hedrick et al., 1959). Abnormally high stress-sensitivity could, therefore, reduce or even prevent quantitative progress in meat production through selection for breeding qualities or carcass composition. This observation is of great concern to producers raising animals like DM cattle, which in continental Europe have a much higher butcher value than normal cattle, due to their greater lean content and more tender meat.

SENSITIVITY TO STRESS IN DM ANIMALS

The stresses experienced most frequently by meat animals before slaughter are fasting, psychic stress (fear, excitement), exercise, muscular fatigue and changes in ambient termperature.

Fasting

The response of DM cattle to fasting has been studied by Holmes et al. (1973). They examined blood lactate, glucose, urea and creatine kinase (CPK) values during two days of fasting, and found no noticeable difference between the values of such parameters for normal and DM cattle. However, fasting for longer periods would probably elicit a differential response in DM cattle, which have been shown to be more sensitive to nutritional stress of long duration, due to their lower ability to mobilise fat stores (Holmes and Robinson, 1970).

Psychic stress

Behaviour of animals before slaughter is of particular interest, since this was shown by Rhodes (1973) to influence greatly the occurrence of DFD meat. Holmes et al. (1973) observed that DM cattle are more excitable and difficult to control than normal cattle. They attributed high excitability to a higher blood lactic acid level in DM cattle. To our knowledge, it has not been observed in France or other European countries that DM cattle are particularly difficult to handle, but more information is needed in this field.

Holmes et al. (1973) simulated psychic stress using adrenaline injections. They observed a much higher increase in blood lactic acid and plasma CPK in DM animals, which led to the conclusion that the muscle of DM cattle was more affected by adrenaline injections than the muscle of normal animals. Therefore, it may be suggested that DM animals are more sensitive to psychic stress than normal animals.

Exercise

Holmes et al. (1973) submitted normal and DM cattle to enforced exercise. Exercise drastically stressed DM cattle, since one of the four cattle developed a condition similar to 'equine paralytic myoglobinuria' and had to be euthanased some hours later, while exercise was stopped for a second animal in order to prevent the same fatal result. It was observed that blood lactic acid increased sharply during stress and in some animals there was a very sharp increase in plasma CPK, indicating severe muscle damage.

Monin and Boccard (1974) examined changes in blood acid/base status brought about by enforced exercise in DM and normal animals. They found that DM cattle exhibited a greater and more slowly compensated metabolic acidosis at the end of a 10 min run. The 'oxygen debt' induced by exercise was more pronounced in DM animals, probably due to both a deficiency in pulmonary ventilation and an inferior blood oxygen-binding capacity. Animals showing an intermediate phenotype between definite double-muscling and normal behaved intermediately with respect to these traits.

Thermal stress

Heat tolerance of DM cattle as compared to normal cattle has been studied by Halipre (1973). Thermal stress was realised by increasing ambient temperature from 25°C to 37°C during an 8 h period. Heat tolerance was lower in DM animals as compared to normal animals. Halipre (1973) attributed this difference to a lower thermoliability in DM cattle. He noticed also that by simply displacing cattle from the shed to the experimental room (adjacent to the shed) he provoked a higher increase in rectal temperature of DM animals than that of normal animals. This observation probably indicates once again the higher susceptibility to stress in DM cattle.

Generally, therefore, DM cattle appear to be more sensitive to stress than normal cattle. However, Menissier (1980) commented that "there are double-muscled cattle relatively well adapted to hard conditions, such as those belonging to the 'Tinima' breed kept in tropical conditions in Cuba (Menendez Butadera, 1977, personal communication) or cows of the Asturiana breed formerly used for agriculture and forest draught although exhibiting some double-muscling expression (Lavin-Arenas, 1964)".

PHYSIOLOGICAL AND METABOLIC CHARACTERISTICS OF DM CATTLE RELATED TO STRESS-SENSITIVITY

DM cattle have reduced heart and lung weights as compared to normal animals (Holmes and Ashmore, 1972; Monin and Boccard, 1974; Ansay and Hanset, 1979; Hendricks et al., 1973). Moreover, they have a lower blood oxygen-binding capacity, due to a lower blood haemoglobin content, without change in oxygen-binding capacity of the haemoglobin (Monin and Boccard, 1974). The ratio of the enlarged muscle mass to the respiratory and circulatory capacities is therefore higher in DM than in normal cattle, and this obviously induces deficiencies in blood supply to muscle in the DM cattle, particularly under stressful conditions.

Holmes and Ashmore (1972) reported that the muscle of DM animals contains larger myofibres and a greater proportion of αW fibres, than the muscle of normal animals. Ouhayoun and Beaumont (1968) and later Hanset et al. (1980) found smaller fibres in the muscles of DM cattle; Hendricks et al. (1973) and West (1974) failed to find any significant difference in the average size of myofibres between normal and DM animals. Biochemical determinations were found to be compatible with the hypothesis of an increased transformation of αR to αW fibres in enlarged muscles of DM cattle (Ouhayoun, 1980). The greater proportion of αW fibres in the muscles of DM animals could favour anaerobic metabolism and lactic acid production in response to stress. Concomitant reduction of organs able to utilise lactic acid such as heart, liver, kidneys, and of red muscle mass, probably promotes metabolic acidosis during stress situations (Holmes and Ashmore, 1972). In this respect, the size of myofibres could be of some relevance. Merkel (1971) hypothethised that in stress-susceptible pigs, the increased size of myofibres could impede diffusion of oxygen into and lactic acid out of myofibres. Difficulty in oxygen diffusion might be reinforced by the low level of myoglobin in the muscles of DM cattle (Ouhayoun, 1980; Boccard and Monin, unpublished data).

On the basis of an osmotic response test on erythrocytes, King et al. (1976) postulated that DM cattle might have a generalised membrane defect. King and Basrur (1979) were able to verify this hypothesis recently, using light and electron microscopy. A membrane defect would explain the very high plasma CPK levels found by Holmes et al. (1973) in DM cattle submitted to stress conditions. King and Basrur (1979) also observed by means of light microscopy gross degenerative changes in the musculature of DM animals. This is in contrast to the observations of Ashmore and Robinson (1969) and Hendricks et al. (1973) who found no such structural alterations.

IMPLICATIONS FOR MEAT QUALITY

Preslaughter stress can modify carbohydrate stores and phosphorylated compounds present in muscles at slaughter, thereby influencing the onset of *rigor mortis* and the ultimate pH of the muscles and consequently affecting meat quality. The more sensitive the animal to preslaughter stress, the more important is the influence on meat quality.

Commenting on observations of Culley (1807), Kidwell (1952) speculated that double-muscling and DFD proneness could have been genetically related characters in the English Shorthorn breed during the last century. He concluded that probably selection had separated these two characters in the breeds currently used in the USA. However, MacKeller (1960) (cited by Holmes et al. 1973) describes the meat of DM cattle from the South Devon breed as dark-coloured, which suggests that these cattle are more prone to DFD condition than normal cattle, and indicates the continued existence of a genetic relation between double muscling and DFD susceptibility. This opinion is strengthened by the results obtained by Holmes et al. (1973) in previously cited experiments designed to study the influence of fasting, adrenaline injection and exercise. These authors concluded that DM cattle are more prone to DFD condition than normal cattle. Bouton et al. (1978), and Boccard and Monin (unpublished results - Table 1), however, found no difference in the ultimate pH of meat from DM and normal steers. In France, DM cattle are not reputed to be particularly prone to the DFD condition. Probably in France as well as in other continental European countries (Italy, Belgium), DM cattle are more carefully handled than other animals before slaughter, due to their higher commercial value and their well known sensitivity to stress, and this helps to reduce the occurrence of DFD meat in these animals.

TABLE 1

ULTIMATE pH IN SOME MUSCLES FROM NORMAL CATTLE AND DOUBLE-MUSCLED CATTLE (MEAN ± s.e.m.)

Muscle	Normal (n = 11)	Double muscled (n = 4)
Psoas major	5.73 ± 0.04	5.76 ± 0.06
Longissimus dorsi	5.76 ± 0.04	5.71 ± 0.04
Semimembranosus	5.64 ± 0.03	5.64 ± 0.04
Semitendinosus	5.69 ± 0.03	5.71 ± 0.05
Pectoralis profundus	5.70 ± 0.02	5.74 ± 0.06
Triceps brachii	5.78 ± 0.04	5.69 ± 0.01

As mentioned previously, preslaughter stress could also influence the rate of onset of *rigor mortis* and therefore the state of contraction of myofibrils and the meat tenderness. Hendricks et al. (1973), however, found no noticeable difference in *rigor mortis* traits (initial extensibility and time to completion) between DM and normal cattle. Bouton et al. (1978) also reported a similar sarcomere length in the two types of cattle. Looking at the rate of *post-mortem* glycogenolysis in muscles of DM animals, it was observed that early post-slaughter pH and phosphocreatine (PC) values were lower in *M. pectoralis* of DM

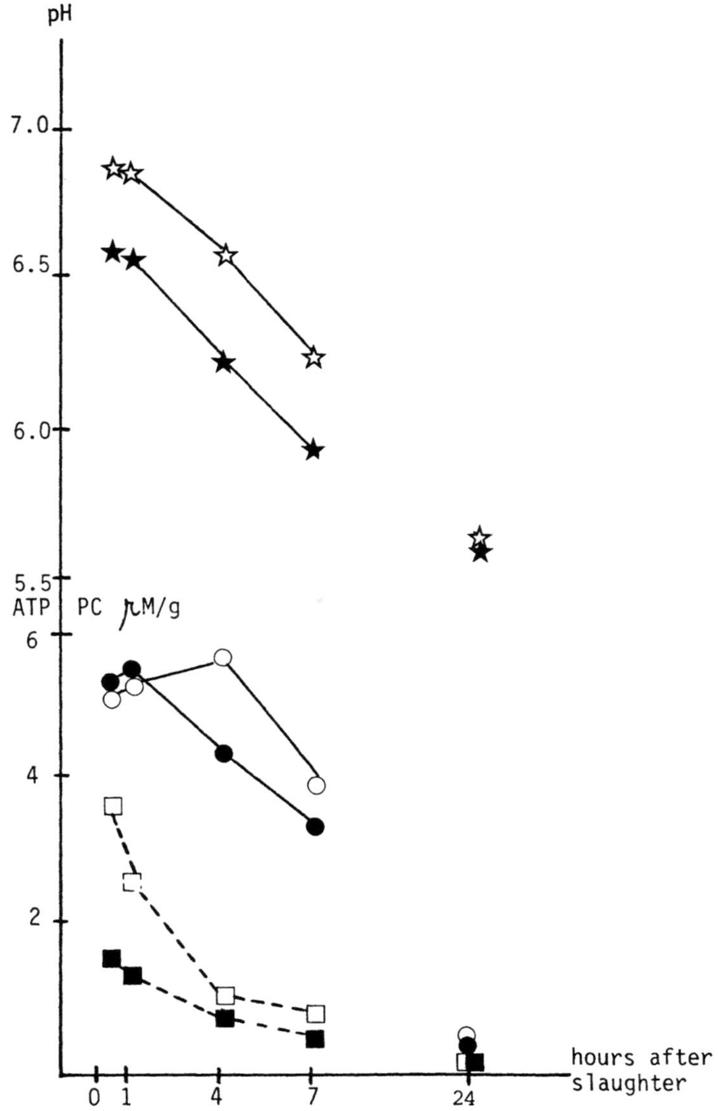

Fig. 1. *Post mortem* fall in pH, ATP and PC values in *M. pectoralis profundus* from normal (n = 11) and DM (n = 4) cattle

pH : normal ☆ DM ★
PC : normal □ DM ■
ATP : normal ○ DM ●

cattle. As a result of the lower PC level, ATP was maintained for a shorter time at its initial level (Figure 1 - Boccard and Monin, unpublished observations). The differences were small and probably of little or no significance with regard to meat quality.

CONCLUSION

Generally, DM cattle are more sensitive to stress than normal animals, because of their physiological and metabolic characteristics. Enlarged 'white' muscle mass and reduced 'red' muscle mass favour anaerobic metabolism. There is a low ratio between muscle mass and respiratory or circulatory capacities, and perhaps a generalised membrane defect which influences muscle homeostasis. However, it is not clear whether this increased sensitivity to stress has a negative influence on meat quality, under current slaughter conditions. From this point of view, it seems that there is some difference between the situation in continental European countries and the USA. Clearly further investigation is needed in this area.

REFERENCES

Ansay, M. and Hanset, R., 1979. Anatomical, physiological and biochemical differences between conventional and double-muscled cattle in the Belgian blue and white breed. Livestock Production Science, 6: 5-13.

Ashmore, C.R. and Robinson, D.W., 1969. Hereditary muscular hypertrophy in the bovine. I. Histological and biochemical characterization. Proc. Soc. exptl. Biol. Med., 132: 548-554.

Bouton, P.E., Harris, P.V., Shorthose, W.R. and Ellis, R.W., 1978. Comparison of some properties of meat from normal steers and steers heterozygous for muscular hypertrophy. Meat Science, 2: 161-167.

Culley, G., 1807. Observations on livestock, 4th ed. G. Woodfall, London.

Halipre, A., 1973. Etude du caractère culard. X. Sensibilité des bovins culards au stress thermique. Ann. Génét. Sél. Anim., 5: 441-449.

Hanset, R., Michaux, C., Dessy-Dore, C. and Burtonboy, G., 1980. Studies on the 7th rib cut in double-muscled and conventional cattle. Anatomical, histological and biochemical aspects. EEC Seminar 'Muscle hypertrophy in cattle', June 10 - 12, 1980, Toulouse, France.

Hedrick, H.B., Boillot J.B., Brady, H.E. and Naumann, H.D., 1959. Etiology of dark-cutting beef. Res. Bull. 717, University of Missouri, Agricultural experiment station, 10 - 60.

Hendricks, H.B., Aberle, E.D., Jones, D.J. and Martin, T.G., 1973. Muscle fibre type, rigor development and bone strength in double-muscled cattle. J. Anim. Sci., 37: 1305-1311.

Holmes, J.H.G. and Ashmore, C.R., 1972. A histochemical study of development of muscle fibre type and size in normal and 'double-muscled' cattle. Growth, 36: 351-372.

Holmes, J.H.G., Ashmore, C.R. and Robinson, D.W., 1973. Effects of stress on on cattle with hereditary muscular hypertrophy. J. Anim. Sci., 36: 684-694.

Holmes, J.H.G. and Robinson, D.W., 1970. Hereditary muscular hypertrophy in the bovine. Metabolic response to nutritional stress. J. Anim. Sci., 31: 776-780.

Holmes, J.H.G., Robinson, D.W. and Ashmore, C.R., 1972. Blood lactic acid and behaviour in cattle with hereditary muscular hypertrophy. J. Anim. Sci., 35: 1011-1015.

Kidwell, J.F., 1952. Muscular hypertrophy and 'black cutter' beef. J. Hered., 43: 157-158.

King, W.A. and Basrur, P.K., 1979. Ultrastructural changes in hereditary muscular hypertrophy in cattle. Acta vet. scand., 20: 245-247.

King, W.A., Basrur, P.K. and Brown, R.G., 1976. Osmotic response tests on erythrocytes for the detection of double-muscle carriers in cattle. Ann. Génét. Sel. Anim., 8: 41-45.

Lavín Arenas, S., 1964. La raza asturiana de los valles como productora de carne. Noticias Neosan, 122: 61-87.

Lawrie, R.A., 1966. Metabolic stresses which affect muscle. In: The physiology and biochemistry of muscle as a food. E.J. Briskey, R.G. Cassens and J.C. Trautman (editors), The University of Wisconsin Press, Madison. 137-164.

MacKellar, J.C., 1960. The occurrence of muscular hypertrophy in South Devon cattle. Vet. Rec., 72: 507-510.

Menissier, F., 1980. General survey about the incidence of double-muscling on cattle performances. EEC Seminar 'Muscle hypertrophy in cattle'. June 10 - 12, 1980, Toulouse, France.

Merkel, R.A., 1971. The relationship of some cardiovascular and haematological parameters to porcine muscle quality. Proceed. 2nd Int. Symp. Condition and meat quality of pigs, Zeist, 1971. Edited: PUDOC, Wageningen, the Netherlands.

Monin, G. and Boccard, R., 1974. Caractéristiques physiologiques respiratoires des bovins culards. Ann. Génét. Sél. Anim., 6: 241-253.

Ouhayoun, J., 1980. Comparative study of muscular tissue of normal and double-muscled Maine Anjou bull calves. DNA and metabolism. EEC Seminar 'Muscle hypertrophy in cattle', June 10 - 12, 1980, Toulouse, France.

Ouhayoun, J. and Beaumont, A., 1968. Etude du caractère culard. III. Anatomie microscopique comparée du tissu musculaire de mâles charolais normaux et culards. Ann. Zootech., 17: 213-219.

Rhodes, D.N., 1973. Some observation on the genesis of dark-cutting beef from bulls and steers. MRI memorandum 6, February; Meat Research Institute, Langford.

West, R.L., 1974. Red to white fibre ratios as an index of double-muscling in beef cattle. J. Anim. Sci., 38: 1165-1175.

DISCUSSION

T.R. Dutson *(USA)*

I would like to refer to your comment on the difference between double muscled cattle in the USA and those in European countries. Our experience with double muscled cattle in Texas is the same as yours. We find that they have a somewhat higher susceptibility to stress but, out of all the cattle we have killed, we have never had any dark-cutting carcass characteristics. Therefore, our data would match yours quite closely and are somewhat different to those of the California group.

P.V. Tarrant *(Ireland)*

I would like to follow on from Dr. Dutson's comment. Dark-cutting is less likely to occur in cattle slaughtered at a university laboratory because these animals are not usually exposed to circumstances that produce dark-cutting. Therefore, Dr. Dutson, have you ever observed dark-cutting in normal animals at the university?

T.R. Dutson

Yes, we do occasionally. Much less than the incidence found in slaughterhouses, particularly those who handle their animals rather badly, but we do occasionally find dark-cutters in our meat laboratory animals.

P.V. Tarrant

I would also like to comment on the ultimate pH values which Dr. Monin showed. I think the double muscled values were based on 4 animals and the values for normal beef were for 11 animals. Therefore, if there was a tendency to DFD in double muscled animals, I do not think it would show up under that type of examination, unless the animals were subjected to stress before slaughter.

G. Monin

The animals were transported from Paris to our research centre at Theix. The journey lasts approximately 10 h. That was 4 - 5 days before slaughter. Between the travel and slaughter they had been submitted to the exercise stress I spoke about. It explains why the ultimate pH was rather high in the two groups; normal pH is about 5.5.

P.V. Tarrant

I see! So there was a pre-slaughter stress of moderate intensity. Thank you.

D.B. MacDougall *(UK)*

The haemoglobin values of the blood in the Charolais calves which you showed as different: was the difference maintained to the maturity of the animals?

G. Monin

I do not have the data here, and they are very old results, but I believe we found a small difference in the haematocrit. I think it was about 35 per cent in double muscled animals and 40 per cent in normal animals at 15 months.

SESSION V

IDENTIFICATION AND PREVENTION OF DARK-CUTTING

Chairman: A. Romita

PREVENTIVE TREATMENTS DURING THE PRE-SLAUGHTER PERIOD

H.B. Hedrick
Food Science and Nutrition Department,
University of Missouri, Columbia, USA.

ABSTRACT

Dark-cutting in beef is caused by cattle being exposed to several hours stress pre-slaughter. The most effective method of preventing dark-cutting beef is careful handling of animals from the time they leave the farm until they are slaughtered. Specific recommendations which will aid in preventing the conditions are:

Market and slaughter well-nourished and healthy cattle.

Avoid exciting cattle while loading, transporting to abattoir, and while holding prior to slaughter. Provision of adequate loading chutes, properly equipped trucks and rail cars and holding-pens will help to minimise excitement and injury.

Avoid overcrowding and mixing of large and small cattle during shipment. If mixed loads are to be shipped, dividers should be used to keep large and small cattle separated.

Avoid mixing strange cattle, females that are in oestrus, or bulls during shipment and particularly in holding pens prior to slaughter.

Reduce time in shipment and holding pre-slaughter to as short a period as possible, preferably less than 12 h.

Protect cattle from heat and high humidity by transporting during the cool portion of the day or night.

Provide protection against wind, rain or snow during shipment and holding pre-slaughter.

When cattle arrive at the market or abattoir always provide water, and if slaughter is scheduled for the following day, provide feed.

Move cattle from holding pens to the slaughter floor with a minimum of excitement.

INTRODUCTION

In order to recommend preventive treatments for dark-cutting beef, one must first consider the characteristics of dark-cutting muscle and then the factors which would likely produce this type of muscle. Dark-cutting beef is unattractive; it is discriminated against by the consumer and therefore has been a problem to the beef industry for many years, particularly when the consumer can exercise a choice of purchase based on visual preference. Although the consumer discriminates against dark-cutting in the fresh form, the evidence is not clear whether the palatability characteristics of dark-cutting differ from normal beef (Hedrick, 1965). In addition to the dark colour, dark-cutting muscle consistently has a high ultimate pH, reflecting a deficiency of glycogen in the muscle at slaughter. Thus, preventive treatments should be directed toward the assurance of an adequate level of glycogen in muscle at slaughter.

Bernard (1878) recognised that the maintenance of a balanced internal environment is a fundamental characteristic of the living animal, and as a result of this, life can continue under varied environments and resist, to a large extent, numerous adverse treatments. Treatments or factors which cause disturbance to the internal environment are called 'stressors', while the loss of stability or homeostasis (Cannon, 1929) caused by 'stressors' is 'stress'. 'Stress' involves muscle because muscle is an integral part of the animal body, providing support and locomotion. The muscle mass of the body expends large amounts of energy, especially during periods of stress. Homeostasis of muscle is influenced by the blood supply, nervous stimuli and by hormones.

Cattle are subject to numerous 'stressors' which bring about a disequilibrium of muscle and the internal environment, particularly during the period prior to and during slaughter (Hedrick et al., 1959). These 'stressors' may include nutrition, emotional excitement, fatigue, trauma, fear, shock, anoxia, temperature and humidity. When Selye (1936) introduced his concept of the stress syndrome he showed that regardless of the specific nature of the 'stressor', a similar 'stress response' was induced in an animal. Specifically, an animal increases the release of hormones from the adrenal gland in an act of resistance to a 'stressor'. These hormones, catecholamines, 17-hydroxycorticosterone and 11-deoxycorticosterone elicit various responses in the animal. One response to catecholamines (epinephrine) is the mobilisation of muscle and liver glycogen. It is not my objective to discuss further the intricate nature of stress and the stress response, but rather to discuss animal-to-animal variation to stressors, the effect of stressors on the incidence of dark-cutting beef muscle and possible preventive treatments.

ANIMAL VARIATION

Whether dark-cutting beef is genetically related has not been established. However, Guilbert (1937) cited reports dating back to 1774 which suggested the dark-cutting condition is caused by hereditary factors. Based on reports which have shown that 'stress-susceptibility' and 'stress-resistance' in pigs (Judge et al., 1967) and pork muscle quality (Christian, 1972) are inherited traits, there is reason to suspect a similar situation exists for cattle. The reports by Kidwell (1952) and Holmes et al. (1972a,b,c) suggest cattle with muscular hypertrophy, an inherited trait, were particularly susceptible to stress. Lawrie (1958) concluded that effective prevention of dark-cutting beef will depend on the concomitant progress of genetics and neuro-endocrinology.

All cattle subjected to a given stressor do not react the same. Temperament and particularly ease of excitement is an inherited trait (Stricklin et al., 1980). Variation in animal temperament is common. Seldom do all animals in a given group or shipment have the same temperament. The incidence of dark-cutting is variable among groups of cattle slaughtered in the US, ranging for zero to 10 per cent. In general, the current average incidence experienced by major processors is less than one per cent. Selection of breeding animals which have no related incidences of dark-cutting and especially animals which have temperament not conductive to ready excitability should be considered as one preventive measure.

MUSCLE VARIATION

Considerable variation may exist in pH, colour and water-holding properties among muscles of a given beef carcass designated as being dark-cutting. Also, considerable variation may exist for these muscle properties among carcasses. Hunt and Hedrick (1977a,b) characterised four quality groups of beef carcasses: dark-cutting (DC); normal in colour, firmness and exudation (NOR); normal in colour, but soft and exudative (NSE); and pale in colour, soft and exudative (PSE). Histochemical and histological characteristics of muscle fibres from DC, NSE and PSE were similar in metabolic potential which suggests that these three aberrant muscle quality groups have a common aetiology. Personal observations over a 25 year period of research related to beef quality indicate that short-term stress is conductive to the PSE condition and long-term stress is conductive to the DC condition. In other words, cattle that are stress-susceptible and if subjected to stress for approximately one hour immediately before slaughter may be NSE or PSE and if subjected to stress for several hours before slaughter may be DC. A similar aetiology for PSE and DC pork muscle has been described (Topel, 1969).

SEX CONDITION

Canadian workers (Munns and Burrell, 1966) reported the incidence of dark-cutting in cow carcasses was higher than that of steer and heifer carcasses. They also reported a lower incidence (3.5 per cent) in Choice steers compared to lower-quality Commercial grade steers (12 per cent). If heifers and cows are in oestrus during the pre-slaughter handling period, the physical activity and stress associated with oestrus will contribute to the incidence of dark-cutting. Fighting and mounting among bulls will also increase the incidence. Augustini and Fischer (1979) reported a greater incidence of dark-cutting in young bulls (housed untethered) compared to heifers and cows. Fischer and Augustini (1980) reported a 50 per cent incidence of dark-cutters in young bulls transported for 4 h and fasted 48 h prior to slaughter.

NUTRITIONAL REGIMEN

Composition of the diet *per se* during growth and development has no direct effect upon the incidence of the dark-cutting condition provided a reasonable level of nutrients is available and cattle are not maintained in a fasting or starvation state. This statement is made even though some industry personnel have attributed dark-cutting to various diets. For example, when corn silage became a common ingredient in some feed-lot rations in the US and when diethylstilbestrol was used, it was quite common to attribute incorrectly the incidence of dark-cutting to these ingredients. The main consideration from the dietary standpoint is fasting during the shipment and holding period prior to slaughter.

The importance of adequate feeding to maintain adequate muscle glycogen and to ensure a low ultimate muscle pH was demonstrated by Callow (1936, 1938, 1939) for pigs, and by Bate-Smith and Bendell (1949) for rabbits. Howard and Lawrie (1956) demonstrated that fasting lowered the glycogen level in *M. longissimus* muscle of steers but the ultimate pH was 'normal'. Fasting for 7, 14 and 28 days did not produce dark-cutting carcasses. The resistance of steers to changes in glycogen level due to fasting was greater than that of the rabbit and pig.

Kauflin et al. (1969) reported the results of a study involving US Choice grade steers and heifers fasted up to four days before slaughter (Table 1). All animals had previously received a concentrate grain diet, were held in their respective

TABLE 1

EFFECT OF PRE-SLAUGHTER FASTING ON THE LIVER OF BEEF CATTLE

Item	Days fasted				
	0	1	2	3	4
	Steers (12 animals per treatment)				
Liver glycogen (mg/gm)	40.76[a]	22.83[b]	10.60[c]	6.24[c]	14.39[c]
Liver weight (per cent carcass weight)	2.07[a]	1.88[bc]	1.73[cd]	1.63[d]	1.64[d]
	Heifers (10 animals per treatment)				
Liver glycogen (mg/gm)	64.88[a]	44.97[b]	14.21[c]	5.98[d]	5.64[d]
Liver weight (per cent carcass weight)	2.20[a]	2.09[a]	1.88[b]	1.73[bc]	1.62[c]

[a,b,c,d]Means on the same line bearing different superscripts are significantly different ($P < 0.05$)

feed-lots during the fasting period (environmental temperature 21 - 33°C) with *ad libitum* water, were transported 3 to 6 km and slaughtered within 3 h of departure from the feed-lot. Liver glycogen and liver weight were significantly reduced after either one or two days fasting. However, all carcasses had normal ultimate pH and colour in *M. longissimus dorsi*. Another similarly designed study conducted at a central market (Kauflin et al., 1969) also resulted in reduction of liver glycogen and all carcasses had normal ultimate muscle pH and colour. A more recent series of studies conducted at the University of Missouri during the months of February, August and October (Asplund et al., 1980), which involved trucking cattle for varied distances (65 to 1 190 km) and fasting without water from zero to two days, resulted in carcass weight losses and some dark-cutting carcasses. However, all dark-cutting carcasses were from animals slaughtered after one day of treatment and from animals that were identified as being very excitable initially while being weighed, restrained for blood sampling and during trucking and handling prior to slaughter. The incidence of dark-cutting in this later study was attributed to the additional stress associated with excitement during at least a period of one day before slaughter. The significance of excitement will be discussed later in this paper.

These studies clearly indicate that fasting reduces glycogen stores of the body but during fasting cattle can maintain muscle glycogen levels for sufficient lactic acid production *post mortem*. Fasting when combined with other stress treatments can be a contributory factor to dark-cutting. Recommendations to producers and processors should include providing *ad libitum* fresh water for animals at all possible times, withhold feed for a few hours immediately prior to transporting followed by providing feed at the slaughterhouse if slaughter is scheduled for the following day or later. Based on numerous personal observations, exhaustive exercise of well-fed cattle for one to two hours immediately before slaughter will not cause dark-cutting muscle.

While exhaustive exercise is known to reduce the quantity of glycogen available at death for the formation of lactic acid and hence the ultimate pH in muscle, training is known to increase the quantity of glycogen (Mitchell and Hamilton, 1932). Cattle that have been reared in close confinement experience less physical activity than animals reared in large lots or pastures and therefore may have lower initial glycogen levels.

Whenever strange cattle are mixed there is usually a fight or struggle to establish the social order of the group; stress-susceptible and more agressive animals involved in the struggle may be unable to adapt to the stress associated with fighting and become dark-cutters: particularly young bulls when mixed will fight and if held for several hours prior to slaughter, or overnight, the incidence of dark-cutters is high (Tennessen and Price, 1980). Grandin (1979) reported a 13 to 17 per cent incidence of dark-cutting in show steers that were trucked about 5 h, group penned and held for 1 to 2 days at the slaughter plant. A similar group of steers trucked about 5 h and slaughtered upon arrival had no dark-cutters. Whenever possible, cattle should not be mixed with strange cattle or overcrowded during transit and during holding prior to slaughter.

The greater the time period cattle are in transit to the slaughter plant the greater the demand for energy and more likely a reduction in glycogen stores. Therefore, long hauls to market should be avoided. If long haul by railroad is necessary, consideration may be given to equipping the rail car with a water tank and feed supply. A report by Friend et al. (1980) indicated that feeder cattle transported for 57 h in a railroad car equipped with a water tank and *ad libitum* feed, compared to cattle transported in a truck for 11.3 h without feed and water, lost less body weight (4.5 *vs.* 10.6 per cent) and were less fatigued at the final destination.

EXCITEMENT

When cattle are moved from the farm or feed-lot to slaughter, they are subjected to more extreme conditions than those to which they are accustomed and usually experience excitement and anxiety. The degree and duration of excitement and anxiety may vary among animals and among the various conditions of pre-slaughter handling. These are variables which have a major effect upon the incidence of dark-cutting. The initial reaction to excitement is the release of epinephrine from the adrenal medulla causing the breakdown of liver and muscle glycogen to glucose and lactic acid respectively. Epinephrine stimulates the anterior pituitary to produce ACTH, which in turn stimulates the adrenal cortex to produce 17-hydroxycorticosterone, which tends to restore the glycogen balance by gluconeogenesis from protein. The ease by which this series of events is initiated in individual animals and the lack of ability to withstand and adapt to these events is directly related to the incidence of dark-cutting.

Data presented in Table 2 illustrate the effect various periods of pre-slaughter excitement had on ultimate muscle pH. Short-term excitement (2 h) did not produce dark-cutting but long-term excitement (24 h) produced the condition. The important point to be derived from these data is that several hours of stress were required to produce the dark-cutting

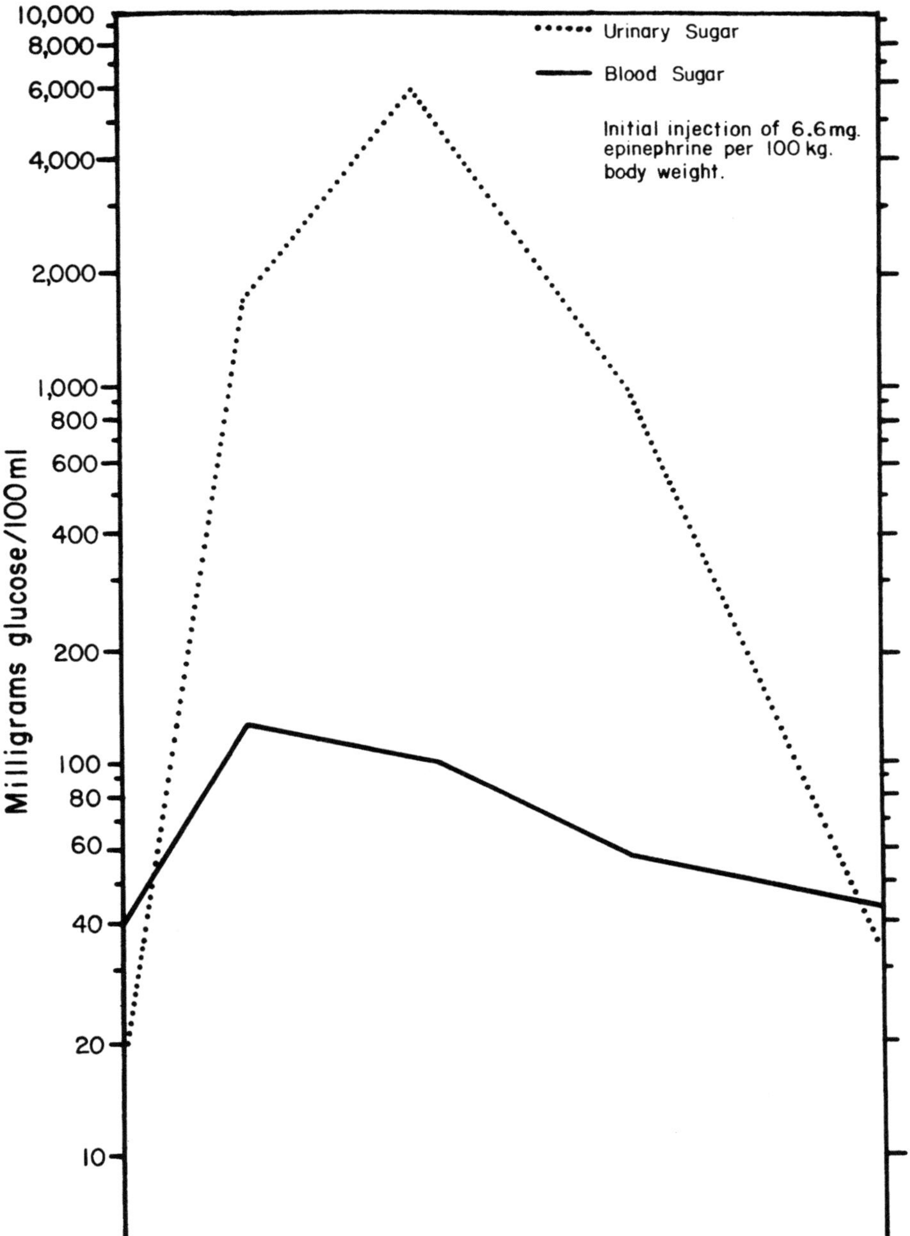

Fig. 1. The effect of a subcutaneous injection of epinephrine on blood and urinary sugar of beef cattle.

condition in well-nourished cattle. The indiscriminate use of electrical devices such as a 'hot-shot' can produce dark-cutting beef.

TABLE 2

EFFECT OF PRE-SLAUGHTER EXCITEMENT ON ULTIMATE BEEF MUSCLE pH

Animal number	Period of excitement (h)[a]	Live weight (kg)	USDA carcass grade	*M. longissimus* pH
12	0	410	Good	5.4
13	0	386	Choice	5.4
33	2	355	Choice-	5.5
44	2	355	Choice	5.5
14	24	348	Choice	6.7[b]
15	24	390	Good+	6.4[b]

[a]Periodic excitement induced with an electric 'hot-shot'.
[b]Dark-cutting.

To determine the effect epinephrine-induced stress had on ultimate muscle pH and colour a number of experiments were conducted with cattle (Hedrick et al., 1957, 1959), lambs (Hedrick et al., 1961) and pigs (Hedrick et al., 1964). Data presented in Table 3 illustrate that a comparatively large dosage of epinephrine was required to produce dark-cutting muscle, that the time interval from injection to slaughter had to be several hours, and that the apparent period to restore glycogen balance was longer than the period of time required to deplete it. As demonstrated previously with excitement (Table 2), a main key to the cause of dark-cutting muscle is a severe and continuous form of stress over several hours before slaughter. Data presented in Figure 1 illustrate the effect injected epinephrine had on blood and urinary sugar levels of a well-nourished steer that yielded a dark-cutting carcass. A precipitous rise in blood sugar and urinary sugar occurred following the injection of epinephrine and the concentrations of both remained high for at least 12 h, stimulating a period of sufficient stress to produce dark-cutting beef.

TABLE 3

EFFECT OF PRE-SLAUGHTER INJECTION OF EPINEPHRINE ON BEEF MUSCLE ULTIMATE pH AND COLOUR

Animal number	Time before slaughter (h)	Live weight (kg)	Epinephrine injected mg/100 kg live weight	USDA carcass grade	*M. longissimus* pH
25	Control	352	0	Good	5.45
17	5	390	11.0[a]	Choice-	5.8[c]
18	5	357	5.5	Choice-	5.6
26	23	318	2.2	Good+	5.55
27	23	318	4.4	Good	5.75[c]
28	23	318	6.6	Good+	6.15[b]
801	Control	359	0	Choice-	5.4
807	Control	318	0	Choice-	5.4
828	24	335	6.6	Choice-	6.0[b]
829	24	345	6.6	Choice	6.2[b]
802	48	404	6.6	Choice	5.75[c]
803	48	354	6.6	Choice	5.95[b]
819	72	375	6.6	Choice-	5.95[b]
806	72	340	6.6	Choice-	6.0[b]
809	96	343	6.6	Choice	5.55
810	96	334	6.6	Choice-	5.9[b]

[a] Intramuscular injection. All other injections were subcutaneous.

[b] Dark-cutters.

[c] Dark colour borderline of being dark-cutters.

TRAUMA

Sorting, loading and hauling cattle to slaughter frequently result in injuries. Nearly every measurable function of the body is affected by trauma. Therefore, an injury can be a major contributing factor toward dark-cutting. Bruised carcasses are often dark-cutting carcasses. Loading and unloading chutes should be designed to move animals easily without injury or excitement. Trucks and rail cars should provide good footing for animals and partitions to separate the load and particularly separate smaller animals from larger animals.

TRANQUILLISERS

Tranquillisers are used extensively in human medicine to relieve anxiety or tension and by the veterinarian to control the behaviour of animals. Huber (1958) pointed out that tranquillisers act to diminish anxiety and reduce the intensity of the 'alarm' reaction, enabling the animal to adjust adequately without going into a stage of hyperexcitement. There is wide variability among animals as to the dosage which can be tolerated without various side effects becoming evident.

Administration of tranquillisers (synthetic phenothiazine derivatives and reserpine) prior to stress did not prevent dark-cutting beef (Hedrick et al., 1959). However, there were indications that these compounds caused a reduction in reflexes and alarm responses and delayed excitement. Oedema was present in the carcass surrounding the site of injection of the phenothiazine derivatives. Reserpine at levels used produced deleterious side effects which would preclude the use of this compound as a preventive measure. The use of tranquillisers is not approved in the US for use in slaughter animals and therefore compounds of this nature cannot be considered as a preventive measure for dark-cutting beef.

ENVIRONMENTAL ELEMENTS

Many elements of the environment can be stressful to animals. Extremes in temperature and humidity are effective 'stressors' and can contribute to the dark-cutting condition. When temperatures become cooler than those to which cattle are acclimatised, they require additional energy to maintain body temperature. On the other hand, unusually high temperatures and relative humidity place heavy demands on the animal's cooler mechanisms. When cattle are transported (unprotected) during cold weather in rain or snow or in hot and humid conditions (Figure 2) the level of discomfort and incidence of dark-cutters increases. Particularly in the fall of the year when sudden changes in environmental temperatures occur the incidence of dark-cutting increases (Munns and Burrell, 1966). During the winter months when cooler temperatures become more constant, the cattle become acclimatised to the cooler temperatures and are better able to withstand inclement weather conditions. However, to minimise the stress of extremes in temperature, cattle should be protected from inclement weather conditions during handling, transporting and holding before slaughter.

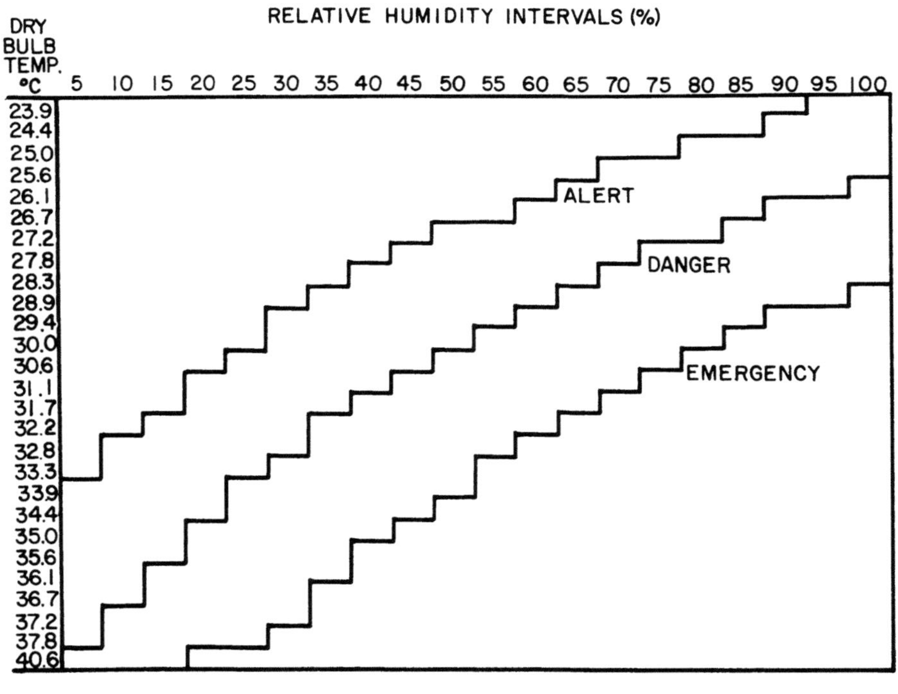

Fig. 2 The temperature-humidity index for estimating the level of discomfort in animals. The chances of death loss during movement of livestock are specified as 'alert', 'danger', and 'emergency'. (Adapted from Livestock Conservation, Inc., Hinsdale, Illinois).

REFERENCES

Asplund, M.R., Anderson, M.E., Hedrick, H.B., Johnson, H.D. and May, H.F., 1980. Unpublished data. Univ. of Mo.-Columbia.

Augustini, Chr. and Fischer, K., 1979. Untersuchungen zum Problem des dunklen, leimigen Rindfleisches (dark cutting beef). 1. Mitteilung: Erscheinungsform und Vorkommen. Fleischwirtsch 59 (12), 1871.

Bate-Smith, E.C. and Bendall, J.R., 1949. Factors determining the time course of *rigor mortis*. J. Physiol. 110, 47.

Bernard, Claude, 1878. Lecons sur les phénomènes de la vie communs aux animaux et aux végétaux. J.B. Bailleire, Paris.

Callow, E.H., 1936. Report Food Invest. Bd., London.

Callow, E.H., 1938. Report Food Invest. Bd., London.

Callow, E.H., 1939. Report Food Invest. Bd., London.

Cannon, W.B., 1929. Organization of Physiological homeostasis. Physiol. Rev. 9, 399.

Christian, L.L., 1972. A review of the role of genetics in animal stress susceptibility and meat quality. The Proc. of the Pork Quality Symposium. P. 91. Univ. Wisconsin Extension Publ. 72-0.

Fischer, K. and Augustini, Chr., 1980. Untersuchungen zum Problem des dunklin, leimigen Rindfleisches (dark cutting beef). 3. Mitteilung: Auseverkungen unterschiedlicher Transport temperaturen und mehrtägiger Nüchterung. Fleischwirtsch 60 (3), 469.

Friend, T.H., Sharp, A.J., Irwin, M.R., Ashby, B.H., Thompson, G.B. and Bailey, W.A., 1980. Behaviour of calves in a railcar modified for feeding and watering in transit. Abstracts 72nd Annual Meeting American Society Animal Science, Cornell Univ., NY, p. 106.

Grandin, T., 1979. The effect of pre-slaughter handling and penning procedures on meat quality. Abstracts 71st Annual Meeting American Soc. Animal Science. Univ. Arizona. p. 147.

Guilbert, H.R., 1937. What causes 'black cutter' beef? A historical basis for the hypothesis that the condition known as 'black cutter' in beef is caused by hereditary factors. J. Heredity 28, 213.

Hedrick, H.B., 1965. Influence of *ante mortem* stress on meat palatability. J. Anim. Sci. 24, 255.

Hedrick, H.B., Boillot, J.B., Brady, D.E. and Naumann, H.D., 1959. Etiology of dark-cutting beef. Mo. Agr. Exp. Sta. Res. Bulletin 717.

Hedrick, H.B., Boillot, J.B., Dyer, A.J. and Naumann, H.D., 1961. Effect of *ante mortem* administration of adrenaline on *post mortem* lamb carcass characteristics. J. Anim. Sci. 20, 558.

Hedrick, H.B., Brady, D.E. and Turner, C.W., 1957. The effect of *ante mortem* stress on *post mortem* beef carcass characteristics. Proc. Research. Conf. American Meat Institute Foundation. 9, 9.

Hedrick, H.B., Parrish, F.C., Jr and Bailey, M.E., 1964. Effect of adrenaline stress on pork quality. J. Anim. Sci. 23, 225.

Holmes, J.H.G., Ashmore, C.R. and Robinson, D.W., 1972a. *Post mortem* changes in the meat of stressed muscular hypertrophied cattle. J. Anim. Sci. 34, 892.

Holmes, J.H.G., Ashmore, C.R. and Robinson, D.W., 1972b. Stress response of cattle with hereditary muscular hypertrophy. J. Anim. Sci. 34, 899.

Holmes, J.H.G., Robinson, D.W. and Ashmore, C.R., 1972c. Blood lactic acid and behaviour in cattle with hereditary muscular hypertrophy. J. Anim. Sci. 35, 1011.

Howard, A. and Lawrie, R.A., 1956. Part II. Physiological and biochemical effects of various pre-slaughter treatments. Studies on beef quality. Tech. Paper No. 2. Div. Food Pres. and Transport. CSIRO Melbourne.

Huber, W.G., 1958. Tranquilization and sedation of livestock. Sixth Annual Res. Conf. Proceedings. Pfizer and Co. Chicago, Illinois.

Hunt, M.C. and Hedrick, H.B., 1977a. Histochemical and histological characteristics of bovine muscles from four quality groups. J. Food Sci. 42, 578.

Hunt, M.C. and Hedrick, H.B., 1977b. Chemical, physical and sensory characteristics of bovine muscle from four quality groups. J. Food Sci. 42, 716.

Judge, M.D., Cassens, R.G. and Briskey, E.J., 1967. Muscle properties of physically restrained stressor-susceptible and stressor-resistant porcine animals. J. Food Sci. 32, 565.

Kauflin, V.R., Hedrick, H.B. and Stringer, W.C., 1969. Effects of pre-slaughter feeding regimen on beef carcass characteristics. Mo. Agr. Exp. Sta. Res. Bul. 953.

Kidwell, J.F., 1952. Muscular hypertrophy and 'black cutter' beef. J. Heredity 43, 157.

Lawrie, R.A., 1958. Physiological stress in relation to dark-cutting beef. J. Sci. Food Agric. 9, 721.

Mitchell, H.H. and Hamilton, J.S., 1932. The effect of long-continued muscular exercise upon the chemical composition of the muscles and other tissues of beef cattle. J. Agr. Res. 46, 917.

Munns, W.O. and Burrell, D.E., 1966. The incidence of dark-cutting beef. Food Techn. 20, 1601.

Selye, H., 1936. A syndrome produced by diverse nocuous agents. Nature 138, 32.

Stricklin, W.R., Heisler, C.E. and Wilson, L.L., 1980. Heritability of temperament in beef cattle. Abstracts 72nd Annual Meeting American Soc. Animal Science, Cornell Univ., NY p. 109.

Tennessen, T. and Price, M.A., 1980. Pre-slaughter management and dark-cutting in young bulls. Abstracts 72nd Annual Meeting American Soc. Animal Science, Cornell Univ., NY p. 110.

Topel, D.G., 1969. In: Recent points of view on the condition and meat quality of pigs for slaughter, ed. Sybesma, W., Van der Wal, P.G. and Walstra, P., Zeist, Holland.

DISCUSSION

Lis Buchter *(Denmark)*

Dr. Hedrick, I noticed in your first Table that the liver glycogen content of the heifers was much higher than in the steers and that the glycogen content in the heifers, after one day of fasting, was at the same level as the initial level of the steers.

H.B. Hedrick *(USA)*

I have no explanation for this. There were two separate feed-lots in the experiment; heifers were in one and steers in an adjacent feed-lot. Both had exactly the same conditions and slaughter was on the same day. Samples were taken and analysed randomly. This is the result; I have no other explanation.

Lis Buchter

In your experience do you think that it occurred only in this particular experiment, or is it something that is commonly found?

H.B. Hedrick

I am afraid I do not know.

Lis Buchter

I am looking for a sex difference which might give some explanation for some of the problems.

J. Wismer-Pedersen *(Denmark)*

You stated that the composition of the diet probably did not have any bearing on the occurrence of the dark-cutting situation. What about the selenium content of the diet? Work with pigs shows that it may have some effect. What is the situation with cattle?

H.B. Hedrick

There is some current research related to selenium in the diet, but what the effect is, I do not know.

E. Dransfield *(UK)*

I was interested to see that you followed up your observations with a publicity promotion to advertise to your market. Can you say whether the incidence of dark-cutting beef has remained stable, is on the increase, or is declining as a result?

H.B. Hedrick

It is my observation that the incidence has decreased in the States. There are a number of factors. One is that a large number of our cattle are moved from the feed-lot to the slaughterhouse for slaughter on the same day. It is a matter of concern for the slaughterer, because a dark-cutting carcass will be down-graded. This means considerable reduction in price. It does not take very many for the plant to become alarmed about this. They keep a record of the source of the animals: where they came from and who trucked them, etc. The better plants begin to check this out immediately.

EARLY IDENTIFICATION OF THE DFD CONDITION IN PRE-*RIGOR* BEEF CARCASSES

C.L. Davey and A.E. Graafhuis
Meat Industry Research Institute of New Zealand (Inc.)
P.O. Box 617, Hamilton, New Zealand.

ABSTRACT

A key to the elucidation of the biochemistry of DFD meat and to its control lies ideally in its ante mortem or early post mortem identification. The present paper examines a way of determining the ultimate pH of carcasses within about 30 min after slaughter by a sensitive method developed to identify DFD meat while still in its pre-rigor state. Through biopsy techniques the method can be extended to ante mortem identification so that it should be a useful tool in achieving control of the unwanted condition. The paper also examines the difficulties and potential errors in identifying DFD carcasses from ultimate pH measurements.

INTRODUCTION

Dark-cutting meat has always been a part of the butcher's lore. That it is due to the meat being of a relatively high ultimate pH has been recognised for 40 years (Winkler, 1939). If the condition is extreme (pH above ∿6.2) the meat, especially beef, is purplish-black in colour, firm in texture, and dry to the touch. For this reason it is now generally referred to as dark, firm, dry (DFD) meat. It occurs in both beef and pork animals, *M. longissimus*, *M. semitendinosus* and *M. gluteus medius* being particularly affected (Augustini and Fischer, 1979). Although the meat is commercially discounted through its colour and texture, and its reduced shelf-life, it has a relatively high water-holding capacity which is a desirable property in most processed meats (Hamm, 1960; Wirth et al., 1976; Bouton et al., 1971).

The condition occurs in carcasses from animals with low stores of muscle glycogen (Potthast and Hamm, 1976). On the death of an animal, the resting aerobic utilisation of glycogen is replaced by glycolysis, with its end-product of lactic acid. Approximately 100 μmol/g lactate is produced in muscle having a normally low ultimate pH (pH 5.5) whereas only 40 μmol/g lactate would be expected in a DFD muscle with an ultimate pH 6.2 (Davey and Gilbert, 1976). In other words the DFD muscle (pH 6.2) has less than half the available glycogen store of normal meat from which to produce lactic acid. Since the purpose of glycolysis is to maintain ATP supplies, muscles with low glycogen reserves enter *rigor mortis* a lot earlier than muscles that have normal levels of glycogen (Davey and Winger, 1979). For this reason high ultimate pH carcasses in a commercial situation may enter *rigor* well before they have been chilled sufficiently for the muscles to cold shorten. The meat from such carcasses is therefore inclined to be tender.

Because of the commercial significance of the DFD condition, much attention has been given to determining its cause. While certain emaciating diseases may lead to a DFD condition, *ante mortem* stress and starvation are the overriding causes in healthy animals (Hall et al., 1944; Howard and Lawrie, 1956). The condition may be induced by sharp climatic changes and also by fighting brought on by an upset in established mob behaviour, especially during confinement in abattoir stockyards (Hedrick, 1958; Fell et al., 1973; Gallwey and Tarrant, 1978). A short burst of activity just prior to slaughter is not in itself important (Howard and Lawrie, 1956). Prolonged starvation is an exacerbating factor, but by itself is not an overriding one in the 1 - 2 days deprivation that may be expected from the extremes of transportation and holding for slaughter (Howard and Lawrie, 1956).

Studies on the microbiology of DFD meat are now being pursued actively (Nicol et al., 1970; Tarrant, 1976; Taylor and Shaw 1977; Gill and Newton, 1979). The reduced shelf-life of such meat is not only due to a high ultimate pH but to the attendant very low concentration of available glucose, the usual substrate for spoilage bacteria (Gill and Newton, 1979). Without glucose, those bacterial species utilising amino acids as a prime energy source will grow to the progressive exclusion of the usual spoilage organisms. Deterioration, such as greening in packaged meat, or the development of objectionable smells and off-flavours then occurs at rather low bacterial counts (10^6/g), substantially reducing acceptable shelf-life.

Considerable effort has been directed to the reliable monitoring of the DFD condition. Subjective procedures have been developed based on colour and feel with the additional use of pH indicator strips (Roemmele et al., 1961; Scheper, 1971; Von Mickwitz, 1971; Honikel, 1976). Although changes in the adenine-inosine ratio measured spectrophotometrically can be used, monitoring pH with glass electrodes is the more usual objective method. In normal practice the ultimate pH value of *M. longissimus* from beef animals for instance, is determined at the 11 - 12th rib (Munns and Burrell, 1965) either by surface or probe electrode. Such investigations reveal considerable variations in ultimate pH values amongst the muscles of beef animals, pigs and sheep (Linke et al., 1976; Sornay and Legras,

1978; Davey, unpublished data). It is clear from these studies that the ultimate pH value of a single muscle does not represent the general pH condition of the carcass. A degree of variation amongst muscles is not unexpected, for, depending on the requirement for sustained aerobic functioning, some muscles will presumably have a lower glycogen need than others and this will be reflected in ultimate pH differences. Variations in ultimate pH within a single muscle are more difficult to explain. In one topographical study seven estimations of ultimate pH were made on a single muscle. While in most muscles the variation was generally small and about 0.1 pH units, in the *M. aconeus* it rose to about ± 0.3 pH units (Sornay and Legras, 1978).

A key to the elucidation of the biochemistry of DFD meat and to its control lies ideally in its *ante mortem* or early *post mortem* identification. The present paper examines a way of determining the ultimate pH of carcasses within about 30 min after slaughter by a sensitive method developed to identify DFD meat while still in its pre-*rigor* state. Through biopsy techniques the method can be extended to *ante mortem* identification so that it should be a useful tool in achieving control of the unwanted condition. The paper also examines the difficulties and potential errors in identifying DFD carcasses from ultimate pH measurements.

EXPERIMENTAL PROCEDURE

Carcass selection and muscle sampling

The animals used in this study were from the normal line of stock slaughtered in a commercial abattoir. The majority of beef animals were good quality Angus steers, 18 months of age, and between 320 and 450 kg live weight. The sheep, largely ewes, ranged in age from 1 - 5 years. The beef *M. sterno-mandibularis* were removed within 10 min of slaughter immediately following pelt-removal and before decapitation, and were trimmed of surrounding tissue. Samples of *M. longissimus* of the beef and sheep animals were cut from the carcasses adjacent to the 10 - 14th ribs within 30 min after slaughter.

To follow the time courses of pH fall, *M. sternomandibularis* of beef carcasses were treated variously as follows. Muscles were held at 15°C under a thin layer of polyethylene film and sampled from their interiors at intervals to obtain the reference time-course of pH fall. To obtain the pH fall in muscle homogenates, 50 g samples of the pre-*rigor M. sternomandibularis* were first minced and then homogenised for 30 sec in a Waring blender with an equal volume of either cold water, 0.17 M KCl or 0.16 M KCl containing 100 mM $CaCl_2$ (Davey and Gilbert, 1974). The homogenates were held in a water-bath at 15°C and periodically stirred. At intervals, 2 ml samples were removed for pH determinations.

For measuring topographical distribution of ultimate pH values within a muscle, beef *M. sternomandibularis* was held at 15°C under thin polyethylene film for 24 h and then at 2°C for a further 24 h to enter *rigor mortis* and to reach a true ultimate pH value. Some muscles were sprayed with aureomycin (100 ppm) and chloramphenicol (100 ppm) to inhibit bacterial spoilage and were further held at 2°C for 10 - 14 days to undergo aging. The muscle tissue remained to all intents sterile throughout the aging period. The unaged (2 days *post mortem*) and aged muscles (12 - 16 days *post mortem*) were sampled throughout their length, breadth and thickness.

Measurement of pH

Meat samples (1 - 2 g) trimmed of the external layer of aerobic tissue were homogenised in 10 ml neutralised sodium iodoacetate (5 mM) Marsh and Snow, 1950). The homogenates were equilibrated to the electrode temperature (15°C) and measurements were made with a Radiometer 26 pH meter. Measurement of pH time-courses in homogenates were carried out on aliquots taken at intervals, of 5 ml homogenate mixed with 5 ml neutralised iodoacetate (5 mM).

The estimation of the ultimate pH by the freeze-thaw technique is the only departure from conventional methodology. The pre-*rigor* samples of muscle (1 - 2 g) were dropped into stainless steel centrifuge tubes (length 89 mm/diameter 25.5 mm) containing ∿5 ml liquid nitrogen. After a freezing period of 5 min, the excess nitrogen was poured off and the tubes were placed immediately in a water-bath at 43°C. Thawing was complete in 5 - 10 min and ultimate pH values were reached in 20 - 30 min from freezing. Cold sodium iodoacetate (10 ml, 5 mM) was then added to the thawed samples and after homogenisation and temperature equilibration, pH values were measured.

RESULTS

Knowledge of the development of *rigor mortis* suggests a number of ways of inducing rapid glycolysis in muscle so that the ultimate pH is obtained in a short time after death. Triggering rapid ATP hydrolysis in muscle is an evident and simple way of achieving this. Figure 1 shows the time-courses of pH fall in whole-tissue muscle and in muscle homogenates under conditions expected to increase the rate of ATP hydrolysis. The reference curve is that of whole-tissue muscle held at 15°C (Curve 1). During the first 4 h of interest there is a small pH decline and the ultimate pH is not reached until about 36 h *post mortem*. Mincing, or homogenising in isotonic KCl effectively doubles the rate of pH decline (Curve 2). Homogenisation of muscle in an equal volume of water again increases the rate (Curve 3) and isotonic salt containing ionic calcium (1 mM) produces a further rate increase (Curve 4). Increasing the calcium ion concentration to 10 mM had no additional effect on either the rate or extent of pH fall. The fact that the pH values of the homogenates virtually stabilised after about 10 min with only a relatively slow decline thereafter, suggests that adenine nucleotides, essential for maintaining glycolysis have been irretrievably lost to the system through deamination of AMP to IMP. Alternatively, through dilution effects, phosphorylase could have been effectively lost to the glycolytic system (Newbold and Lee, 1965). The figure shows that the most effective way of identifying the ultimate pH values of muscle early *post mortem*, is to take whole-tissue muscle through a rapid freeze-thaw cycle (Curve 5). The ultimate pH of the muscle is then reached in little more than 10 min. The maximum acceptable

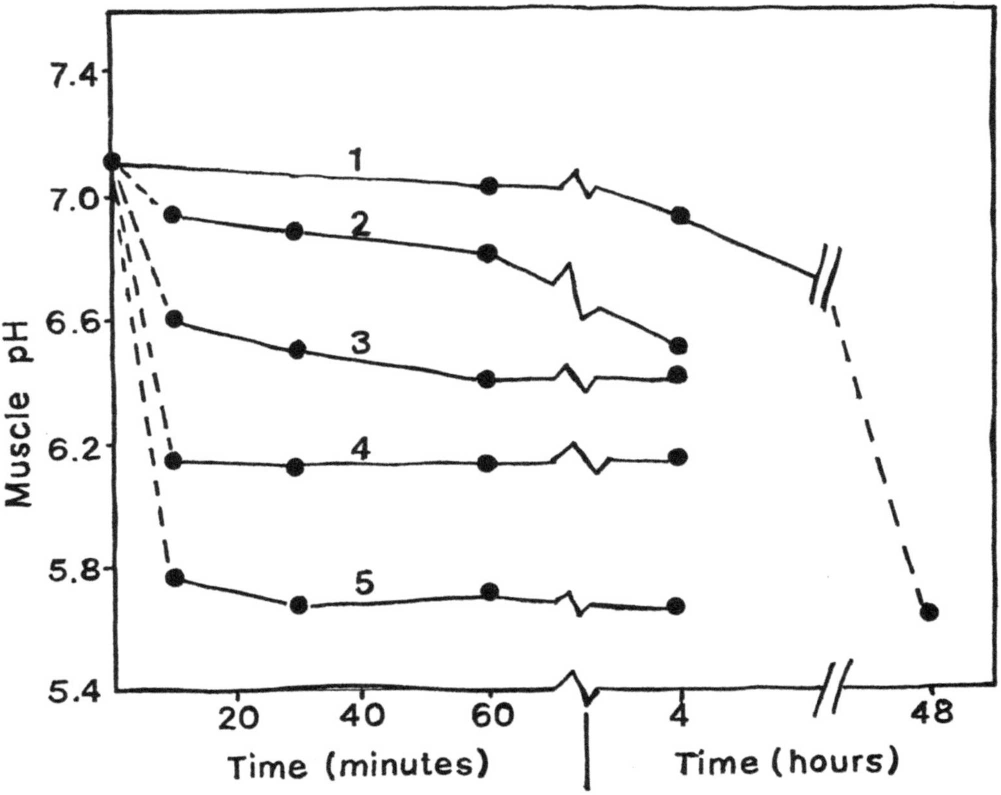

Fig. 1. Time courses of pH fall in beef *M. sternomandibularis* either as whole muscle tissue or as homogenates. The pH fall in whole-muscle tissue held at 15°C, (Curve 1). Falls in pH in homogenates of muscle made from equal volumes of muscle with KCl, 0.16M (Curve 2); water, (Curve 3); KCl, 0.15 M $CaCl_2$, 1mM (Curve 4). The pH fall in whole-muscle tissue frozen in liquid nitrogen and then thawed at 43°C (Curve 5).

temperature for thawing was 43°C, since at higher bath temperatures the muscle began to denature and the ultimate pH values achieved were respectively ∿0.2 pH units higher at 50°C and 0.5 pH units higher at 80°C. Ultimate pH values were also, on average, 0.2 pH units higher if freezing was carried out at -23°C in propylene glycol. *Post mortem* delays in freezing the samples did not appreciably affect the value of the ultimate pH obtained (Figure 2). However, in two of three experiments the freeze-thaw values determined within the first hour *post mortem* were higher by about 0.1 pH units than values obtained with longer delays.

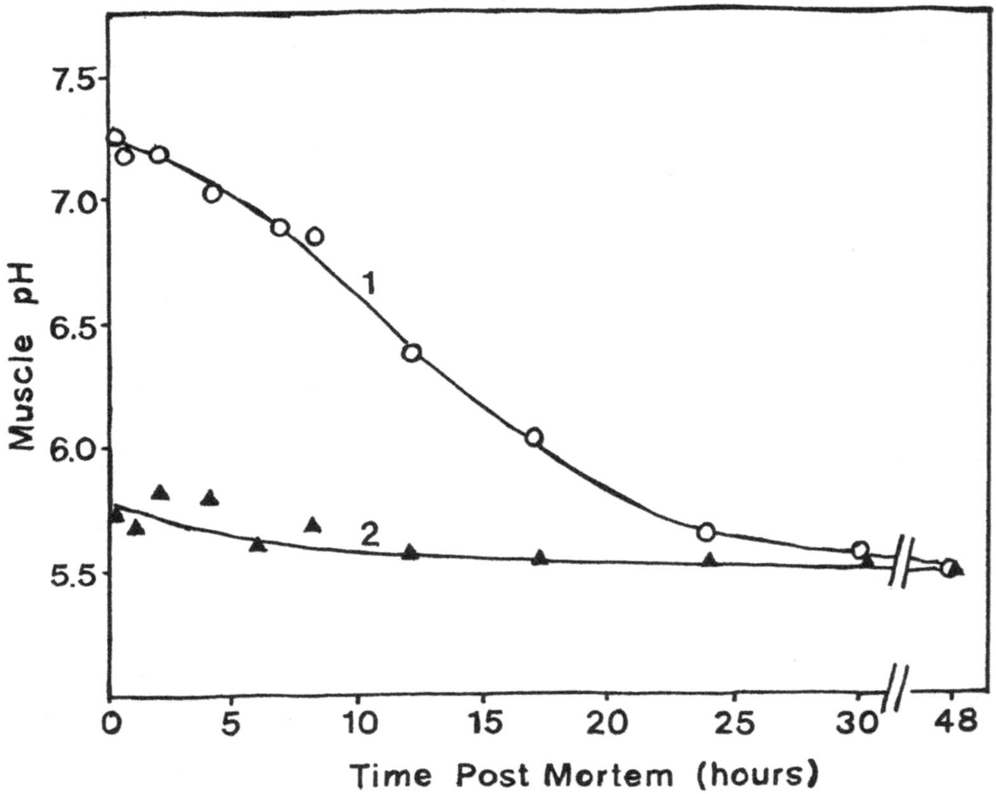

Fig. 2. The effect of delaying the determination of the freeze-thaw pH on its value in beef *M. sternomandibularis*. Curve 1, the typical time course of pH fall in muscle held at 15°C. Curve 2, the effect of *post mortem* delay on the freeze-thaw pH values.

Correlations between true and freeze-thaw determinations made over the range of ultimate pH values expected in muscle, confirm the merit of the technique. Relationships between the two sets of pH values for *M. longissimus* of sheep and beef animals and for *M. sternomandibularis* of beef animals are shown in Figure 3. Linear relationships were obtained for all three muscles over the extreme range of ultimate pH (5.5 - 7.1). The statistical analyses are also given in Figure 3 including the linear regression equations. At a certain level of statistical confidence these allow true ultimates to be predicted from the freeze-thaw values. The correlations between the pH values for *M. longissimus* for both sheep and beef animals were very high and

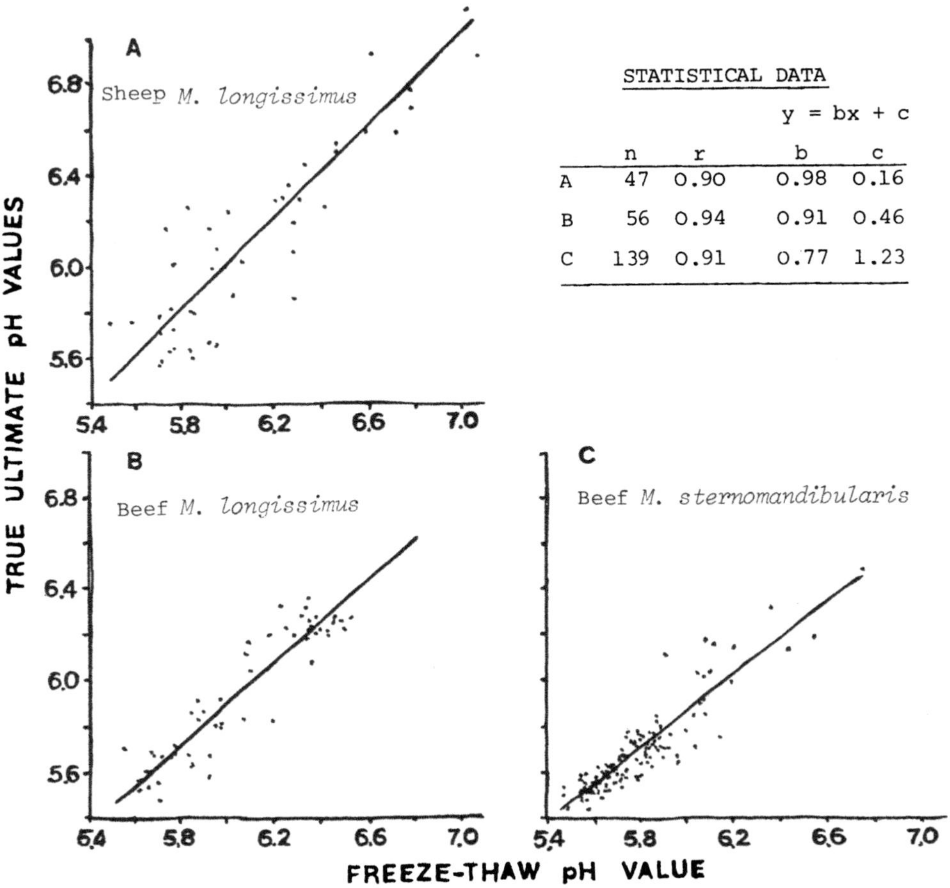

	n	r	b	c
A	47	0.90	0.98	0.16
B	56	0.94	0.91	0.46
C	139	0.91	0.77	1.23

Fig. 3. The relationships between ultimate and freeze-thaw pH values for muscles from sheep and beef animals.

the departure from 1 to 1 relationships was small (regression coefficients, respectively 0.98 and 0.91). On the other hand, the correlation for *M. sternomandibularis* although high, departed considerably from an equivalent relationship (regression co-efficient 0.77). Since *M. sternomandibularis* rarely had a high ultimate pH value, the relationship in Figure 3 is weighted heavily towards the lower end of the range (pH 5.5 - 5.8). However this does not account for the greater departure from pH correspondence in this muscle since the regression co-efficient is virtually unchanged by excluding values above pH

5.8. Since the muscle can be obtained almost immediately on the death of the animal, frozen samples shrink very actively on thawing, exuding the juices that contain enzymes and substrates. This probably accounts for the slightly higher freeze-thaw pH values in the very early stage of *rigor* development (see Figure 2) in this muscle and the greater departure from correspondence of the true ultimate and freeze-thaw pH values (Newbold and Lee, 1965).

The considerable scatter in pH values around the regression lines in Figure 3 does not indicate an error in the measurement of muscle pH. In this respect variations were found to be as high as 0.3 pH units or as low as 0.1 per unit in contrast to the 0.02 pH units found in a large number of measurements of the pH of a muscle homogenate containing iodoacetate (1 mM) as a glycolytic poison. The considerable pH scatter is therefore a true indication of variations existing in muscle. There is no consistent pattern in the topographical distribution of pH values in beef *M. sternomandibularis* and these same variations were encountered in pre-*rigor* muscle, in muscle which had just entered *rigor mortis*, and to a lesser degree in aged muscle. In the last, the distribution shifted by 0.15 pH units to higher values with a small narrowing of the range. A much narrower range might have been expected through the slow equilibration of ions, especially hydrogen ions, within the muscle tissue. Presumably ionic separations were maintained across the muscle membranes which remained largely intact throughout the ageing period (Swatland, 1980).

The pH variation is further analysed in Figure 4, which illustrates the distributions of values in *M. sternomandibularis* in a number of *post mortem* states. To obtain a clear picture of the shape of the pH distribution in a muscle the number of ultimate pH values in each 0.05 unit range has been expressed as a percentage of the total number of measurements made on the muscle. The results from a number of muscles have then been combined by centering the distributions on the mean pH values of the individual muscles. The results show that the pH dist-

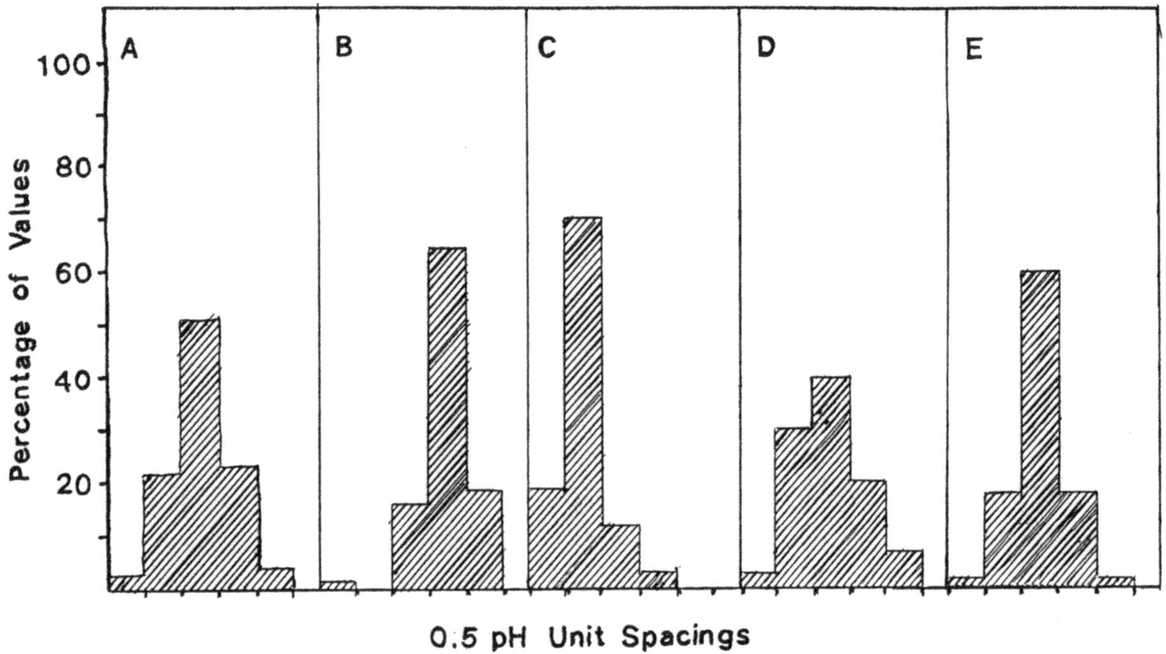

Fig. 4. Percentage distributions about the mean of ultimate pH-values in beef *M. sternomandibularis* covering various pH ranges and treatments. The number of ultimate pH values in each 0.05 unit range have been expressed as a percentage of the total number of measurements made on a muscle. The results from a number of muscles have then been combined by centering the distributions on the mean pH values of the individual muscles.

A. *Rigor* muscles, mean ultimate pH values < 5.8.
B. *Rigor* muscles, mean ultimate pH values > 5.8.
C. Aged muscles, mean ultimate pH values < 6.0.
D. Pre-*rigor* muscles, the ultimate pH values of which were estimated by the freeze-thaw technique. Mean ultimate pH values 5.6 to 6.4
E. All muscles and treatments combined from Figure 4 A to D.

ributions for two sets of *rigor* muscles with mean ultimate pH values respectively below and above pH 5.8 (Figure 4a and b) were essentially the same. In contrast to its unaged counterpart, (Figure 4a) the distribution for aged muscle (Figure 4c) was slightly skewed to lower values but with a general upward shift of all values by about 0.15 pH units. The same distribution pattern was obtained with pre- *rigor* muscle by the freeze-thaw technique (Figure 4d). The results for all muscles irrespective of *post mortem* condition or method of measuring the ultimate pH have been combined in Figure 4e. The pH distribution is then seen to be symmetrically disposed about the mean pH value.

DISCUSSION

The identification of DFD beef carcasses with a considerable degree of certainty within 30 - 40 min after death is the main emphasis of the present work. Such an early *post mortem* diagnosis is of potential importance to the meat processor. He can then decide, before chilling, to divert such carcasses to a more profitable end use in which the DFD condition is no detraction and may even be an advantage. A significant and evidently profitable departure from normal processing would be to hot bone the DFD carcasses, the meat being used in comminuted products requiring a good water-holding capacity (Schmidt and Gilbert, 1970).

The advantages of the method to basic studies of the DFD condition are even more evident. The method supplies the ultimate pH value of carcasses while these are still in a pre-*rigor* state. It therefore becomes possible to examine the biochemistry, and the physiological responses of high ultimate pH carcasses as they progress into *rigor*. Of even more significance is the use of the method in miniature, as a biopsy technique to identify those live animals predisposed to produce high ultimate pH meat. Such an adaptation has been used in New Zealand in animal behavioural and handling studies that form part of wider investigations into the causes and control of the DFD condition

(Holmes, R.J., personal communication). It is imagined that DFD animals through their *ante mortem* identification could be selectively fed to overcome the condition (Fernandes et al., 1979).

The present results have highlighted the considerable variability in ultimate pH values existing within muscles (Sornay and Legras, 1978). Such variations occur independently of whether the pH values have been determined by conventional or freeze-thaw techniques. The observations emphasise that caution is required in using a single pH measurement, no matter how precise, as a guide to the pH condition of a muscle. Based on the ultimate pH distributions shown in Figure 4 and assuming a mean ultimate pH 6.0 as being the DFD threshold, then the hazard of a single pH measurement is exposed. In these circumstances 2 per cent of muscles with a true, mean ultimate of pH 5.90 would be classified DFD and 24 per cent would be so classified having a true, mean ultimate of pH 5.95. Conversely 24 per cent and 2 per cent would be classed as having an acceptably low pH despite having respectively true, mean ultimates of pH 6.05 and pH 6.10. Consider further the reported variations existing in the mean ultimate pH values amongst the muscles of a carcass and the hazard is then even greater of using a single pH measurement at a set location within a single muscle to judge the ultimate pH condition of the whole carcass. In other words, to the meat processor's disadvantage, a significant proportion of carcasses could be erroneously classified as DFD. Conversely, an equal proportion of DFD carcasses could be erroneously considered to have a suitably low ultimate pH and acceptable standards of appearance and keeping quality.

The microbiological condition of the carcass from a healthy animal is largely related to the standard of carcass dressing, and statistical sampling techniques have been developed as a quality-assurance aid. In contrast, the DFD condition of a carcass is an *ante mortem* predisposition requiring individual rather than statistical identification of incidence. For both commercial and regulatory reasons therefore, there is a need to have a reliable and easy method for DFD identification. This requirement becomes more necessary with the trend towards large-scale production of chilled, packaged meats. Present knowledge indicates that there is no reliable criterion for the classification of DFD carcass. Certainly a single muscle pH is a very doubtful guide while the alternative of an extensive topographical mapping is quite unrealistic and impracticable.

REFERENCES

Augustini, C. and Fischer, K., 1979. Untersuchungen zum Problem des dunklen, leimigen Rindfleisches ('dark-cutting beef') 1. Mitteilung: Erscheinungsform und Vorkommen. The problem of dark-cutting beef. 1. Manifestation and incidence. Fleischwirts. 59, (12), 1871-1873.

Bouton, P.E., Harris, P.V. and Shorthose, W.R., 1971. Effect of ultimate pH upon the water-holding capacity and tenderness of mutton. J. Fd. Sci. 36, 435-439.

Davey, C.L. and Gilbert, K.V., 1974. The mechanism of cold-induced shortening in beef muscles. J. Fd. Technol. 9, 51-58.

Davey, C.L. and Gilbert, K.V., 1976. Thaw contracture and the disappearance of adenosinetriphosphate in frozen lamb. J. Sci. Fd. Agric. 27, 1085-1092.

Davey, C.L. and Winger, R.J., 1979. The structure of skeletal muscle and meat toughness. In Fibrous Proteins: Scientific Industrial and Medical Aspects. Vol. 1, p 97. Academic Press, London.

Fell, H.R., Boughey, R. and Lucas, I.A.M., 1973. Report on Bull Beef. Advisory Council for Agriculture and Horticulture in England and Wales.

Fernandes, T.H., Smith, W.C., Ellis, M., Clark, J.B.K. and Armstrong, D.G., 1979. The administration of sugar solutions to pigs immediately prior to slaughter. II. Effects on carcass yield, liver weight and muscle quality in commercial pigs. Anim. Prod. 29, 223-230.

Gallwey, W.J. and Tarrant, P.V., 1978. An investigation of high pH_u pigmeat in Irish bacon factories. Ir. J. Fd. Sci. Technol. 2, 21-30.

Gill, C.O. and Newton, K.G., 1979. Spoilage of vacuum-packaged dark, firm, dry meat at chill temperatures. Appl. Environ. Microbiol. 37, 362-364.

Hall, J.L., Latschar, C.E. and MacKintosh, D.L., 1944. Part IV. Characteristics of dark-cutting beef survey and preliminary investigation. Kansas Agric. Expt. Sta. Tech. Bull 58, 55.

Hamm, R., 1960. Biochemistry of meat hydration. Adv. Fd. Res. 10, 355-488.

Hedrick, H.B., 1958. Etiology and possible preventive measures in the dark cutter syndrome. Vet. Med. 53, 466-472.

Honikel, K.O., 1976. Überlegungen und Vorschläge zur Früherkennung von PSE- und DFD-fleisch in Schlachttierkörpern. (The early recognition of PSE- and DFD-meat in animal carcasses). Fleischwirts. 56 (8), 1143-1146.

Howard, A. and Lawrie, R.A., 1956. Studies on beef quality. Spec. Rpt. Fd. Invest. Bd., Lond., No. 63.

Linke. H.. Jankowitsch, H., Murke, M. and Eigner, U., 1976. Topographie des DFD-fleisches. (The topography of DFD-meat). Fleischwirts. 56 (7), 973-975.

Marsh, B.B. and Snow, A., 1950. A simple tissue homogenizer. J. Sci. Fd. Agric. 1, 190.

Mickwitz, Von G., 1971. Die Ursachen des Transportverlustes bei Schlachtschweinen. Hülsenberger Gespräche S.91.

Munns, W.O. and Burrell, D.E., 1965. The use of rib-eye pH for detecting dark-cutting beef. Fd. Technol. 19, 126-128.

Newbold, R.P. and Lee, C.A., 1965. *Post mortem* glycolysis in skeletal muscle. Biochem. J. 19, 1-6.

Nicol, D.J., Shaw, M.K. and Ledward, D.A., 1970. Hydrogen sulphide production by bacteria and sulfmyoglobin formation in prepacked chilled beef. Appl. Microbiol. 19, 937-939.

Potthast, K. and Hamm, R., 1976. Biochemie des DFD-fleisches (The biochemistry of DFD-meat). Fleischwirts. 56 (7), 978-982.

Roemmele, O., Scheper, J. and van der Wall, B., 1961. Ein praktisches Geräl zur dokumentarishchen Feststellung des pH-wertes, der Durchsaftung und des Blutgehaltes von Fleisch und Fleischwaren. Fleischwirts. 13, 208-209.

Scheper, J., 1971. Research to determine the limits of normal and aberrant meat quality (PSE and DFD) in pork. Proc. 2nd Int. Symp. Condition Meat Quality Pigs, Zeist, PUDOC, Wageningen, 271-277.

Schmidt, G.R. and Gilbert, K.V., 1970. The effect of muscle excision before the onset of *rigor mortis* on the palatibility of beef. J. Fd. Technol. 5, 331-338.

Sornay, J. and Legras, P., 1978. Cartographie du pH dans les carcasses des gros bovins. (Mapping pH in beef carcasses). Ind. Aliment. Agric. 95, 392-397.

Swatland, H.J., 1980. Membrane survival in pre-*rigor* beef muscle. Can. Inst. Fd. Sci. Technol. J. 13, 45-46.

Tarrant, P.V., 1976. The occurrence of dark-cutting beef. 22nd Eur. Meat Res. Wkrs. Conf., Malmö, Vol. 1, B8:1-B8:6.

Taylor, A.A. and Shaw, B.G., 1977. The effect of meat pH and package permeability on putrefaction and greening in vacuum packed beef. J. Fd. Technol. 12, 515-521.

Winkler, C.A., 1939. The colour of meat: I. Apparatus for its measurement, and relation between pH and colour. Canad. J. Res. 17, Sect. D. 7.

Wirth, F., Bohm, H. and Salziger, G., 1976. Technologie bei DFD-fleisch. (The technological approach to DFD-meat). Fleischwirts. 56 (7), 988-994.

DISCUSSION

E. Dransfield *(UK)*

You used *M. sternomandibularis* and calculated the within-muscle variation. Can you say what the prediction of pH is, within a carcass from muscle to muscle? How accurately does one single muscle represent the carcass?

C.L. Davey *(New Zealand)*

I believe our French colleagues would be able to answer that more successfully than I. However, our views are based upon studies with a large number of muscles in sheep (I do not have the information with me), and based upon *M. longissimus* and other muscles in beef, as well as *M. sternomandibularis*. One is in a very doubtful position if one wishes to get any indication of the pH condition of a carcass based upon pH measurement within *M. longissimus*, let's say between the 11th and 12th rib. There is no real consistency.

There is one additional point. You may have noticed that the variation in pH within an aged muscle was just about as wide as the muscle that had just gone into *rigor mortis*. This is a rather curious situation. One would think that there was sufficient opportunity for hydrogen ions to equilibrate reasonably through the muscle tissue. It can only be assumed that membranes form ionic barriers, which remain intact in the muscle tissue, and the scatter in pH still persists in the aged muscle.

P.V. Tarrant *(Ireland)*

Perhaps I may refer to a slide (Figure 1).

This figure illustrates intermuscular variability in commercial dark cutters in Ireland. In considering the method that Dr. Davey has outlined, we think that there is a major problem in trying to predict carcass ultimate pH from a value in a neck muscle or elsewhere in the forequarter. The dark cutting problem in our carcasses seems to be centred around

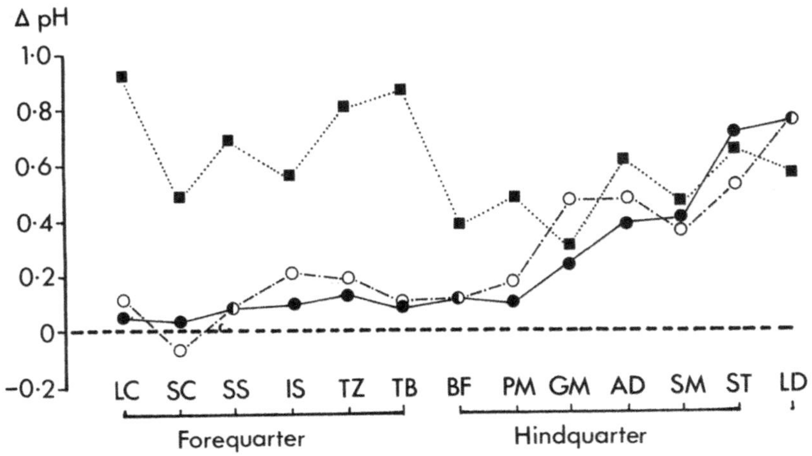

Fig. 1. (Reproduced by courtesy of Applied Science Publishers Ltd. Originally published in Meat Sience Vol. 4, No.4, p.294.)

M. longissimus dorsi and the hindquarter muscles. The base-line represents normal ultimate pH in factory-killed beef. The ordinate represents the difference in pH for 13 muscles between normal beef and dark-cutting carcasses. The 3 curves refer to adrenaline-treated animals and two groups of commercial animals. The closed circles are factory-killed steers and heifers, and the open circles are factory-killed young bulls. In the commercial animals the forequarter muscles are relatively normal. Many hindquarter muscles in steers, heifers and young bulls show high ultimate pH. Of course, in adrenaline treated animals (squares) it is quite a different picture; quite dissimilar to the commercial situation. Therefore, the point I would like to make in relation to Dr. Dransfield's question and Dr. Davey's paper is that, if you take a neck muscle and use this excellent technique, which is obviously a very useful one for a particular muscle, it will not indicate the pH_u in the more valuable cuts in *M. longissimus dorsi* and the muscles of the round and rump.

C.L. Davey

What I am presenting is a methodology which can be extended to all muscles. I doubt that we will be preoccupied with attempting to get an accurate measure of the DFD condition of a carcass.

I think our work will go more into the biochemistry and physiology; I simply feel that this is crude, quick indicator which will be useful to us.

H.B. Hedrick *(USA)*

I recall that Canadian workers reported some work on early measurement of pH *post mortem*, with hindquarter muscles. They found a fairly good relationship between the pH at about an hour after slaughter with ultimate pH.

C.L. Davey

It is a useful approach, but as we have indicated throughout our discussions, yesterday and today, it is very difficult to predict the initial pH that you can obtain after a carcass is slaughtered; it could be pH 7.0 to pH 7.3; quite often it is down around pH 6.5 initially, and this relates very much to a death struggle etc. Therefore, to get some indication of DFD, based upon the progressive decline of pH over the first hour, is very suspect in my view.

G. van Logtestijn *(The Netherlands)*

Some 15 years ago we made a number of pH measurements in different animals and observed three main groups. In normal animals - well rested and well fed - there may not be very big differences in pH values between muscles, only 0.2 or so. Also, in extreme DFD animals, the differences were not great; not more than 0.2. However, in PSE pigs and in animals that were not well rested, there may be very big differences between muscles - 0.5 or 0.6 would not be unusual!

C.L. Davey

Our experience in the field has indicated that there is no real consistency in these sorts of pictures at all. I would think that they scatter all over the place and any value of ultimate pH can be achieved, within physiological boundaries.

G. van Logtestijn

In my opinion, you have to measure at least three muscles. If you want to say something about the whole carcass, you must measure the LD, one muscle from the forequarter and one muscle from the hindquarter.

J.J.A. Heffron *(Ireland)*

Dr. Davey, as far as the methodology is concerned, why did you get a lower ultimate pH with the freeze-thawed sample than with the calcium?

C.L. Davey

My colleague Dr. Chrystall has shrugged his shoulders - and that is all I can do too! One can only theorise at this stage. My inclination is to believe that there are a number of requirements for the glycolytic process and any of them can, perhaps, be rate limiting. One of them is the supply of adenosine diphosphate as an appropriate substrate for the glycolytic processes. If this is not obtainable, glycolysis will not go on. One can imagine, in a muscle where the ATP is being hydrolysed by the actomyosin ATPase, and so on, that you would get such a rapid splitting of the ATP, resulting in the irretrievable loss of the nucleotide through the combined action of myokinase, AMP deaminase and adenosine deaminase to IMP and inosine, respectively. Under these circumstances, you would run out of ATP before glycolysis was completed. Therefore, glycolysis just stops. That may be the case - but we have not really examined it.

P.V. Tarrant

Could Dr. Davey speculate on a simple non-destructive technique which could be applied to the live animal. From your paper, it does not appear that such a technique is available, so I am asking you to speculate.

C.L. Davey

Our work is still very formative and we have not obtained any positive results from it as yet. However, we imagine that without the sustaining energy supplies, and recognising that there must be some sort of upset in the biochemistry of the DFD animal, we will be looking at the time-tension decays with electrical stimulation: the onset of fatigue, etc. We have set up a methodology and have done some work on this already to see if we can demonstrate a more rapid rate of decay of tension, once it has developed, in the DFD animals. With the live animal condition, one can think of all sorts of possibilities. I don't know if ruminants suffer from ketosis, which would suggest that they are trying to metabolise other components; perhaps just breath tests and such may be possible! There is also elevated body temperature, if it is properly measured. The feeling is that there is never going to be anything else but a wise judgement supported by a few facts of whether you have got what you can necessarily define as a DFD carcass. Therefore, any method that is reasonably accurate and simple will be as good as any other. If we can get correlations between ultimate pHs with these *ante mortem* tests that we are doing, then we will consider it a useful tool for the work we wish to do.

ELECTRICAL STIMULATION OF *ANTE MORTEM* STRESSED BEEF

T.R. Dutson, J.W. Savell and G.C. Smith

Meat and Muscle Biology, Department of Animal Science.
Texas Agricultural Experiment Station, Texas A&M University,
College Station, Texas 77843, USA.

ABSTRACT

Six heifers of approximately 375 kg were stressed before slaughter and one side of each animal was electrically stimulated. Electrical stimulation had no effect on muscle colour, ultimate pH, shear force or any of the sensory characteristics of muscle fibre tenderness, overall tenderness, connective tissue amount, juiciness, flavour desirability or overall desirability. The data from this study indicate that rapid pH decline is necessary for electrical stimulation to produce its desired effects and that the process of stimulation itself or the contractions produced are not the causative factors in improved quality of electrically stimulated beef.

INTRODUCTION

Electrical stimulation has been shown to improve and brighten muscle colour, increase tenderness, improve flavour, reduce 'heat-ring' (dark ring adjacent to subcutaneous fat of the ribeye) and reduce variable ribeye colour in beef (Smith et al., 1980; Hall et al., 1980; Savell et al., 1978; Smith et al., 1979). Since electrical stimulation has such a marked effect on the colour of beef muscle by improving the brightness and reducing dark colour, it may also have an effect on reducing the dark colour of dark-cutting beef. Thus, an experiment was conducted to determine the effect of electrical stimulation on the colour of *ante mortem* stressed beef.

EXPERIMENTAL PROCEDURE

Six heifers weighing approximately 375 kg were removed from feed, shipped to the slaughter plant (200 km) and held unfed for an additional 36 h. Stress to the animals consisted of handling during shipment, movement in pens at the slaughter plant and cold stress due to a change in ambient temperature overnight from 12°C to -5°C.

Animals were then slaughtered in the normal manner and the left side was electrically stimulated with 18 two-second pulses of 550 V (AC current) with a one second delay between pulses. Stimulation occurred at approximately 35 min after stunning.

Both sides of each carcass were ribbed at 48 h after slaughter and evaluated by a three-member panel for muscle colour on an eight-point scale, with one being very light cherry-red and eight being very dark red.

Duplicate samples (10 g) were removed from *M. longissimus dorsi* and homogenised in neutralised 0.005 M sodium iodoacetate (100 ml). The pH of the homogenate was measured using an Orion 801A digital pH meter.

Two steaks (2.54 cm) were removed from the region of the 10th to 13th rib of *M. longissimus dorsi* of each side for sensory panel analysis of juiciness, muscle-fibre tenderness, overall tenderness, connective tissue amount, flavour desirability and overall desirability and for shear-force measurement. An eight-point scale was used for each sensory parameter with one being extremely dry (juiciness), extremely tough (muscle fibre and overall tenderness), abundant (connective tissue amount), extremely undesirable (flavour desirability and overall desirability) and eight being extremely juicy (juiciness), extremely tender (muscle-fibre and overall tenderness), none (connective tissue amount) and extremely desirable (flavour and overall desirability). Steaks were cooked to an internal temperature of 70°C on Farberware open-hearth grills and presented to the sensory panel while hot, or cooled to room temperature, cored (1.3 cm diameter) and sheared (at least eight shears/steak) using a Warner-Bratzler shear-meter.

RESULTS AND DISCUSSSION

M. longissimus dorsi from each side of each animal received a colour score of eight, indicating that each animal was considered a dark-cutter and that the electrical stimulation treatment had no effect on improvement of muscle colour of dark cutting beef. This is probably due to the fact that electrical stimulation produces its effect by a rapid lowering of pH from the accelerated breakdown of glycogen to lactic acid (Carse, 1973; Locker et al., 1975; McCallum and Hendrickson, 1977; Bowling et al., 1978). If glycogen had been depleted (as was probably the case due to the high ultimate pH; Table 1) in these animals due to stress, then electrical stimulation could not cause a rapid pH decline and the desired effects on the muscle. All animals in this study exhibited marked contractions during the electrical stimulation treatment. Thus sufficient ATP must have been present for the contraction response. In non-stressed animals there is a 35 to 60 per cent reduction in ATP levels in one half-hour after electrical stimulation (McCallum and Hendrickson, 1977;

Bowling et al., 1978). However, some of the ATP present after stimulation must have necessarily resulted from breakdown of glycogen via glycolysis, an avenue not available for the stressed animals in the present study.

TABLE 1

ULTIMATE pH VALUES, SENSORY SCORES AND SHEAR VALUES OF *M. longissimus dorsi* FROM STIMULATED AND NON-STIMULATED SIDES

Trait	ES	Significance	C
Ultimate pH	6.65	NS	6.56
Shear force[a]	4.40	NS	4.30
Muscle fibre tenderness[b]	6.10	NS	6.35
Overall tenderness[b]	5.96	NS	6.31
Connective tissue[b]	6.28	NS	6.45
Juiciness[b]	4.85	NS	4.85
Flavour desirability	3.35	NS	2.86
Overall desirability	3.55	NS	3.26

ES = Electrically stimulated C = Non-stimulated control
NS = Non-significant ($P > 0.05$)

[a]Shear force in kg

[b]Sensory panel traits were evaluated on an 8 point scale.

Ultimate pH values for stimulated and non-stimulated sides were not significantly different (Table 1). The high ultimate pH of animals in this study is consistent with the colour evaluations of the muscle and indicates that the stress treatments were effective in depleting the glycogen content of the muscles before slaughter. There were no significant differences in ultimate pH of stimulated and non-stimulated sides, indicating that sufficient glycogen in the muscle at the time of stimulation is necessary for the stimulation treatment to reduce muscle pH. The data presented in Table 1 also indicate that breakdown of ATP by contractions, at least in quantities sufficient to produce normal contractions, does not appreciably alter *post mortem* pH in itself.

Data presented in Table 1 indicate that electrical stimulation of animals stressed *ante mortem* does not affect palatability traits in the same manner as for non-stressed animals (Smith et al., 1980). Thus the pH decline associated with electrical stimulation is apparently necessary to produce the increase in tenderness and flavour; the stimulation itself or the contractions produced are not the causative factors in producing the desirable effects on palatability. It is interesting to note from data presented in Table 1 that although tenderness of *ante mortem* stressed animals is in the acceptable range, the flavour of steaks from these animals is unacceptable. The lowered flavour scores also result in overall desirability scores that are unacceptable.

REFERENCES

Bowling, R.A., Smith, G.C., Dutson, T.R. and Carpenter, Z.L. 1978. Effects of pre-rigor conditioning treatments on lamb muscle, pH and ATP. J. Food Sci. 43, 502.

Carse, W.A. 1973. Meat quality and the acceleration of *post mortem* glycolysis by electrical stimulation. J. Food Tech. 8, 163.

Hall, L.D., Savell, J.W. and Smith, G.C. 1980. Retail appearance of electrically stimulated beef. J. Food Sci. 45, 171.

Locker, R.H., Davey, C.L., Nottingham, P.M., Haughey, D.P. and Law, N.H. 1975. New concepts in meat processing. In: Advances in Food Research 21, 157. Academic Press, New York.

McCallum, P.D. and Henrickson, R.L. 1977. The effect of electrical stimulation on the rate of *post mortem* glycolysis in some bovine muscles. J. Food Quality 1, 15.

Savell, J.W., Smith, G.C., and Carpenter, Z.L. 1978. Effect of electrical stimulation on quality and palatability of lightweight beef carcasses. J. Anim. Sci. 46, 1221.

Smith, G.C., Dutson, T.R., Cross, H.R. and Carpenter, Z.L. 1979. Electrical stimulation of hide-on and hide-off calf carcasses. J. Food Sci. 44, 335.

Smith, G.C., Savell, J.W., Dutson, T.R., Hostetler, R.L., Terrell, R.N., Murphey, C.E. and Carpenter, Z.L. 1980. Effects of electrical stimulation on beef, pork, lamb and goat meat. Proc. European Meat Res. Workers Conf. 26 : Vol II, 19.

DISCUSSION

H. Ruderus (*Sweden*)

I have no question, just a comment. We did a similar experiment for much the same reason, and our results are consistent with Dr. Dutson's. There is no difference in ultimate pH of DFD animals after electrical stimulation.

T.R. Dutson (*USA*)

Do you have any data on these borderline dark animals?

H. Ruderus

Figures 1 to 4 may help, they illustrate the effect of electrical stimulation immediately after exsanguination on pH/time curves in normal and DFD beef carcasses. *Post mortem* pH decline in individual carcasses is shown for unstimulated DFD carcasses (Figure 1), stimulated DFD carcasses (Figure 2), unstimulated normal carcasses (Figure 3) and stimulated normal carcasses (Figure 4).

It can be seen from Figure 2 that electrical stimulation does not, of course, change the ultimate pH in DFD carcasses. More interesting, if you compare the pH values one hour after slaughter for DFD (Figure 2) and normal carcasses (Figure 4) it is clear that there is a fairly large scatter of pH values at this time in DFD carcasses ranging from pH 5.9 to 7.0 in contrast to normal carcasses, all of which go down below pH 6.0 within one hour of slaughter. I cannot say whether this is the basis of a good method for identification of DFD carcasses, but it might be possible.

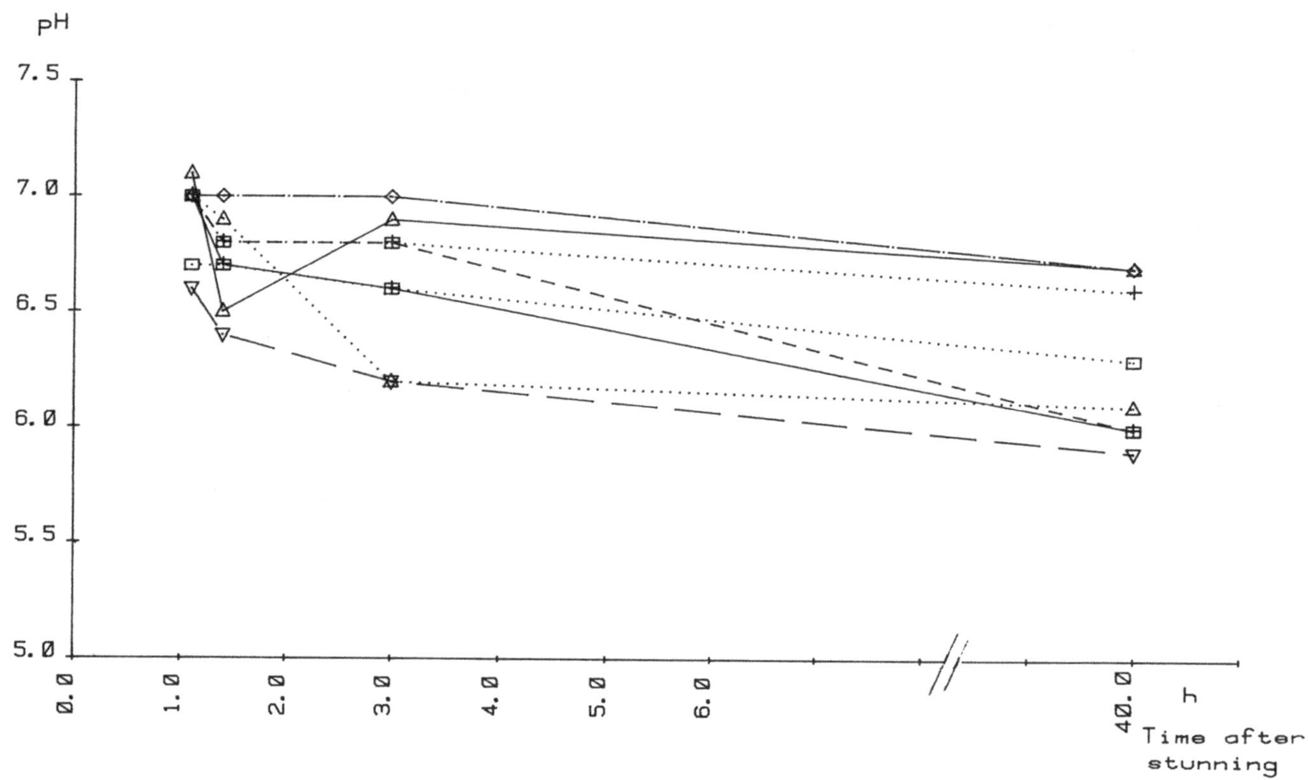

Fig. 1. The pH-values in *M. longissimus dorsi* from 8 young bulls, who were fatigued and stressed before slaughter. The measurements of pH were made 1.1, 1.4, 3 and 40 h respectively after the bulls were stunned.

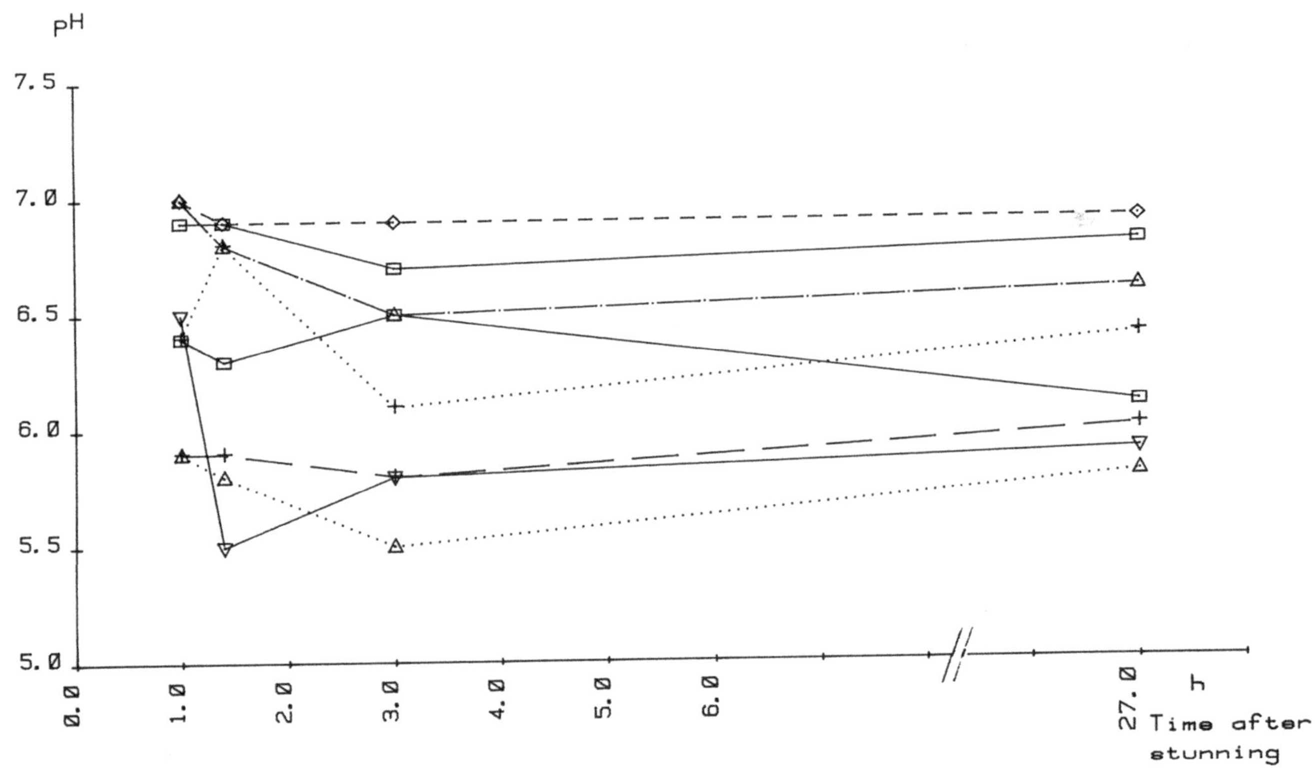

Fig. 2. The pH-values in *M. longissimus dorsi* from 8 young bulls, who were fatigued and stressed before slaughter. The carcasses were electrically stimulated (85 V, 32 s) immediately after the exsanguination. The measurements of pH were made 1.1, 1.4, 3 and 27 h respectively after the bulls were stunned.

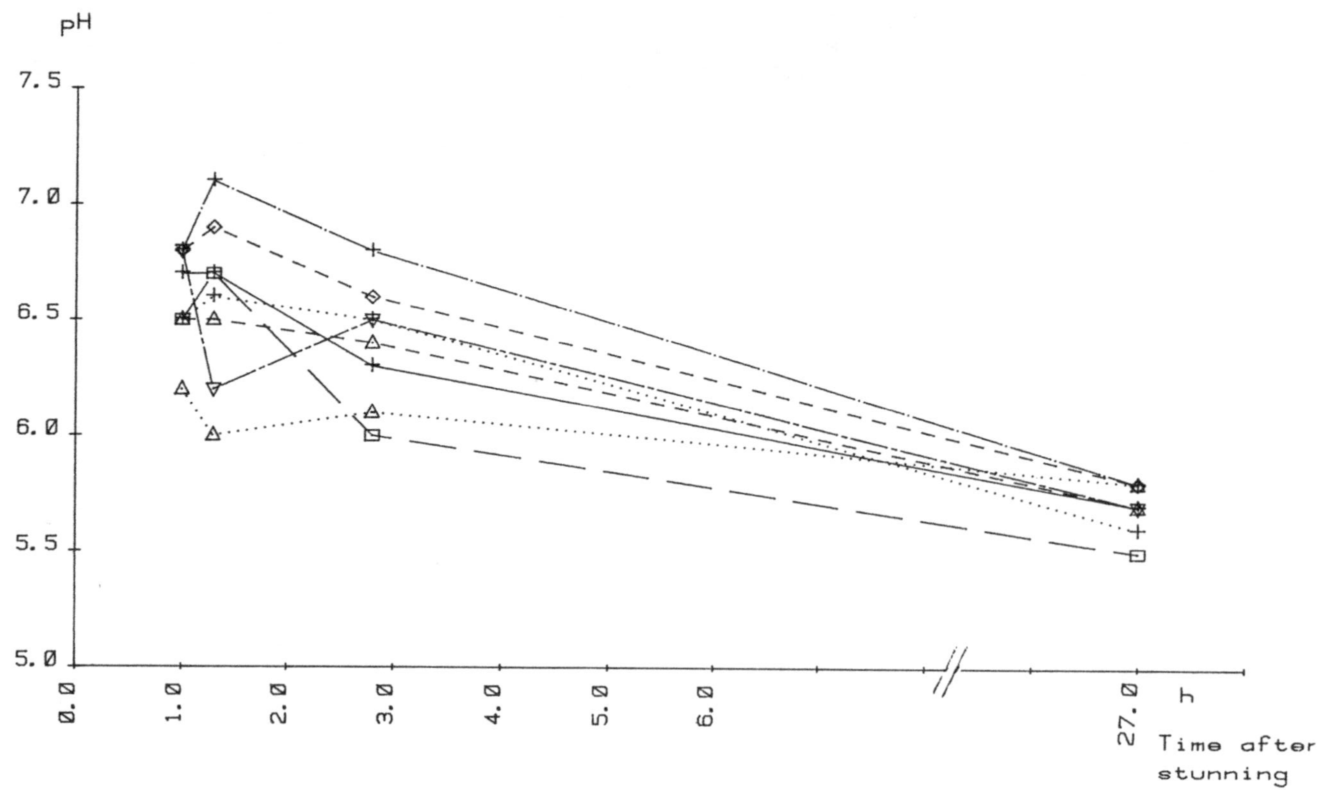

Fig. 3. The pH-values in *M. longissimus dorsi* from 8 young bulls. The measurements of pH were made 1.0, 1.3, 2.8 and 27 h respectively after the bulls were stunned.

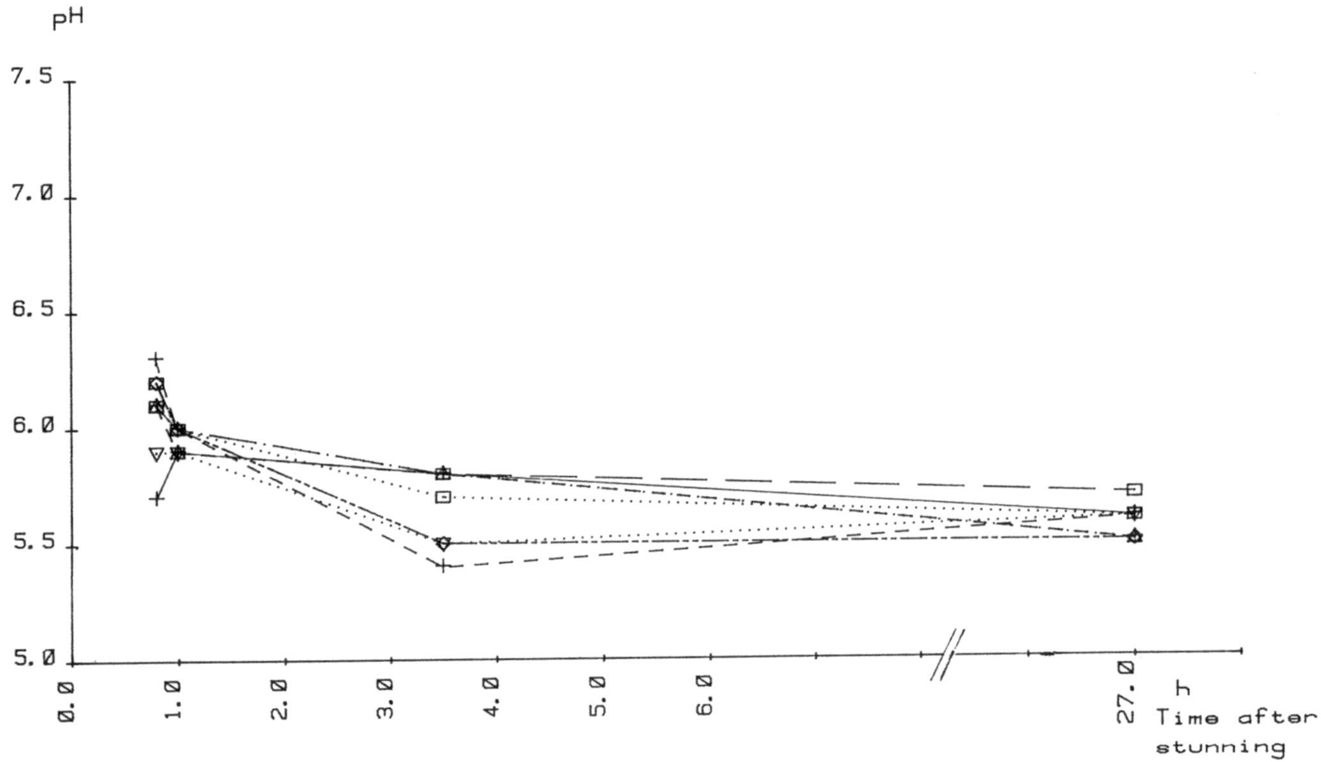

Fig. 4. The pH-values in *M.* longissimus dorsi from 8 young bulls. The carcasses were electrically stimulated (85 V, 32 s) immediately after the exsanguination. The measurements of pH were made 0.8, 1.0, 3.5 and 27 h respectively after the bulls were stunned.

H.B. Hedrick *(USA)*

I have a question regarding flavour differences. A number of years ago the literature referred to flavour differences and it was quite varied. Some reports stated that there is no difference in flavour between DFD animals and normal; others said there is a difference. You show there is a difference. My own observations are that with broiled DFD steaks (which is what you were using), you do not get the same 'browning' reaction or change as you would with the normal. This 'browning' difference could possibly be associated with the difference in flavour because it is generally assumed that the 'browning' reaction influences the flavour.

T.R. Dutson

This might well be the case. We did not expect this low flavour score, therefore we were not really prepared to evaluate it properly. All we have is the evaluation of the score. In our next experiment we will conduct some flavour profiling to characterise the flavour. We will have controlled experiments with the same types of animals. Furthermore, we have to compare this flavour score on this group of animals with the general flavour score that we have in our laboratory. There could have been something else wrong with these animals, but I do not suspect that. They were out of a group that we had conducted another experiment on, and the flavour on those animals was acceptable.

H.B. Hedrick

There was also a report from Tennessee which related to flavour differences due to water-soluble carbohydrate. The lower the amount of carbohydrate, the less desirable the flavour.

B.L. Dumont *(France)*

The maximum score for flavour was 8, so the level of flavour was below average.

T.R. Dutson

Normally, in our experiments, we get flavour scores from 5 - 7 in most of our beef of this type. These scores were in the range of 3, which is considerably lower than we normally get with our panel and our type of beef.

Lis Buchter *(Denmark)*

Can the introduction of electrical stimulation be used for the purpose of identifying DFD animals at an early stage, because you bring the pH in the animals down to a stage where you could take away some of the dark-cutters? This has been suggested by the Swedish Meat Research Institute and I would like to know if you have tried this to pick out really serious DFD carcasses?

T.R. Dutson

We have not conducted any experiments on this, but I feel that this is a very likely possibility. However, you would need to measure the pH within the first 2 - 3 h after death. If you did that within one hour, particularly if you had a good stimulation technique, I think you could predict whether or not that animal was going to drop in pH to the normal values. I think that Dr. Davey's suggestion of determining the amount of muscle fatigue, and the time at which that muscle fatigues, by stimulation may be a possible technique; or perhaps that in combination with some pH measurements too. In this group of animals we found that we still had almost normal types of contractions. However, we have conducted some experiments with electrical stimulation where we stimulated the animals to fatigue, gave the carcass a rest period, and then went back to restimulate. If we increased the voltage after the initial stimulation, then there was a little more activity, and if we gave them a little time they were able to replenish enough ATP to go through some contractions again. We did not try that on the dark-cutting beef, but I have an idea that once you burn up the ATP there will not be a recovery phase where enough ATP is regenerated to cause an additional contraction. We find that if we stimulate an animal immediately after slaughter to fatigue - perhaps this is just fatigue of the membrane, but I believe it is probably exhaustion of the ATP. Then, after about 30 min, just before they go into the coldroom, if we shock them again with high voltage, we can cause another almost complete cycle of stimulation; they have had time to regenerate enough ATP. With the dark-cutting situation, the animals would not be able to do that. That may be a technique that could be used.

C.L. Davey *(New Zealand)*

I was interested in the colour differences with which you identified the stimulated and non-stimulated carcasses. I understand that, as a consequence of colour grading, those carcasses which have been stimulated will, therefore, gain a certain premium. If there was a convergence of the colours, consequent to this, it would seem to be a rather imprudent retailer who would pay a premium for beef under those circumstances. The desirable colour will not be retained.

T.R. Dutson

I agree with what you say. The system in the United States is rather artificial because the grading has to be done on the carcass at this early stage. Then the carcass is sold through the rest of the marketing system, based on the grade it received at that early stage. If the retailer has something that has the same colour, he does not care but he has to pay more for the higher grade. Therefore, it is the packer who actually receives the benefit. We have conducted some studies on the colour of electrically stimulated beef and there is an advantage at the later stage, and even in the retail appearance of electrically stimulated beef at 4 days *post mortem*. However, it is not as great as at the earlier stage.

E. Kallweit *(FRG)*

Does electrical stimulation increase the temperature in the carcass, and is there a difference between normal and DFD beef

T.R. Dutson

We did not measure the temperature of the DFD beef, but we did in our normal electrical stimulation experiments. We got as high as a 4°C increase in the temperature of the muscle of the stimulated side as compared to the non-stimulated side. On an average it was about 2°C, but occasionally it jumped to 4°C immediately following stimulation. However, we did not measure the temperature of the DFD carcasses, so I cannot say. There may be a difference there, but the muscle activity appears the same so we would expect some temperature rise also.

G. Eikelenboom *(The Netherlands)*

As you did not find any effects on tenderness with electrical stimulation, can we exclude myofibre disruption, caused by electrical stimulation, as a specific cause of the tenderising effect?

T.R. Dutson

That had occurred to us. In our next experiments we hope to investigate that a little closer. We did not do electron microscopy of these dark-cutting animals either and it may be that they do not have the structural damage. The structural damage may be caused by the physical action, the pH and the temperature, all combined. I would say that the actual physical activity of the muscle - the contractions that the muscle goes through - may not be so important as far as tenderisation is concerned; it is more the biochemical aspect of lower pH and higher temperature combined. We observed physical activity, but no change in tenderness. There is also another factor which confounds the issue and that is the high water holding capacity of DFD beef. There may be some differences there that are not detected by the panel because of the high pH and 'mushy' condition of the muscle.

J. Wismer-Pedersen *(Denmark)*

Returning to the effect of electrical stimulation, has anyone done colour stability tests, as to whether conversion to metmyoglobin takes place at a faster rate after electrical stimulation, compared to controls?

T.R. Dutson

We are conducting some of those studies now. Our preliminary evidence indicates that there is no increase in the oxidation of myoglobin to the metmyoglobin state. In the retail case, one could get as good a case life, or sometimes better or longer life, in a retail display of stimulated beef compared with normal beef. Based on our biochemical experiments to date, and our observations of the steaks in the retail display, I would say no.

A. Romita

Thank you, Dr. Dutson, We will now go on to the next paper.

ANIMAL STRESS AND ITS EFFECT ON *RIGOR MORTIS* DEVELOPMENT IN LAMBS

B.B. Chrystall, C.E. Devine, C.L. Davey and A.H. Kirton
Meat Industry Research Institute of New Zealand (Inc.)
P.O. Box 617, Hamilton, New Zealand.

ABSTRACT

The effect of transport and physical stress on ultimate pH of lambs was determined in two stages of experimentation. In the first stage transport and light exercise were shown to have very little effect on mean ultimate pH values but there was an increase in inter-animal variability. In the second stage the recovery from severe stress was followed by serial slaughter of groups of animals. Ultimate pH values were still slightly elevated after 24 h recovery. The inter-animal variability in the stressed groups was very high with some animals being relatively insensitive to stress and others recovering very rapidly. Other metabolites showed the expected changes.

INTRODUCTION

Meat quality can reflect differences in rate and/or extent of *post mortem* glycolysis. Muscles in which glycolysis is slow will remain in a *pre-rigor*, cold-sensitive state for much longer than those entering *rigor* more rapidly, thus increasing the probability that an imposed chilling regime will cause cold-shortening. Muscles in which glycolysis is restricted due to lack of glycogen enter *rigor mortis* at a high pH. Although these muscles are unlikely to cold-shorten, they may be dark in colour, which may itself be considered objectionable. If they are stored as a vacuum-packaged chilled product, they will have a poor shelf-life due to deterioration and early greening (Gill and Newton, 1979).

Animals presented for slaughter have been subjected to varying degrees of exercise during mustering and pre-slaughter handling. The animals may also be exposed to the stresses of long transport.

The effect of some stresses and exercise on muscle glycogen levels has been studied in humans and animals. Exercise-induced depletion of muscle glycogen occurs readily in swine (Callow, 1938, 1939), but not so readily in cattle. Mitchell and Hamilton (1933) were able to deplete glycogen stores in cattle by exercise, whereas Howard and Lawrie (1956) found that 1.5 h exercise on its own was insufficient to cause a significant reduction in muscle glycogen levels. Exercise combined with a long train journey did, however, cause a slight elevation of the ultimate pH. Feeding cattle for four days after a long journey caused a reduction in muscle pH compared with only two days rest and feeding (Shorthose et al., 1972). Glycogen depletion through exercise in humans and rats has been extensively studied (Terjung et al., 1974; Ahlborg et al., 1967; Hultman, 1967). Exhaustion coincided with almost complete depletion of muscle glycogen. Resynthesis of muscle glycogen appeared to be much more rapid in fast red muscles than white muscles (Terjung et al., 1974) although other workers have claimed no differences in resynthesis rates (Armstrong and Ianuzzo, 1977).

Build-up of glycogen levels after depletion in meat animals has been recently reported (McVeigh et al., 1979). Complete replenishment in muscles of cattle subjected to 6 h of behavioural stress (even with food and water) took 7 days.

This paper presents results showing the influence of various stresses on pH fall and some muscle metabolites in lambs. Of particular interest is the recovery of muscle glycogen after exhaustive stress, in animals from which food and water was withheld.

MATERIALS AND METHODS

Animals

Well fed, mature lambs obtained from experimental flocks were used in this study, which was conducted in 2 stages.

Stage 1 : Transport stress and light exercise

Twenty (20) lambs were trucked approximately 400 km (9.5 h journey) with average temperatures near 18°C. On arrival at the abattoir 10 were slaughtered (A); the remainder were allowed to rest for 24 h, then slaughtered (B).

A further 20 lambs obtained locally were rested in yards for 24 h, 10 of these were transported to the abattoir by truck (C), the others walked slowly 2 km to the abattoir (D). All the animals were slaughtered immediately on arrival at the abattoir.

Stage 2 : Exhaustion and recovery

This stage consisted of two trials as follows:

a) In the first trial 18 lambs were weighed and randomised on a restricted-weight basis to three treatment groups. One group was transported by truck to the abattoir and rested overnight before slaughter. The other two groups were moved rapidly over a 5 km course to the abattoir. On arrival there was a marked variation in apparent condition of these animals, some appearing exhausted, others barely panting. One group of six exhausted animals was slaughtered immediately on arrival at the abattoir. The remaining exhausted group was held without food or water for 24 h and then slaughtered.

b) The second trial was undertaken to follow the time course of recovery. Forty-two (42) lambs were weighed and randomised on a restricted-weight basis to seven treatment groups. One group was quietly transported by truck to the abattoir and rested overnight before slaughter. The other six groups were subjected to the same physical stress as those in Trial (a). On arrival at the abattoir one of these groups was slaughtered immmediately and the others held without food or water until slaughter at 1, 2, 4, 8 or 17 h later.

Slaughter

All animals were slaughtered without stunning by severing the spinal cord and blood vessels in the neck.

Sampling

M. longissimus dorsi of animals in Stage 1 were sampled at the level of the 13th rib for initial (5 min) and 24 h pH measurements.

Samples from animals in Stage 2 of the experiment were taken as follows: a 4 cm length of *M. longissimus dorsi* was removed within 5 min of slaughter from the 11 - 13th rib area. From this sample, a 1 g portion was used for pH measurement, while another sample (∿2 g) was wrapped in aluminium foil and frozen in liquid nitrogen for subsequent biochemical analysis. The remainder of the muscle sample was immersed in liquid paraffin, gassed with nitrogen to displace dissolved oxygen, and held at 15°C. Samples were removed periodically from this sample for pH measurement. At 24 h *post mortem* a further sample (∿2 g) for biochemical analysis was frozen in liquid nitrogen.

Biochemical assay

A number of biochemical parameters were determined to monitor *post mortem* biochemical changes associated with *rigor* development. Lactate, the end product of anaerobic glycolysis, reflects muscle pH and initial glycogen reserves. Adenosine triphosphate (ATP) and creatine phosphate (CP) were considered as indications of stress levels.

All pH measurements were made on ∿1 g samples of muscle tissue homogenised in 10 ml ice-cold 5 mM sodium iodoacetate (pH 7.0). The homogenate was equilibrated at 15°C and the pH read with a Radiometer pH meter.

For all other analyses the frozen samples were powdered in liquid nitrogen and ∿2 g samples accurately weighed into 0.5 N perchloric acid (20 ml) at -8°C. The mixtures were homogenised with a Polytron (Kinematica), centrifuged at 10 000 g for 5 min and a 5 ml aliquot of the supernatant neutralised with KOH, and made to volume. After 30 min at 15°C the supernatant was decanted off and frozen for later analysis. ATP and CP were determined by modifications of the method of Lamprecht and Trautschold (1974), using creatine kinase, hexokinase and glucose-6-phosphate dehydrogenase. Lactate was determined by the method of Noll (1974). Adenine/inosine (AN/IN) ratios, total nucleotide and total soluble phosphate were determined by the methods of Newbold and Scopes (1967) and Davey (1957).

RESULTS

The initial and 24 h *post mortem* values for *M. longissimus dorsi* from animals subjected to transport and light exercise prior to slaughter in Stage 1 are shown in Table 1. Differences between the initial pH values for all four treatment groups were non-significant, although the values were lower for the rested groups (C and D) than for the groups that had been transported 400 km (A and B).

TABLE 1

INITIAL AND 24 h pH VALUES FOR STAGE 1 OF THE EXPERIMENT

Group treatment	Muscle pH*	
	Initial (5 min *post mortem*)	Ultimate (24 h *post mortem*)
A. Slaughtered immediately after 9.5 h journey	7.01 ± .19[a]	5.83 ± .16[a]
B. Rested for 24 h after 9.5 h journey	7.01 ± .14[a]	5.68 ± .17[b]
C. Rested 24 h	6.87 ± .22[a]	5.56 ± .08[b]
D. 24 h rest, light exercise immediately prior to slaughter	6.84 ± .22[a]	5.63 ± .20[b]

a, b Mean values in any column with the same superscript do not differ significantly

* The results are mean values and standard deviations for 10 animals

Ultimate pH values also showed no significant difference between the two transported groups, A and B, or between the rested groups, C and D. The transported group (A), however, differed significantly from the two rested groups C and D. The order of ultimate pH values from highest to lowest is that which would be predicted on the basis of increasing stress causing a reduction in glycogen reserve and hence a reduction in lactate production.

The pH/time curves for well-fed animals which were slaughtered at various times after strenuous exercise in Stage 2 are presented in Figure 1 (the rate of pH fall in isolated samples held in nitrogen-gassed paraffin at 15°C was identical with that of muscles left on the carcass and held at 15°C). Lowest initial pH values were obtained from the well-rested groups, whilst the groups slaughtered immediately after exercise gave the highest mean initial pH values. This was rather unexpected but may be expkained by the fact that the rested group kicked and moved vigorously at slaughter whereas the exhausted groups were relatively immobile and unresponsive. As expected, the ultimate pH values were highest in animals slaughtered immediately after exhaustion and decreased with increasing periods of rest. Within each group of animals the range of values was high, reflecting in part the differences in animal fitness and response to physical stress.

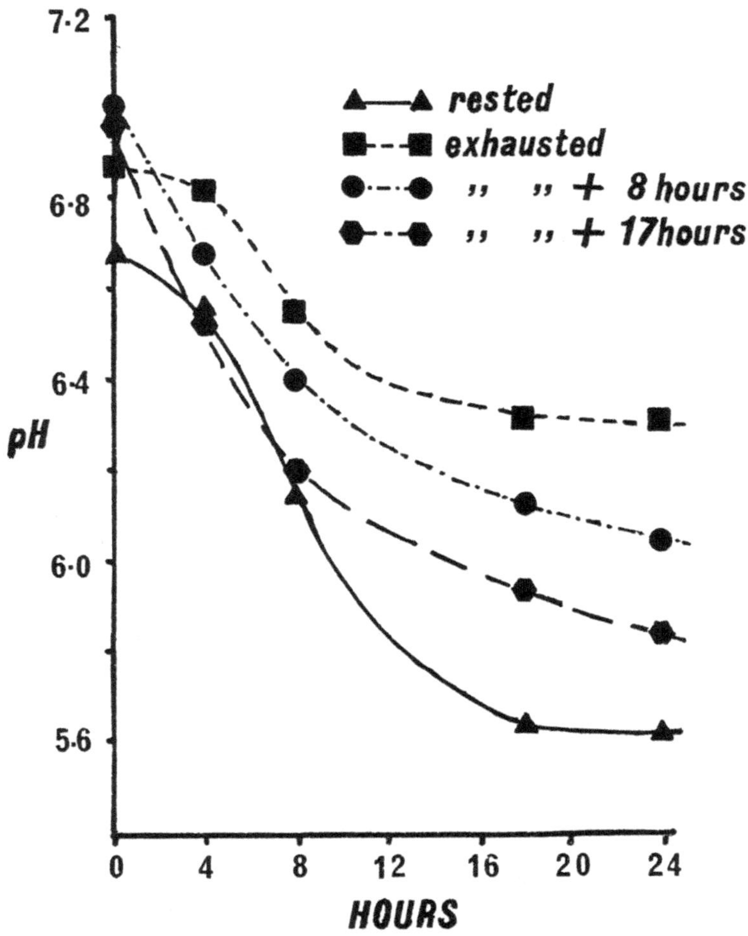

Fig.1. *Post mortem* fall in pH of *M. longissimus dorsi* samples from some of the groups of rested, exhausted and exhausted/rested animals.

Initial and ultimate lactate, ATP levels and adenine/ inosine nucleotide ratios are presented in Table 2 for the rested, exhausted and exhausted-recovered groups of Stage 2.

TABLE 2

INITIAL AND 24 H pH VALUES, LACTATE, ATP, CP AND ADENINE/INOSINE RATIOS IN RELATION TO EXERCISE AND RECOVERY

		Initial µmol/g wet weight					24 h post mortem µmol/g wet weight			
		pH	Lactate	ATP	CP	AN/IN	PH	Lactate	ATP	AN/IN
Control (a)	$\bar{X}$	6.84	16.14	5.20	4.09	1.14	5.51	96.50	-	0.59
	SD	0.12	4.27	0.32	1.66	0.33	0.05	15.36		0.05
Control (b)	$\bar{X}$	6.68	15.55	5.59	5.76	1.12	5.62	86.35	0.39	0.59
	SD	0.09	3.71	0.76	2.08	0.02	0.02	11.43	0.10	0.01
Exhausted (a)	$\bar{X}$	7.06	16.72	5.30	-	0.90	6.38	45.33	-	0.58
	SD	0.14	7.35	1.20		0.09	0.45	18.69		0.09
Exhausted (b)	$\bar{X}$	7.05	9.64	5.72	3.91	1.15	6.31	51.51	0.47	0.59
	SD	0.09	5.29	0.48	2.01	0.03	0.38	16.90	0.21	0.25
Exhausted + 1h recovery	$\bar{X}$	6.91	12.12	4.99	4.59	1.09	5.89	51.64	0.51	0.69
	SD	0.12	3.18	0.75	2.45	0.06	0.52	16.59	0.18	0.22
Exhausted + 2h recovery	$\bar{X}$	6.89	10.32	5.24	4.32	1.16	6.20	47.59	0.37	0,60
	SD	0.15	3.88	2.18	4.18	0.04	0.41	13.41	0.13	0.22
Exhausted + 4h recovery	$\bar{X}$	6.75	17.45	5.22	3.95	1.04	5.90	48.43	0.53	0.60
	SD	0.09	4.87	0.39	1.54	0.22	0.20	13.52	0.27	0.14
Exhausted + 8h recovery	$\bar{X}$	7.02	14.04	4.76	3.76	1.12	6.06	53.33	0.44	0.59
	SD	0.09	3.17	1.26	2.07	0.01	0.53	20.34	0.06	0.02
Exhausted + 17h recovery	$\bar{X}$	6.96	20.80	5.66	3.39	1.17	5.85	61.90	0.39	0.61
	SD	0.16	10.68	0.62	2,29	0.05	0.24	15.66	0.15	0.56
Exhausted + 24h recovery	$\bar{X}$	6.92	19.70	6.20	-	0.85	5.71	83.70	-	0.56
	SD	0.17	7.5	2.26		0.09	0.23	13.43		0.02

Mean values and standard deviations for six animals in each group

Both groups of rested animals have normal, low ultimate pH values and high lactate contents reflecting high initial glycogen stores. The exhausted animals from Trial (a) and (b) of Stage 2, which were slaughtered immediately, were surprisingly similar for two groups of lambs obtained from different sources but subjected to very similar treatments. The mean ultimate pH values (near pH 6.3) in both cases include one animal which was relatively unaffected by the exercise and exhibited a low ultimate pH value.

Despite denial of food and water the exhausted animals were able to replenish their muscle glycogen stores, as evidenced by the decreasing ultimate pH values shown in Table 2. After 17 17 h rest, the mean ultimate pH 5.85, is, however, still significantly higher than the unstressed control animals. It is important to note that three carcasses had an ultimate pH value above 6.0. After 24 h rest, only one of the six carcasses in the group exhibited an ultimate pH above 6.0 (Table 3).

TABLE 3

MEAN ULTIMATE pH, RANGE OF VALUES AND NUMBER OF CARCASES WITH ULTIMATE pH ABOVE 6.0. EACH GROUP CONSISTED OF SIX ANIMALS.

	Mean	Range	Number > pH 6.0
Control (a)	5.51	5.45 - 5.58	0
Control (b)	5.62	5.59 - 5.66	0
Exhausted (a)	6.38	5.74 - 6.95	5
Exhausted (b)	6.31	5.85 - 6.91	5
Exhausted + 1h recovery	5.89	5.59 - 6.87	2
Exhausted + 2h recovery	6.20	5.78 - 6.91	4
Exhausted + 4h recovery	5.90	5.65 - 6.11	3
Exhausted + 8h recovery	6.06	5.60 - 6.91	2
Exhausted + 17h recovery	5.85	5.61 - 6.21	3
Exhausted + 24h recovery	5.71	5.57 - 6.15	1

Adenine/inosine ratios were largely unaffected by treatment, but changed from 1.1 to about 0.6 over the 24 h period.

DISCUSSION

The first stage of the experiment clearly shows that the 'stress' treatments likely to be encountered under normal circumstances are not detrimental to meat quality since mean ultimate pH values were all low. The variation between animals within a group, however, can be very high. The group transported 400 km on a warm day (mean temperature 18°C) and slaughtered immediately on arrival included one animal with an ultimate pH of 6.20, although the mean ultimate pH was not affected. The group rested for 24 h and not subjected to further physical exercise was the only group in which all animals had low ultimate pH values.

The initial pH values showed very slight differences between the transported and locally-obtained animals. Although small, these differences reflect the differences in behaviour of the animals at slaughter. The well-rested, locally-obtained animals (groups C and D) kicked violently at slaughter, whereas the transported groups (A and B) were very still at slaughter.

The same pattern emerges from the results of both trials in the second stage of the experiment. The initial pH values of both groups of well-rested animals were lower than most of the exhausted and recovered animals. There was a general downward trend as recovery proceeded. This corresponded to a progressive increase in activity of the animals at and immediately after slaughter, suggestive of an effect on either the sensitivity of the nervous system or perhaps purely the responsiveness of the muscles.

Initial ATP concentrations, as expected, did not vary between groups as the muscle's metabolism was able to maintain levels until death. The CP level showed a marked drop with exhaustion. The initial values for control groups were substantially below the 20 μm/g expected in resting muscle.

The mean ultimate pH values of exhausted animals declined progressively as the recovery period increased. However, the range of values and number of carcasses with an ultimate pH above 6.0 (Table 3) is perhaps more meaningful. The carcasses in the well-rested groups, besides having the lowest mean ultimate pH values, were relatively uniform in rate and extent of glycolysis. The exhausted groups, however, show extreme variability, probably as a result of variable response to both stress and in recovery. The extreme variability between animals makes the use of a repeated muscle biopsy technique such as that used by Tarrant and McVeigh (1979) very attractive. It may be that closer study of the animals during recovery using serial sampling of muscles, liver and blood from the same animal would enable a more complete and meaningful understanding of the recovery process.

The ruminant has large stores of food in its stomachs even after several days of starvation. For the animals used in these studies we have no information on stomach contents, although other studies have shown a marked reduction in dry-matter during short periods of starvation (Devine et al., 1980).

It is likely that energy needed for replenishing muscle glycogen could come from the liver, or from volatile fatty acids of the rumen. In an isolated muscle sample there is a 1 : 2 ratio between glycogen used (glycosyl units) and lactate produced, but *in vivo* this ratio will not normally be apparent. It is likely that during recovery blood glucose levels would be elevated and could contribute to the pool of hexose phosphates which can be metabolised to lactate or resynthesised to glycogen.

The 'stress' treatments used in this study cover the range from normal good practice (Stage 1) to rather extreme physical stress (Stage 2). However, it is likely that during mustering a degree of exhaustion will occur, depending on terrain and distance the animals are driven. The animals may recover in yards at the farm or slaughterhouse and during transport.

Although the present results suggest that the stresses normally encountered (e.g. Stage 1) have no effect on quality as determined by ultimate pH, there is a possibility that further slight increases in applied stresses have a pronounced effect on ultimate pH.

It is assumed that the major stress applied in Stage 2 is physical, but the increased noise and excitement while being driven to the abattoir could also have been a rather severe psychological stress. Adrenaline, noradrenaline and glucocorticoid levels might have helped define the level of stress to which these animals were subjected. The variability in response to stress and recovery was not unexpected since even in humans there are marked differences in degree of fitness and excitability As in humans there may be an influence of degree of training on muscle glycogen content and amount of exercise before metabolism becomes anaerobic. Further investigation is warranted.

REFERENCES

Ahlborg, B., Bergström, J., Ekelund, L.G. and Hultman, E. 1967. Muscle glycogen and muscle electrolytes during prolonged physical exercise. Acta. Physiol. Scand. 70, 129-142.

Armstrong, R.B. and Ianuzzo, C.D. 1977. Exercise-induced muscle glycogen depletion and repletion in diabetic rats. Life Sci. 20, 301-308.

Callow, E.H. 1938. The "Ultimate pH" of the muscle tissue. Ann. Rept. Fd. Invest. Bd. p.46.

Callow, E.H. 1939. Muscle Fatigue and pH. Ann. Rept. Fd. Invest. Bd. p.29

Davey, C.L. 1957. MS Thesis, Cambridge.

Devine, C.E., Chrystall, B.B., Davey, C.L. and Kirton, A.H. 1980. *Ante mortem* effects on *rigor mortis* in lambs. 2. Nutritional plane (submitted to Meat Sci.)

Gill, C.O. and Newton, K.G. 1979. Spoilage of vacuum-packaged dark, firm dry meat at chill temperatures. Appl. Environ. Microbiol. 37, 362-364.

Howard, A. and Lawrie, R.A. 1956. Studies on beef quality. Spec. Fd. Invest. Bd. London. No. 63.

Hultman, E. 1967. Studies on muscle metabolism of glycogen and active phosphate in man with special reference to exercise and diet. Scand. J. Clin. Lab. Invest. Suppl. 94, 1-63.

Lamprecht, W. and Trautschold, I. 1974. Adenosine-5-triphosphate. Determination with hexakinose and glucose-6-phosphate dehydrogenase. In: Methods of Enzymatic Analysis. Ed. H.U. Bergmayer, 2nd English Edition, Academic Press.

McVeigh, J.M., Tarrant, P.V. and Harrington, M.G. 1979. Influence of behavioural stress on bovine skeletal muscle glycogen content. Biochem. Soc. Trans. 7, (3), 539-541.

Mitchell, H.H. and Hamilton, J.S. 1933. Effects of long-continued muscular exercise upon the chemical composition of the muscles and other tissues of animals. J. Agric. Res. 46, 917-920.

Newbold, R.P. and Scopes, R.K. 1967. *Post mortem* glycolysis in ox skeletal muscle. Biochem. J. 105, 127-136.

Noll, F. 1974. L(+)Lactate - Determination with LDH, GPT and NAD. In: Methods of Enzymatic Analysis. Ed. H.U. Bergmayer. 2nd English Edition. Academic Press. p.1475.

Tarrant, P.V. and McVeigh, J.M. 1979. Physiological responses during percutaneous needle biopsy of bovine skeletal muscle. Biochem. Soc. Trans. 7 (3), 537-539.

Terjung, R.L., Baldwin, K.M., Winder, W.W. and Hollosky, J.O. 1974. Glycogen repletion in different types of muscle and in liver after exhausting exercise. Am. J. Physiol. 226, 1387-1391.

Shorthose, W.R., Harris, P.V. and Bouton, P.E. 1972. The effect on some properties of beef of resting and feeding cattle after a long journey to slaughter. Proc. Aust. Soc. Anim. Prod. 9, 387-391.

DISCUSSION

G. Monin (*France*)

I do not think *M. Longissimus dorsi* is the easiest muscle to work with. In our experience it is one of the less sensitive muscles to stress in the sheep carcass.

B.B. Chrystall (*New Zealand*)

I tend to agree. I think some of the hind leg muscles are more affected by stress than the LD. However, the LD is certainly the easiest to sample. We have looked at *M. triceps brachii* in the fore leg and at several other muscles. I would tend to use hind leg muscles.

G. Monin

When you have a pH of about 6.0 in *M. longissimus dorsi*, all the muscles of the carcass have a very high pH. In my experience, *M. longissimus dorsi* is one of the muscles with the lowest pH in every situation.

B.B. Chrystall

That would not agree with our experience. Quite often we find that the LD can be high and some of the other muscles can have a low ultimate pH. Our experience with sheep ties in with what Dr. Tarrant has found with cattle. It has also been found with cattle in one of the works in New Zealand, where they have found that if the LD is affected there are many muscles in the carcass which will have normal to only slightly elevated pHs.

B.L. Dumont (*France*)

How do you explain the range that you found? Some of the animals were exhausted, and yet were quite normal as far as pH was concerned.

B.B. Chrystall

I think this can be explained by the fact that we submitted these animals to a standard treatment. We have a range of fitness in these animals. Some are like the trained athlete and these appeared quite fit at slaughter, and they are the ones which tended to have lower ultimate pHs. Those that were exhausted have higher ultimate pHs. There is also a difference in recovery rates: the fitter animal recovers more quickly. You will have noticed that there were some animals with normal pHs after much less than 24 h, whereas others, even after 24 h, still had high ultimate pHs. Therefore, there is a difference both in response to the physical stress that was imposed and a difference in the recovery rate.

B.L. Dumont

Were all your animals of the same breed and age and did they come from the same flock?

B.B. Chrystall

They were the same age, same weight and they were assigned to their groups on a restricted weight basis. Therefore, mean weights per group were identical. But there is still a difference in the response to exercise; they are not all exactly the same genotype; they had different sires and different ewes.

C.L. Davey *(New Zealand)*

I would like to point out that these animals recovered their reasonably low ultimate pHs without having access to any food at all. Obviously there was a slow replenishment of muscle glycogen from liver sources, etc., which is interesting in itself. One of the reasons why we use sheep in New Zealand is because there are a lot of them, but also there is no problem with the DFD condition in this species as far as we can see. We can, however, induce it by these means and this is a useful tool for further study of the condition.

In the normal line of animals going through a standard form of processing in our fairly automated conditions, there are some carcasses which respond markedly differently from the bulk of them; some going into *rigor mortis* quite slowly and others quite quickly. This is very important from our point of view because we are imposing a standard regime of chilling or freezing on those carcasses, which reduces toughness. We are very interested to know why some sheep animals, when the biochemistry etc. seems right, go through the process of chilling and freezing, and yet the meat comes out tender; it does not appear to be related to pH or anything else. Therefore, these studies are not really related to DFD beef, they are related to the physiological and biochemical studies which we are doing in lambs.

J. Wismer-Pedersen *(Denmark)*

Looking at your results reminds me of figures published by Canadian workers on pigs. In about 1950 they did the same type of experiments which you have done and their results were remarkably similar. Were the lambs that you were using so young that they could be regarded as pre-ruminants?

B.B. Chrystall

No. Definitely not!

J. Wismer-Pedersen

In that case the effect of ruminant metabolism has not had any bearing on their capabilities to stand up to stress situations?

B.B. Chrystall

In an associated experiment we were looking at starvation, and as part of that we looked at stomach contents. It was obvious that these animals were eating almost entirely grass. An interesting point about starvation was that, even after 4 days without food or water, these animals would give a normal ultimate pH. However, in the stomach, there was a large amount of dry matter initially. But, after the 4 days, the contents were very liquid and there had been a marked decrease in dry matter content. Therefore, as you would expect, the rumen is still supplying a lot of energy.

G. Monin

I use sheep as an experimental model because they are very cheap, but after some years of experience I do not think this is the right model because of the large species differences.

C.L. Davey

Yes, I would agree with that. It was just a useful initial model.

E. Kallweit *(FRG)*

If you measured the intramuscular fat content of these different groups, it might indicate whether some of the fat has been mobilised or metabolised during the recovery time. Do you have any idea about the intramuscular fat?

B.B. Chrystall

We did not measure it, but I agree that the lipid deposits are quite significant during recovery, not only the muscle deposits of fat but also the fatty acids coming from the rumen. I would like to add a comment on DFD in sheep. Although the DFD condition is not readily seen, there are problems associated with the use of meat from exhausted animals. One example of this is the case of a baby food manufacturer who was using meat from a country where the animals were relatively undernourished. He found problems with 'greening' in his baby food. Dr. Gill's paper on microbiology, which I will present later, explains that the 'greening' relates to reduction in glucose and also the higher pH. The baby food manufacturer has overcome the problem by adding glucose and also adjusting the pH, etc. Therefore, something similar to DFD can be manifest in sheep meats.

P.V. Tarrant *(Ireland)*

I am rather puzzled about the discrepancy between the rapid rates of recovery that Dr. Chrystall has observed in his sheep, which were held at the slaughterhouse under fasting conditions, but which show remarkable recovery in 24 h, and the much slower rates of glycogen that we observed (the poster with Mr. McVeigh) in beef heifers fasted for 9 days. Our rates of glycogen resynthesis, determined by muscle biopsy, are of the order of 1.5 micromoles per gram per day which is only about 2.0 per cent of total muscle glycogen. In fact, the increase in muscle glycogen over a 7 day period just achieves statistical significance. This is in marked contrast to the rapid rates of recovery that you observed in your lambs. In our case the rumen was empty when muscle glycogen depletion was induced with adrenaline. Therefore, the animals did not have a reserve of food inside. I wonder whether, in your case, the sheep had full rumens and a store of carbohydrate material available?

B.B. Chrystall

Our lambs certainly would have had a full rumen, and this would contribute quite significantly to the recovery. There would be quite a large store of food material and therefore volatile fatty acids and such would continue to be absorbed.

P.V. Tarrant

We measured muscle glycogen and you measured pH. Even a small increment of muscle glycogen will have quite a marked influence on ultimate pH. I would imagine that if you measured muscle glycogen you probably would not have found a total recovery in a short period.

B.B. Chrystall

I think that is true. In lambs generally, there is an excess of muscle glycogen in a normal, well-fed, unstressed animal. Therefore, there is quite a margin to get rid of without really affecting the ultimate pH. Once it has been depleted, it need not get back to the original level before an apparent low ultimate pH is obtained.

G. Monin

I think I have one explanation for the fast resynthesis in sheep. It may be that transport stress does not deplete glycogen in the liver of the sheep. After transport I have always found a normal glycogen level in the liver. Therefore, there is a store of glycogen in the liver which can be used for muscle resynthesis.

B.B. Chrystall

Another point is the behavioural difference between sheep and cattle. Although sheep are in flocks cattle tend to keep more on their own. When the sheep are mixed together they are probably less susceptible to interaction stress than cattle. Sheep probably have less problems, therefore they can recover quickly. It is probably purely a physical stress, perhaps with a little excitement from the shouting to drive them along.

H.B. Hedrick *(USA)*

I have a comment related to recovery during the fasting condition. Stress releases corticosteroids which have a gluconeogenic action. This action would eventually enable the animal to replenish its depleted muscle glycogen stores. I believe this answers your question: an animal could replenish sufficient glycogen under fasting conditions all through the stress period, but it would take a long time. The recovery would not be entirely dependent on the contents of the food in the rumen.

IDENTIFICATION AND MINIMISATION OF DFD IN YOUNG BULLS IN DENMARK

Lis Buchter

**Danish Meat Research Institute,
Maglegaardsvej 2, DK-4000 Roskilde, Denmark.**

ABSTRACT

The paper describes the main results and experiences concerning the DFD problem in beef obtained by the Danish Meat Research Institute in the period 1966 - 1980.

DFD has been found to be a problem in meat from calves and young bulls, while it has not yet been seen in meat from cows.

For young bulls, which are kept tied during transport and when held in lairages at markets and slaughterhouses, the main cause of DFD is without doubt the duration of transport and the length of time spent in lairages, in new environments together with strange animals.

The occurrence of DFD meat can be kept to a minimum by giving the animals a short, careful transport from the farm to the slaughterhouse and by slaughtering them soon after arrival.

Carcasses that develop DFD in spite of these precautions can be identified by measuring the pH in the loin muscle 2 days after slaughter or later using a pH meter or indicator strips.

INTRODUCTION

The aim of the present paper is to describe some results and experiences obtained by the Danish Meat Research Institute concerning the incidence, identification and avoidance of DFD problems in beef, so that this information can supplement the information given by other participants in this seminar.

BACKGROUND

As it is now known that the occurrence of DFD is closely related to the type of animal and to the systems used when sending the animals to be slaughtered, it might be useful as a start to summarise the cattle production systems commonly used in Denmark.

The main source of income from cattle is milk, and most of the cattle are therefore of the dual purpose Black and White (now heavily crossed with Holstein-Friesian) and Red Danish Cattle. Females are raised for milk production, while the male calves are intensively fed to be slaughtered as calves or young bulls. Almost all male calves are kept indoors either individually tied or in boxes. Steers constitute as little as 1 per cent of the cattle population and their number is constantly declining. Slaughterhouses and cattlemarkets can be reached within 100 km from any farm. The proportion of animals sent direct to the slaughterhouses is slowly but steadily increasing and passed 50 per cent in 1979.

Regulations for transport of cattle for slaughter ensure that the animals are humanely treated. Since 1965 all motor vehicles used for transport of cattle have to be officially approved. It should be noted that except for small calves, all beef animals have to be individually tied during transport or when kept in lairages at market-places and slaughterhouses. Furthermore, there is no tradition for resting animals 12 h before slaughter.

THE PERIOD 1966 - 1970

From the mid-fifties Denmark has had an important export of veal to Italy, where carcasses are expected to have a light meat colour and where dark-coloured meat is regarded as being of inferior quality. Yet it was in 1966 that it was first 'discovered' that high ultimate pH values could be a problem in calves and young bulls.

The 'discovery' came by coincidence. At that time the Institute worked intensively to establish the relation between chilling rates and tenderness in cows, calves and young bulls. In these experiments it was found that some of the calves (250 kg live weight) did not develop tough meat even when exposed to very rapid chilling. This was puzzling.

In the same experiments the ladies who prepared the meat for taste-panel evaluation noticed that some of the steaks reacted peculiarly during frying. That gave the clue. By measuring pH in all samples it was found that a considerable number of the calves had high ultimate pH values in *M. longissimus dorsi*.

The results from calves with pH $\geq$ 5.8 were then omitted from the chilling experiments, and the general relationship between chilling rates and toughness induced by cold shortening became logical. But why did almost 25 per cent of the calves used in the chilling experiments have pH $\geq$ 5.8, when all the calves regularly investigated by the Institute from feeding experiments etc., had normal ultimate pH values of 5.5? The most evident difference between the animals used in the chilling experiments and the animals coming from the experimental farms was that the calves in the chilling experiments were commercial animals often bought by the slaughterhouse in markets, while the calves from the experimental farms were brought directly from the farm to the slaughter plant. This had, of course, to be investigated further. The finding that DFD could be found in calves resulted in the following activities:

1) In several series, meat from calves with high pH values was compared to meat with normal pH values. These comparisons confirmed that high pH meat was much darker, showed less bloom, had better WHC, and had lower keepability (the high pH meat developed very putrid odours). The taste panel mostly found that high pH meat was very tender, often too tender with a mealy consistence, and that the flavour, colour and juiciness in the high pH meat was inferior to normal meat.

2) The pattern of the development of ultimate pH values in the different muscles of the carcass was investigated, and it was found that in cattle - as opposed to pigs - *M. longissimus dorsi* could be used as an indicator muscle, because it normally showed increased ultimate pH values before any of the other big muscles both in the hind- and forequarter. Only when the pH was close to or above 6.5 did the value in the thigh muscles sometimes exceed the value in the loin muscle.

3) The relationships between ultimate pH values and meat quality traits such as colour, WHC, tenderness etc. were established, and it was decided in the future to omit results from meat having an ultimate pH value of 5.8 or above, because in such cases the pH in the meat had a noticeable or dominant influence on the meat quality. For commercial carcasses it was recommended that meat with pH $\geq$ 6.2 should be considered as DFD.

4) A survey of the incidence of DFD in commercial calves was carried out by measuring the pH value in the loin muscle of carcasses slaughtered at a typical Danish plant. The investigation was repeated three times i.e. in November 1967, February 1968, and May 1968. Each time it was planned to cover almost a week's production, but the experimental conditions were very difficult, and the number of animals from which results were finally obtained was rather low. The transportable instruments and electrodes available at that time for measuring pH in meat were unreliable and all measurements had therefore to be

repeated several times with intervals to avoid erratic readings. Furthermore, the carcasses were constantly changed around or removed from the chilling rooms. The results which have been published previously in part (Buchter, 1970; 1975) are shown in Table 1. The results of the survey left little doubt that transport via markets or overnight stays in the slaughterhouse lairages had an adverse effect on the ultimate pH values in the meat.

5) The establishment of the progeny-testing station for beef 'Egtved' in 1967 meant that the number of experimental calves and young bulls being investigated for meat quality by the Institute increased drastically. All animals from Egtved were transported according to a standardised procedure directly from the experimental station to the slaughterhouse and slaughtered within ½ h of arrival. In the period 1967 - 1970 a total of 1500 animals were slaughtered and only 0.5 - 1.0 per cent had ultimate pH values in the loin muscle of 5.8 or above (Buchter, 1970).

6) The meat industry was informed about the DFD problem and consequences and the following advice was given:

DFD in calves and young bulls is most effectively prevented when the animals are transported directly from the farm to a nearby slaughterplant and slaughtered on the day of arrival.

TABLE 1
FREQUENCY OF DARK-CUTTING MEAT IN THE LOIN MUSCLE OF 250 kg LIVE WEIGHT COMMERCIAL CALVES AS RELATED TO TRADE ROUTE AND HOLDING TIME IN THE SLAUGHTERHOUSE LAIRAGE (1967 - 68)

Slaughter plant	Trade route	Holding time on slaughterhouse	Number of animals	Per cent calves with $pH_{ult.} \geq 6.2$ in *M. longissimus dorsi*
A	Direct farm to slaughterhouse	0 nights	296	2
		1 night	34	9
	Via market	0 nights	187	9
		1 night	353	9
		2 nights	95	3

THE PERIOD 1971 - 1975

The above mentioned recommendation of direct transport from farm to slaughterhouse meant by-passing the markets. This had several disadvantages and the discussion for and against markets turned out to be so controversial that further investigations of DFD problems had to be kept at a very low level for a number of years. During this period new knowledge connected with the DFD issue was obtained indirectly from other experiments.

1) In extensive investigations of meat quality in commercial carcasses of mature beef it was found that none of the cows had ultimate pH values as high as 5.8. DFD could be found among steers and in rare cases in heifers. DFD was frequent among 2 year old bulls.

2) Transportable pH meters and spear electrodes to measure directly in the carcasses were improved and reliable readings could now be obtained easily.

3) At the same time the use of indicator strips for measuring pH in meat was investigated on pig carcasses (Yndgaard, 1973).

4) The incidence of high pH values in animals from the experimental stations was still very low. This is illustrated by the figures in Table 2. Among the animals with pH values close to 5.8 some abnormalities were found. The most noticeable characteristics were very low contents of dry matter and protein. In the abnormal animals the content of fat-free dry matter was 20.0 per cent and the protein content 19.4 per cent as opposed to ca 23 per cent dry matter and ca 22 per cent protein in normal meat. The meat from the abnormal animals was also light and had low WHC. Besides the three abnormal animals in Table 2, three more animals with similar qualities have been found among animals with pH $\geq$ 5.8 from Egtved slaughtered in the period 1967 - 1970.

TABLE 2

FREQUENCY OF HIGH ULTIMATE pH VALUES IN THE LOIN MUSCLE FROM CALVES AND YOUNG BULLS FROM THE PROGENY TESTING STATION FOR BEEF 'EGTVED'

Year	Live weight kg	Number of animals	Number with ultimate pH ≥ 5.8	Description of high pH values and meat types[1]
1971	450	222	0	
1971	250	288	5	5.83(N), 5.87(A), 5.88(s.DFD), 6.05(s.DFD), 6.72(DFD)
1972	450	219	3	5.82(N), 5.93(A), 6.50(DFD)
1972	250	261	0	
1973	250	282	2	5.83(A), 6.34(DFD)
1974	250	225	3	5.84(s.DFD), 5.85(s.DFD), 5.95(s.DFD)
1975	320	221	0	
1976	300	212	0	
1977	300	228	0	
1978	340	227	1	6.08(DFD)
1979	340	280	0	
1980	340	270	1	6.32(DFD)

[1]N = normal meat colour, consistency, WHC etc.
A = abnormal (very low dry matter and protein content, light meat colour, low WHC.
s.DFD = slightly DFD
DFD = dark meat colour, tender meat, high WHC.

THE PERIOD 1976 - 1980

This last period has been a transitional one. The Institute has again worked with DFD problems and the interest from the industry has been steadily increasing. The following activities have been undertaken:

1) In the summar of 1976 a minor survey of the incidence of DFD meat in young bulls from two commercial plants confirmed the previous results of the influence of trading route and lairage time. The results are shown in Table 3.

2) A study in 1977 on yields, meat quality and keepability of vacuum-packed primal cuts from young bulls showed an

TABLE 3

FREQUENCY OF DARK CUTTING MEAT IN THE LOIN MUSCLES OF 350 kg LIVE WEIGHT COMMERCIAL YOUNG BULLS AS RELATED TO TRADE ROUTE AND HOLDING TIME IN THE SLAUGHTERHOUSE LAIRAGE (1976)

Slaughter plant	Trade route	Holding time in slaughter house	Number of animals	Average pH ultimate *M. longissimus dorsi*	Percentage of young bulls with the following ultimate pH			
					5.45 - 5.79	5.80 - 6.19	6.20 - 6.59	6.60 - 7.10
B	Direct	0 nights	52	5.50	100	0	0	0
	Via market	0 nights	18	5.58	94	0	0	6
		1 night	44	5.75	77	7	7	9
		2 nights	63	5.87	60	13	14	13
		3 nights	43	6.05	30	40	16	14
		4 nights	1	6.42	-	-	-	-
C	Direct	0 nights	53	5.55	100	0	0	0
		1 night	66	5.61	97	2	0	2
	Via market	0 nights	1	5.55	-	-	-	-
		1 night	158	5.68	84	6	4	6
		2 nights	1	5.60	-	-	-	-

even lower keepability of DFD meat than expected. The DFD meat was spoiled within 1 - 2 weeks while the normal meat kept fresh for 4 - 6 weeks at 2°C and 4°C.

3) In the same study the use of indicator strips for sorting out DFD carcasses was tested, and the indicator strips were found to be well suited. The following method was recommended to the industry:

Time of measurement:	2 days after slaughter or later.
Place:	The loin muscle at the first lumbar vertebra.
Method:	Make a 2 cm deep slit in the muscle sheath and insert an indicator strip (Merck Special-indikator pH 5.2 - 7.2 Art. 9547). Press with fingers to make good contact between meat and indicator paper. After ca 2 min remove strip and read pH on the indicator scale.

4) Investigation of the possibilities of decreasing the DFD problem in young bulls, which are held overnight in the slaughterhouse lairage, by feeding special diets were initiated in 1978. Details of these experiments are presented elsewhere (Kousgaard, 1980).

CONCLUSION

DFD is a problem which in healthy animals is induced by pre-slaughter treatment. It results in meat of inferior quality and causes the meat industry financial losses mainly because of the dark and unpleasant colour, but also - and increasingly so - due to the low keepability especially of vacuum-packed meat.

In Denmark the structure of the trade, the short distances to slaughterhouses and market places, and the traditions for transport of animals for slaughter are all favourable for keeping the incidence of DFD low. The knowledge of how to minimise the occurrence of DFD, as well as the knowledge of how to identify it in carcasses where it could not be avoided, is available, and it should therefore be possible within the foreseeable future to regard 'the problem of dark-cutting in beef' as a very small one.

REFERENCES

Buchter, L., 1970. Development of a standardized procedure for the slaughter of experimental beef animals from the Danish progeny station 'Egtved'. 16th European Meeting of Meat Research Workers. Varna, Bulgaria Vol. 1, 45-56.

Buchter, L., 1975. Slaughter of meat animals. In 'Meat' ed. Cole D.J.A. and R.A. Lawrie. Butterworths, England p. 133-148.

Kousgaard, K., 1980. Development of special feeds for young bulls kept in overnight lairages. Proc. EEC Seminar 'The Problem of Dark Cutting in Beef', Brussels, 7-8 October.

Yndgaard, C.F., 1973. Technical note: A routine procedure for pH measurements in pig carcasses. J.Fd. Technol. 8, 485-488.

DISCUSSION

H.B. Hedrick *(USA)*

I was interested in your comment regarding abnormal meat types (Table 2). Was colour uniform throughout *M. longissimus dorsi*, or was it two-tone, dark spots, light areas and very watery?

Lis Buchter *(Denmark)*

I cannot say. I have gone back through my laboratory books. When the meat was available for inspection we did not know about the low protein content. Therefore, I cannot remember looking at the meat as such.

H.B. Hedrick

I have seen the same situation myself when judging a group of carcasses. As that time I did not have the equipment available to make any measurements and could only make subjective observations. I recall vividly instances similar to those you have described.

E. Kallweit *(FRG)*

I understand that all animals were tied during transportation. Is this the practice with animals from a group which were loosely housed before?

K. Kousgaard *(Denmark)*

It is so, yes. The regulations insist that all animals must be tied during transportation. We hope the regulations will be changed in the future.

H. Ruderus *(Sweden)*

Do you find the use of indicator strips is precise enough to decide on the exact pH value?

Lis Buchter

Not the exact pH values, but the difference between the normal, intermediate and the very bad groups. I do not think that we can ever teach the people on the slaughter line to use the pH meter correctly. Taking that into consideration, indicator strips are unbreakable and do not need adjusting. One can sort out the worst cases and a skilled person from the laboratory can do the fine sorting afterwards.

T.R. Dutson *(USA)*

With the calves and young bulls, what are their ages? Are they marketed as veal?

Lis Buchter

At the beginning, in 1965, the live-weight and age of the animals exported to Italy was 250 kg live-weight and 6 - 7 months old. However, now they have increased to 400 kg and 7 - 12 months. Therefore, we have had a range of animals.

P.V. Tarrant *(Ireland)*

I think that Mrs. Buchter's paper provides us with a very good opportunity to investigate the problem of dark cutting in cows. In my paper, most respondants found 6 - 10 per cent dark-cutting in cow beef and some found it to be as high as 15 per cent. However, 3 countries reported zero incidence of DFD in cow beef: West Germany, Denmark and Poland. We are lucky to have Denmark represented on the rostrum at the moment. Perhaps you could describe the way in which cows are brought to slaughter in Denmark because they are a category which causes many problems in other countries. It is possible that the differences between cows in these 3 countries and elsewhere are due mainly to environmental factors rather than any basic physiological differences.

Lis Buchter

Most of our cows come from milk farms and they are used to being tied and handled by men. They are transported just as carefully as the rest of the cattle. In many cases there is a lift at the end of the transport vehicle. When they get into the slaughterhouse, they are tied individually in the lairage and they might be slaughtered on the day of arrival or the following day.

P.V. Tarrant

If they are held overnight, what are the conditions?

Lis Buchter

Water.

K. Kousgaard

Perhaps we should add that more than half of the culled cows are delivered via the market place.

Lis Buchter

Yes, they follow the same pattern; the proportion being sent via markets and by direct route is almost the same for young bulls and cows.

G. van Logtestijn *(The Netherlands)*

On another topic do you have any idea of the minimum time necessary for the development of DFD meat in pigs and in veal calves compared with young bulls. Would it be one hour or two hours perhaps?

Lis Buchter

In our earlier surveys the actual live-weight of the carcasses was 250 kg. If the animals were brought directly from the farm and slaughtered on the day of arrival they did not develop DFD. That gives an indication that we have 2 - 5 h if the animals are treated in an agreeable fashion. However, with pigs it can occur much more quickly but this is not really my field.

SESSION VI

MICROBIOLOGICAL, TECHNOLOGICAL AND ORGANOLEPTIC PROPERTIES

Chairman: D.E. Hood

MICROBIOLOGY OF DFD BEEF

C.O. Gill and K.G. Newton*

Meat Industry Research Institute of NZ (Inc.),
P.O. Box 617, Hamilton, New Zealand.

*Australian Government Analytical Lab.
P.O. Box R176, Royal Exchange 2000
Sydney, Australia.

ABSTRACT

DFD meat is characterised by a high ultimate pH (>6.0) but it also contains little or no glucose. In normal meat, glucose is preferentially utilised by meat bacteria. Aerobic spoilage is delayed until glucose is exhausted and amino acids are attacked. In the absence of glucose, amino acids are attacked without delay and spoilage odours can be detected when bacterial densities are still low. Early aerobic spoilage of DFD meat can be prevented by addition of small quantities of glucose.

The high pH of DFD meat allows growth of species inhibited at the normal ultimate pH of meat. One such organism, Alteromonas putrefaciens, is responsible for 'greening' of vacuum-packaged meat. This type of spoilage is not prevented by addition of glucose but can be controlled by addition of small quantities of citrate to vacuum-packs of meat.

INTRODUCTION

There are a number of problems associated with DFD meat. One of the most important is that such meat, and products made from it, spoil more rapidly than normal meat (Nicol et al., 1970; Bem et al., 1976). It has been generally supposed that the accelerated rate of spoilage is due to the spoilage bacteria growing faster at the high pH (>6.0) of DFD meat than at the normal ultimate pH 95.5) of red meat. This simple explanation can at best be only partially correct. It is true that the high pH of DFD meat will allow a greater proportion of the initial psychrotrophic flora to commence growth (Figure 1). Some species, notably *Alteromonas putrefaciens*, cannot grow at all at the pH of normal meat. Most other species of importance to the aerobic spoilage flora include strains which are inhibited at pH 5.5. However, it is notable that the pseudomonads, the major aerobic spoilage organisms of fresh meat, are unaffected by pH changes within the range occurring in meat (Newton and Gill, 1980). Moreover, for most species, strains which can initiate growth at pH 5.5 do not grow faster at a high pH (Table 1). To understand why DFD meat is subject to early spoilage, it is necessary to consider the normal course of spoilage and how this is affected by the different composition of normal and DFD meat.

TABLE 1

MEAN GROWTH RATES OF FIVE LACTIC ACID TOLERANT STRAINS OF EACH GENUS ON MEAT SLICES HELD AT $2^{\circ}C$ UNDER AEROBIC CONDITIONS

Meat pH	Generation time (h)	
	5.5 to 5.7	>6.0
Pseudomonas	11.8	11.4
Enterobacteriaceae	21.2	20
Moraxella	13	13.2
Aeromonas	25	17.6
Acinetobacter	15.2	15.5
Flavobacterium	20.3	21

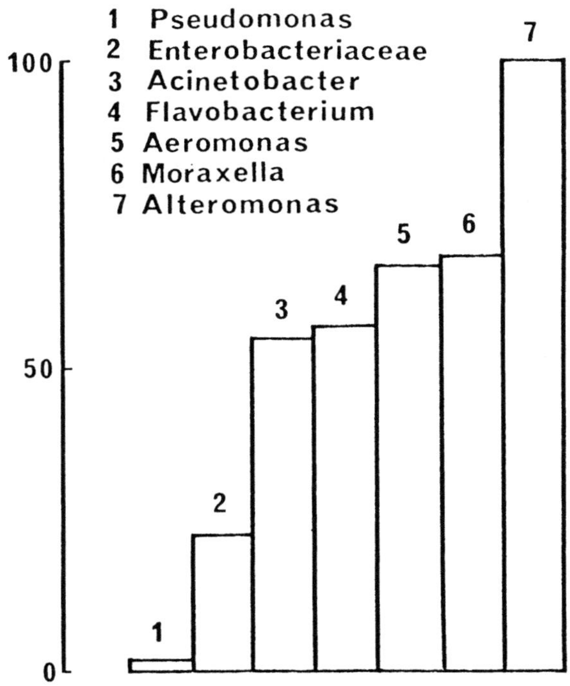

Fig. 1. Percentage of strains of Gram negative bacteria from meat, which are able to grow on DFD meat but are unable to grow at 2°C and pH 5.5.

The DFD condition arises because of depletion of muscle glycogen prior to slaughter. The DFD muscle therefore has a reduced concentration of lactic acid, which is the end-product of the glycolytic breakdown of glycogen during *rigor* onset. Normal muscle usually has some residual glycogen after glycolysis ceases, but this is absent in DFD muscle. In addition, the small quantities of glucose and glycolytic intermediates usually present in muscle are absent in the DFD condition (Fischer and Augustini, 1977; Newton and Gill, 1978). The effects of the altered meat composition on spoilage onset will be separately considered for aerobic and anaerobic storage as there are differences in the development of spoilage under these two storage conditions.

AEROBIC SPOILAGE

Most of the bacteria which grow on meat preferentially utilise glucose for growth (Table 2). The exception is *Acinetobacter*, which cannot metabolise hexoses. When glucose is exhausted amino acids are attacked, except in the case of *Enterobacter*, which will first consume any available glucose-6-phosphate. Lactic acid will only be utilised when available amino acids have been consumed. Although the concentration of glucose in meat can be very low, about 100, 300 and 900 μg/g in beef, mutton and pork respectively, it is far from negligible in terms of bacterial growth, as 100 μg of glucose would allow the growth of at least 10^7 bacteria under aerobic conditions.

During the development of the spoilage flora, bacteria are confined to the meat surface (Gill and Penney, 1977). As the cell density at the surface increases, the glucose concentration in the outer layers declines and a concentration gradient of glucose develops in the meat (Figure 2). Eventually the rate of diffusion of glucose from the interior becomes too slow to meet the requirements of the developing flora, which then begin degrading the secondary substrates, amino acids (Gill, 1976). In normal meat this occurs when the bacterial cell density is in excess of 10^8 cells/cm^2, which has long been established as the bacterial load required for spoilage odours to become detectable. That amino acids are attacked is shown by the rise in ammonia concentration and pH, which can be detected at the meat surface soon after glucose is exhausted (Figure 3).

Aerobic spoilage is therefore a result of amino acid degradation, which is delayed until the glucose available to the spoilage bacteria has been consumed. It has often been suggested that protein degradation is a necessary part of spoilage. In fact, the spoilage flora has no need to degrade protein, as there are still high concentrations of amino acids and lactic acid at the meat surface when growth ceases due to

TABLE 2

ORDER OF UTILISATION OF SUBSTRATES BY AEROBIC SPOILAGE BACTERIA

	Non-fluorescent *Pseudomonas*	Fluorescent *Pseudomonas*	*Enterobacter*	*Acinetobacter*	*Bronchothrix thermosphacta*
Glucose	1	1	1	-	1
Glucose-6-phosphate	-	-	2	-	-
Amino acids	2	2	3	1	2
Lactic acid	3	3	4	2	-

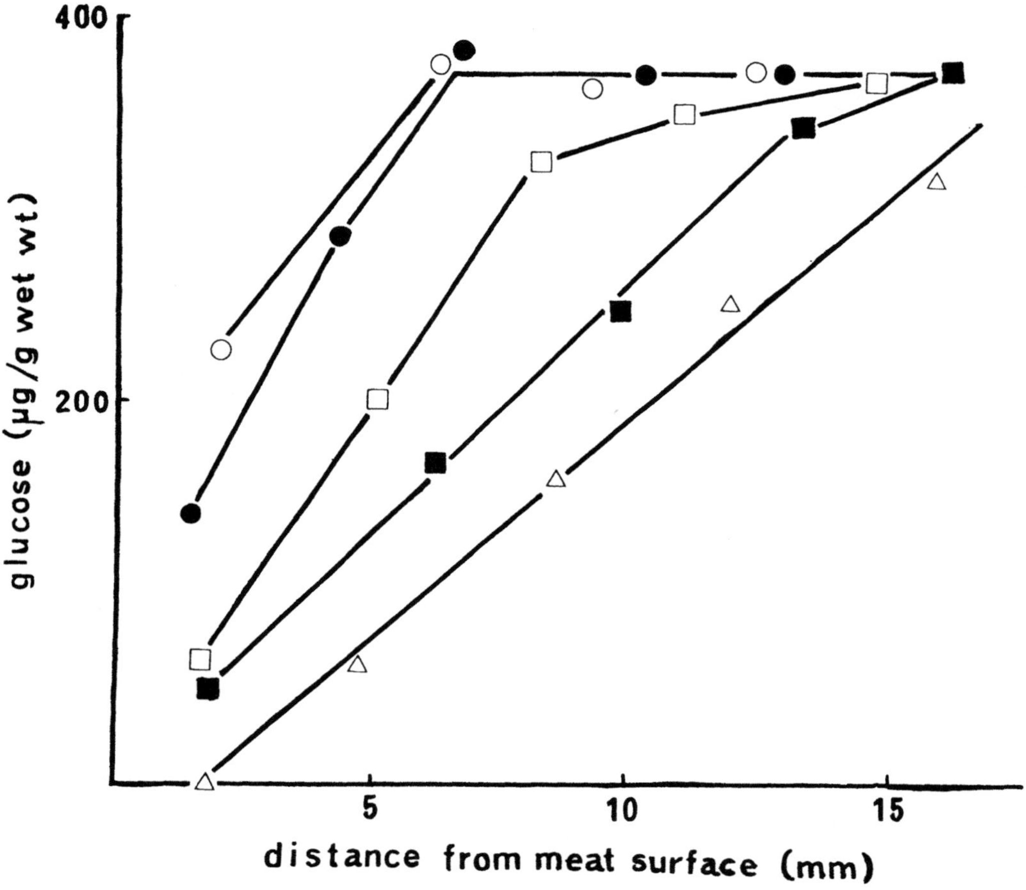

Fig. 2. Concentration gradients of glucose in meat with a *Pseudomonas* on the surface at numbers/cm^2 of 2.7×10^7 (o), 6.3×10^7 (●), 3.2×10^8 (□), 1.1×10^9 (■) and 2.8×10^9 (Δ).

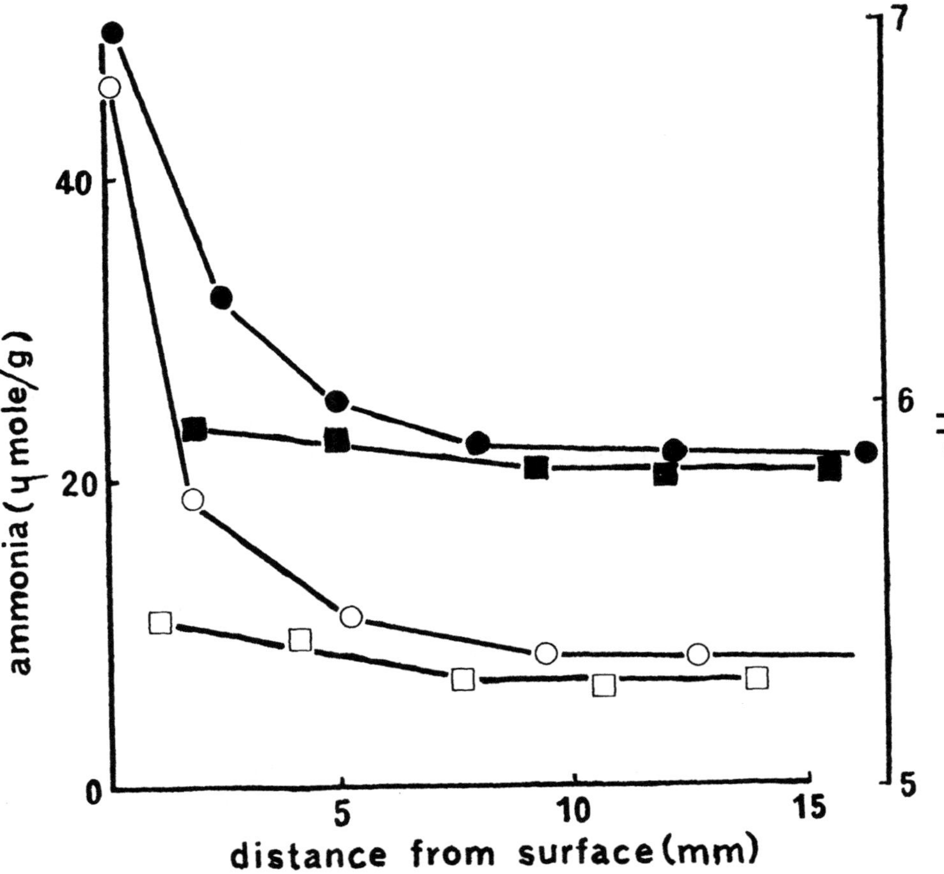

Fig. 3. Ammonia and pH gradients in meat with a *Pseudomonas* on the surface at numbers 2.8×10^9 (o NH_3, ● pH), 5×10^8 (□ NH_3, ■ pH).

oxygen limitation (Gill, 1976). Non-proteolytic strains are capable of causing spoilage and proteolytic bacteria only produce extracellular proteases towards the end of the growth phase when spoilage is already far advanced (Gill and Penney, 1977).

Since DFD meat is devoid of glucose, the pseudomonads degrade amino acids without delay. Under these conditions the onset of spoilage is simply a function of the time necessary to accumulate detectable quantities of the bacterial metabolites responsible for spoilage odours. This occurs when the cell density exceeds $10^6/cm^2$ (Figure 4). Spoilage can be delayed by adding glucose to the meat to give a final concentration similar to that in normal meat, but reduction of the pH to 5.5 by addition of lactic acid has no significant effect upon the time of spoilage onset (Newton and Gill, 1978).

The presence of spoilage organisms which do not grow on meat of normal pH generally has little effect upon the onset of aerobic spoilage of DFD meat, as they too produce spoilage odours only when metabolising amino acids. *Acinobacter* species would be expected to cause spoilage when their density exceeds $10^6/cm^2$ as they do not utilise glucose, but fortunately these bacteria appear to have little potential for producing the metabolites of unpleasant aroma that are responsible for spoilage (Lerke et al., 1965).

The fat surfaces of meat of normal pH are also prone to early spoilage for the same reasons that apply to DFD meat. Like DFD meat, the pH of fat surface is high (Table 3). Although there is a significant glucose concentration at the surface, the rate of diffusion is very much lower than with muscle so the supply of glucose is very limited. The water-soluble components present at fat surfaces are probably derived from the serum in cut blood vessels.

The fat surfaces of carcasses are usually too dry to allow bacterial growth, whereas in packages the fat surfaces are bathed in drip from the muscle and so spoil at the same

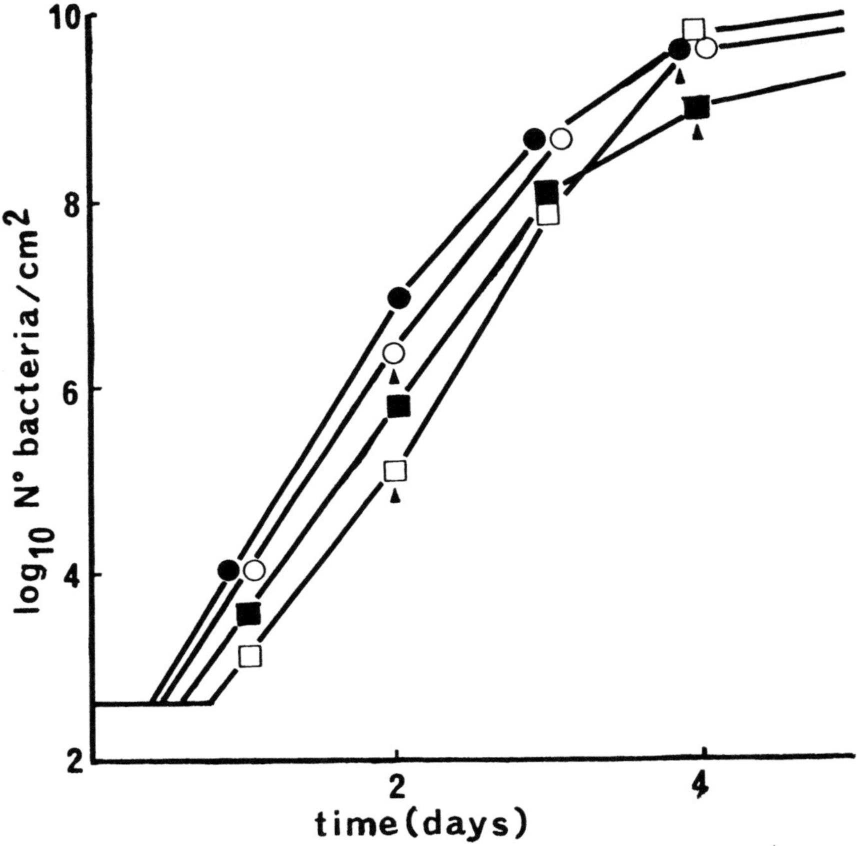

Fig. 4. Growth of *Pseudomonas fluorescens* at 10°C on meat slices of different pH and glucose content. (o) pH 6.3, glucose absent; (●) pH 6.3, glucose at 100 µg/g wet tissue; (□) pH 5.6, glucose absent; (■) pH 5.85, glucose at 100 µg/g wet tissue; (▲) spoilage odours detected.

rate as that tissue. In a domestic refrigerator fat surfaces will often be kept moist by the periodic entrance of warmer air. Under these conditions bacteria grow and cause spoilage when the cell density reaches $10^6/cm^2$ (Figure 5). Fat degradation plays no part in the spoilage at fat surfaces of meat.

ANAEROBIC SPOILAGE

The anaerobic storage of meat in vacuum-packages can greatly extend the shelf-life of chilled meat. To obtain the

TABLE 3

CONCENTRATIONS OF LOW MOLECULAR WEIGHT, WATER-SOLUBLE SUBSTANCES AND PH in 1 mm THICK AGAR LAYERS ON THE SURFACES OF ADIPOSE TISSUE FROM SIX LAMB LOINS

	Glucose (μg/g)	Amino acids (μg/g)	Lactic acid (μg/g)	Ammonia (μmole/g)	pH
	41	210	597	2.5	7.30
	33	180	488	2.9	7.25
	43	234	570	2.8	7.20
	66	158	813	3.2	7.10
	39	203	1058	3.9	7.15
	37	202	705	2.9	7.20
Average	43	198	705	3.0	7.2

maximum effect, the oxygen permeability of the packaging film must be sufficiently low to prevent growth of psuedomonads, which will otherwise spoil the meat in the manner previously described (Newton and Rigg, 1979). When anaerobic conditions are maintained, the flora of vacuum-packaged normal meat is dominated by the strictly anaerobic lactobacilli. The factult-ative anaerobes *Brochothrix thermosphacta* and *Enterobacter* are usually present as minor components. The substrates available in meat for fermentation by these bacteria are very restricted (Table 4). All three species can use glucose and in addition *Enterobacter* can ferment glucose-6-phosphate. Otherwise only one or two amino acids are available to each species. The maximum cell density is therefore determined by the amounts of fermentable substrates available (Gill and Newton, 1978). This is usually about 10^8 bacteria/cm^2. It might be expected that the *Enterobacter* could compete successfully with *Lactobacillus* because they alone can use glucose-6-phosphate. However, the *lactobacilli* not only outgrow *Enterobacter*, but produce an antimicrobial substance which prevents the *Enterobacter* from overgrowing them when the *lactobacilli* have reduced the surface concentrations of glucose and arginine to zero (Figure 6). Anaerobic spoilage of normal meat seems to be due to the slow accumulation of some products of fermentation. The absence of glucose in DFD meat means that

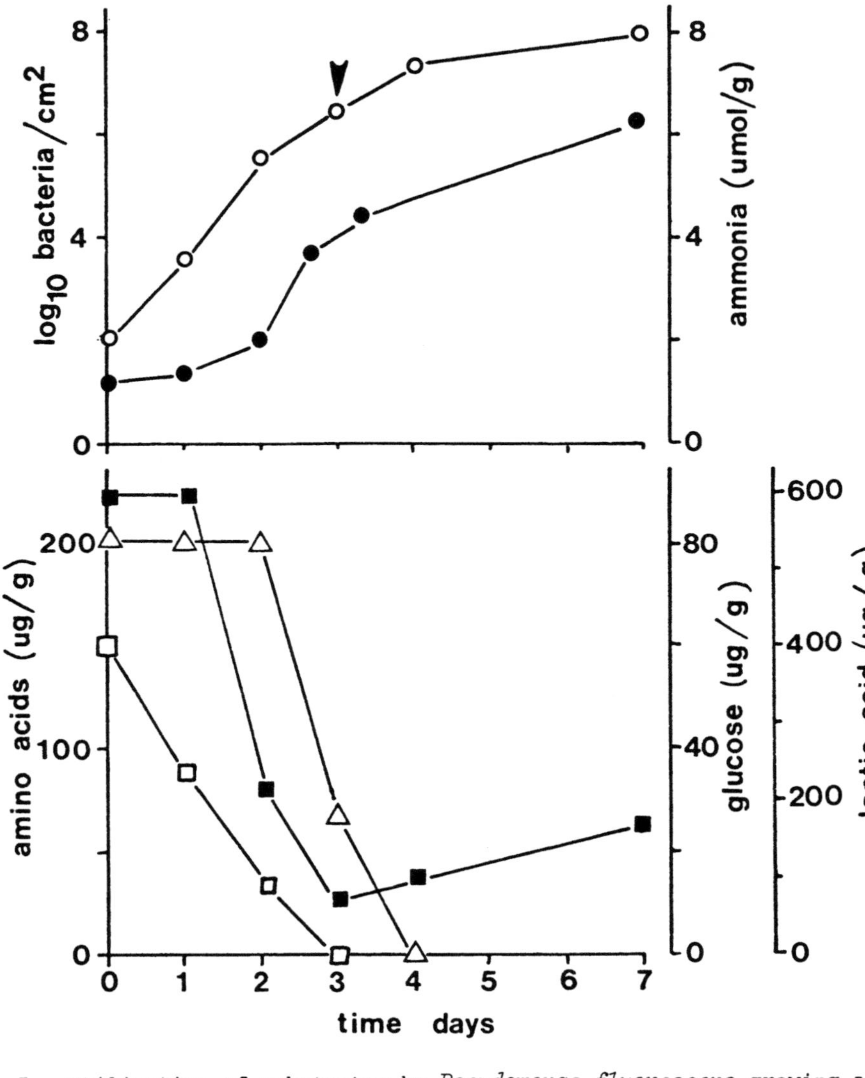

Fig. 5. Utilisation of substrates by *Pseudomonas fluorescens* growing at 10°C on a 1 mm thick agar layer on the surface of lamb adipose tissue. Symbols: Log_{10} bacterial cell density (O); concentration in the agar of: ammonia (●), glucose (□), amino acids (■), lactic acid (Δ); spoilage (▼).

TABLE 4

ORDER OF UTILISATION OF SUBSTRATES BY ANAEROBIC SPOILAGE BACTERIA

	Lactobacillus	*Enterobacter*	*Bronchothrix thermosphacta*
Glucose	1	1	1
Glucose-6-phosphate	-	2	-
Amino acids	arginine only	-	-

the only substrate available to the *lactobacilli* is arginine, and this limits the cell density that can be attained by these organisms. They are, therefore, unable to reach a density rapidly which is sufficient to prevent the growth of competing species.

The high pH of DFD meat allows the growth of three facultative anaerobes which do not usually form a significant part of the anaerobic spoilage flora. The three species are *Yersinia enterocolitica*, *Enterobacter liquifaciens* and *Alteromonas putrefaciens*. *Y. enterocolitica* is usually present on vacuum-packaged meat as a minor contaminant. The increased numbers on DFD meat do not seem to cause any spoilage problem, but certain strains are known to be pathogenic, which may be cause for concern. However, the strains found on meat occur widely in meat works and so probably form part of the normal bacterial population (Newton, 1979). It is, therefore, unlikely that any pathogenic properties would have escaped recognition. *E. liquefaciens* is an important spoilage organism which produces spoilage odours at low cell densities on DFD meat as a result of amino acid degradation (Gill and Newton, 1979). The third organism, *A. putrefaciens*, is responsible for the green discolouration which usually limits the storage life of vacuum-packaged DFD meat.

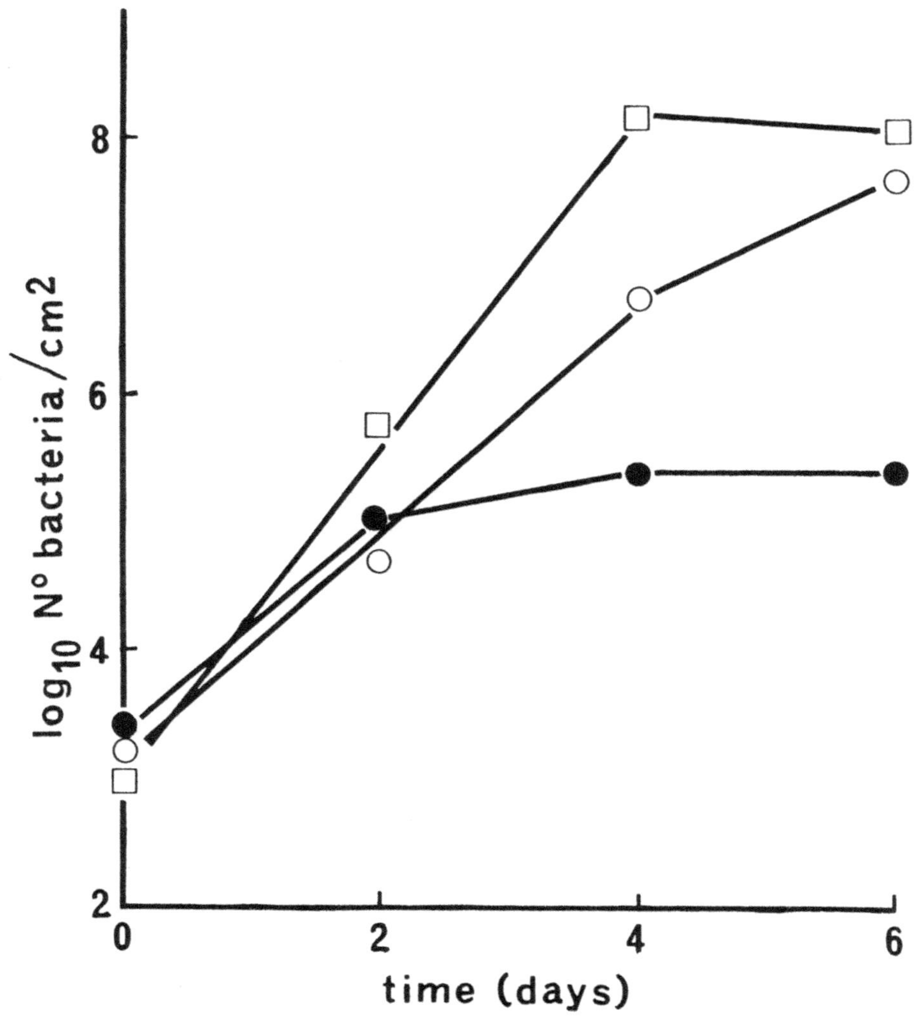

Fig. 6. Growth on meat, at 10°C under anaerobic conditions, of *Enterobacter* alone (o) and *Enterobacter* (●) in mixed culture with *Lactobacillus* (□).

Greening is caused by the reaction of hydrogen sulphide with the muscle pigment to produce green sulphmyoglobin. Under anaerobic or oxygen-limited conditions, *A. putrefaciens* produces large amounts of hydrogen sulphide by degradation of cysteine or glutathione, a cysteine-containing tripeptide present in meat. Although *E. liquefaciens* has a weak ability to produce H_2S, it does not seem to make any significant contribution to visible greening.

Since early anaerobic spoilage of DFD meat is a result of amino acid degradation, it might be expected to be prevented by the addition of glucose. This is true with respect to the prevention of spoilage odour by *E. liquifaciens*, but unfortunately it does not prevent greening. Even in the presence of glucose, *A. putrefaciens* will still utilise serine and cysteine (Figure 7).

To prevent greening it is therefore necessary to reduce the pH of DFD meat to below 6.0 to stop the growth of *A. putrefacien* This can be done by addition of glucose and a *lactobacillus* starter culture or by addition of buffers (Table 5). The first method not only prevents the growth of *A. putrefaciens* but also produces a marked improvement in the appearance of the meat (Newton and Gill, 1980). Unfortunately, the high numbers of *lactobacilli* cause early spoilage by imparting to the meat the dairy flavour which develops in normal vacuum-packaged meat after extended storage. However, addition of a small amount of citrate buffer (1.9 M, pH 4.8, 6 ml/kg of meat) prevents greening and gives a normal shelf-life. This small quantity of buffer does not permanently alter the pH of the bulk of the meat. It seems to reduce the surface pH for a sufficient time for other species to grow to high enough densities to prevent growth of *A. putrefaciens* when the surface pH rises. The citrate is utilised preferentially to amino acids by *E. liquifaciens* and so spoilage by this organism is also prevented.

TABLE 5

EFFECT OF DIFFERENT TREATMENTS OF VACUUM-PACKAGED DFD MEAT SLICES ON GROWTH OF *Alteromonas putrefaciens*

	Generation time	Final counts ($\log_{10}$ No/cm^2)
Untreated control	4.2	7.5
Glucose	4.2	8.0
Lactobacillus	15.6	5.4
lactobacillus + glucose	NG	< 4.0
Citrate buffer	NG	< 4.0

NG = no growth

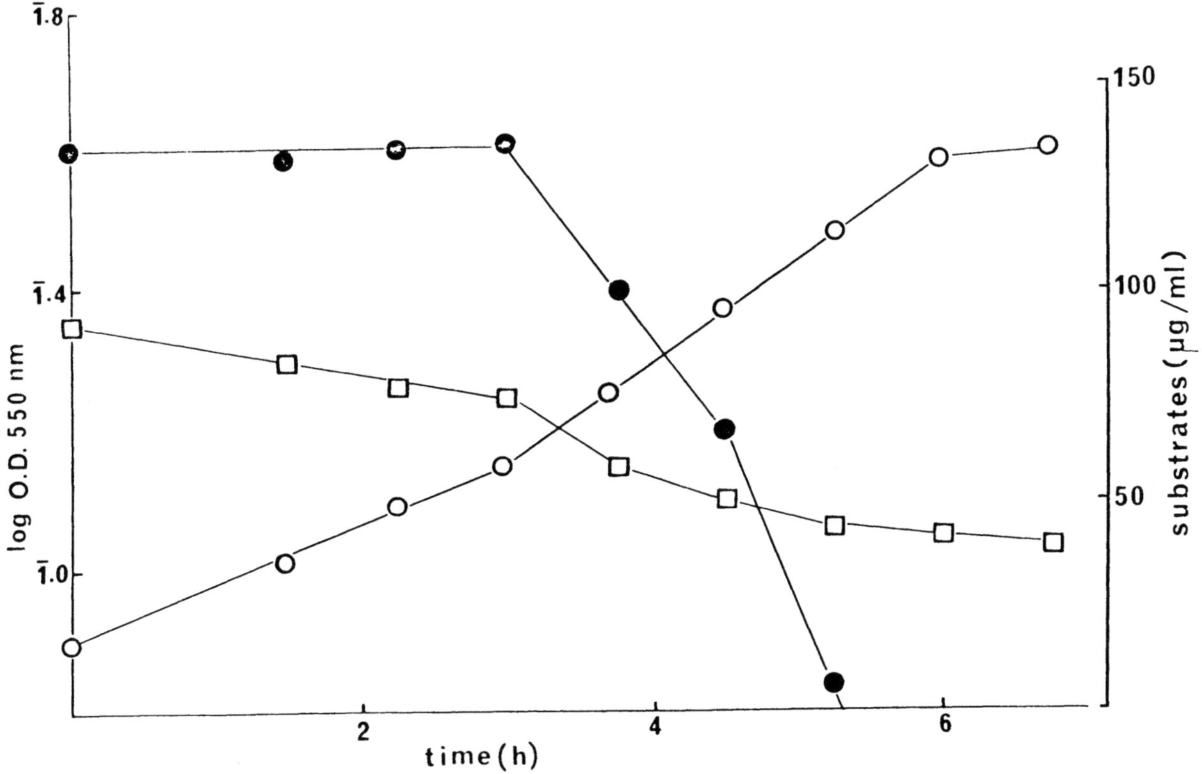

Fig. 7. Anaerobic growth of *Alteromonas putrifaciens* at 30°C. Optical density 550 nm (o), glucose (●), and serine (□).

CONCLUSIONS

The early spoilage of DFD meat is becoming an increasing problem with the greater use of vacuum-packaging to extend the storage life of chilled prime cuts. It would obviously be best to resolve the problem by preventing development in the animal of the muscle state which results in DFD meat. However, even with good control over stock for an extended period prior to slaughter, it may well be impossible to eliminate the condition and certainly it will continue to be present in a proportion of the carcasses produced under current commercial practice. It is therefore worthwhile considering prophylactic measures to prevent the early spoilage of such meat.

The altered composition of DFD meat has important effects upon the composition and metabolism of the bacterial flora. Changes that affect bacterial metabolism and growth are relatively minor ones and can be readily reversed. The spraying of carcasses with a small quantity of glucose solution would ensure that early aerobic spoilage did not occur. Spoilage in vacuum-packages can be prevented by addition of a few ml of citrate buffer to the pack before the vacuum is drawn. Neither of these additions could be to the detriment of the consumer, while they could prevent considerable wastage of perfectly sound meat. It does seem ridiculous that such treatments may not be possible because of some legalistic interpretation of the word 'fresh' applied to meat with the supposed objective of safeguarding the consumer, who will in the end pay for all unnecessary wastage of sound meat.

(Paper read by Dr. B. Chrystall)

REFERENCES

Bem, Z., Leistner, L. and Dresel, J., 1976. Schnellmethoden zur Keimzchlbestimmung bei Fleisch. (Quick methods of determining bacterial counts in meat) Fleischwirts. 56 (12), 1803-1804.

Fischer, K. and Augustini, C., 1977. Stadien per *post mortem* Glykogenolyse bei unterschiedlichen pH_1-werten in Schweinefleisch. (Stages of *post mortem*glycolysis at various ph_1-values in pigmeat). Fleischwirts. 57, 1191-1194.

Gill, C.O., 1976. Substrate limitation of bacterial growth at meat surfaces. J. Appl. Bacteriol. 41, 401-410.

Gill, C.O. and Newton, K.G., 1979. Spoilage of vacuum-packaged dark, firm, dry meat at chill temperatures. Appl. Environ. Microbiol. 37, 362-364.

Gill, C.O. and Penney, N., 1977. Penetration of bacteria into meat. Appl. Environ. Microbiol. 33, 1282-1286.

Lerke, P., Adams, R. and Farber, L., 1965. Bacteriology of spoilage of fish muscle. Appl. Microbiol. 13 (4), 625-630.

Newton, K.G., 1979. Value of coliform tests for assessing meat quality. J. Appl. Bacteriol. 47, 303-307.

Newton, K.G. and Gill, C.O., 1978. Storage quality of dark, firm, dry meat. Appl. Environ. Microbiol. 36, 375-376.

Newton, K.G. and Gill, C.O., 1980. Control of spoilage in vacuum packaged dark, firm, dry (DFD) meat. J. Fd. Technol. 15, 227-234.

Newton, K.G. and Rigg, W.J., 1979. The effect of film permeability on the storage life and microbiology of vacuum-packed meat. J. Appl. Bacteriol. 47, 433-441.

Nicol, D.J., Shaw, M.K. and Ledward, D.A., 1970. Hydrogen sulphide production by bacteria and sulphmyoglobin formation in prepacked chilled beef. Appl. Microbiol. 19, 937-939.

DISCUSSION

D.E. Hood *(Ireland)*

Thank you, Dr. Chrystall, for presenting the paper on microbiology of DFD beef. Are there any questions?

J.J. Sheridan *(Ireland)*

I am intrigued by one thing in particular. We have made many isolates from DFD meat in Ireland and we have never found *Alteromonas*. This may be a problem of taxonomy. I note that Gill and Newton describe the organisms as facultative anaerobes. If *Alteromonas* was formally *Pseudomonas*, this is not a facultative anaerobe; it is a strictly aerobic organism. We think that what we are looking at is *Aeromonas*. I believe Dr. Patterson's experience is more or less the same as mine in that he, like me, has never found *Alteromonas*.

B.B. Chrystall *(New Zealand)*

I would not like to go into the taxonomy of that. However, I will certainly convey that back to Dr. Gill. It will be interesting to get his comments - which will probably be quite dry!

J.T. Patterson *(UK)*

I would be inclined to agree with Dr. Sheridan on this. It may be a question of dealing with a different environment, but we found, in our paper of 1977, that *Aeromonas* was certainly there in high pH meat and had the ability to produce sulphide-type odours. It may be a taxonomic thing, I am not sure. *Alteromonas putrefaciens* has a side flagellum. One can only pick this up by electron microscopy. I am inclined to think it is *Aeromonas* that is possibly the problem here. However, I do not think this matters too much in terms of the overall conclusions which I think are good.

B.B. Chrystall

It is still a point which I will convey to Dr. Gill for clarification.

J.T. Patterson

There is another point which I would like to raise regarding the use of citrate buffer. While in the laboratory it seems to work very well, it is being used at 2 molar, which would probably not be used under commercial conditions. Therefore, commercially, it might not be viable at that concentration.

B.B. Chrystall

We were adding 6 ml/kg which is not a great quantity. If you wished to decrease that concentration of citrate you could always add a greater volume to the given weight. I am not sure whether the whole approach would be commercially viable at the moment. I am not sure what the regulatory situation is anyway. Adding something moves it out of the 'fresh' category into the 'processed meat' category.

J.T. Patterson

One could possibly get away with adding lactic acid as opposed to citrate buffer. I am not sure about that, but lactic acid is being produced anyway by the lactobacilli.

B.B. Chrystall

But that doesn't make much difference to regulations, does it?

J.T. Patterson

There are quite a number of organisms which utilise citrate, and this is probably why it is being used. It probably works very well, but I just do not know how it would work in practice.

J.J. Sheridan

The molarity of the citrate could be reduced quite considerably. We used a 0.2 molar citrate and got a delayed greening. Therefore, you can reduce the molarity and the ionic strength.

H. Ruderus *(Sweden)*

In this context we are talking about glucose as opposed to free glucose. In another DFD context we were talking about the glycogen that is left in the meat. Is there any strict correlation between free glucose and glycogen content? Are there any factors which influence the proportion of these?

B.B. Chrystall

One can end up with virtually no glycogen and still have free glucose. With DFD there is very little glycogen to start off with, it is all used and there is no glucose left at the end. Whereas with the non-DFD muscle there could be quite a lot of glycogen left at the end plus quite a bit of free glucose. Dr. Augustini may be able to answer Dr. Ruderus.

Chr. Augustini *(FRG)*

We did not find a close correlation between them. The glucose level was very variable.

P.V. Tarrant *(Ireland)*

We found glucose indicator strips were very useful for weeding out dark-cutters. In most cases one could find carcasses with *M. longissimus dorsi* pH values above 6.0 by simply testing their reaction to a glucose indicator strip. Normal beef reacts strongly and dark-cutters give a negative reaction on the glucose test. It is a simple, rapid test and can be performed by non-technical people.

J.T. Patterson

I wonder if Dr. Tarrant could tell us a little more about

these strips. I do not know how they work; it is the first time I have heard about them.

P.V. Tarrant

We have not got any hard data. We have used them in factories where pH meters were not available but where the management needed to have some means of identifying dark-cutting carcasses other than on visual judgement, which is notoriously unreliable in artificial lighting and dim lighting. Therefore, I provided glucose indicator strips of the standard variety which are available through any pharmacist and they were found to be satisfactory on these occasions. We have not collected data on them, but my observations indicate that about 90 per cent of carcasses with pH values above 6.0 in *M. longissimus dorsi* could be identified using glucose indicator strips.

J.T. Patterson

Is there a colour change?

P.V. Tarrant

There is. Thirty seconds or one minute is sufficient time to allow the strip to become saturated with meat juice. After a further wait of about 30 s we judge the colour using a colour standard on the case. It is quite a useful technique and compares with the pH indicator strip which was developed at Roskilde for one of the German chemical companies.

Lis Buchter *(Denmark)*

How soon after slaughter can you use the glucose strips?

P.V. Tarrant

They should be used at the same time as a normal ultimate pH measurement would be taken.

B.L. Dumont *(France)*

In the case of high pH, is there always sufficient juice to have a good contact?

P.V. Tarrant

If the meat is very DFD it may be difficult to get the strip saturated. If the meat is that dry it would be rejected anyway. In intermediate cases, around pH 6.0, there is sufficient loose water in the meat to cause saturation.

J.J.A. Heffron *(Ireland)*

So they are enzyme-based tests?

P.V. Tarrant

Yes. Some of the strips contain dyes which are involved in the colour reaction and would not be suitable for use on food stuffs. Others do not contain any dyes.

J.J.A. Heffron

For the urinary glucose tests glucose oxidase and orthodianisidine is used, which is not a very safe dye.

P.V. Tarrant

In that case the sample of meat would have to be destroyed. Some of the chemical companies have developed glucose indicator strips for use on food stuffs, if there was a demand from the meat industry I think they could produce a suitable indicator strip.

C.L. Davey *(New Zealand)*

It seems to me that the glucose strip and the pH strip are measuring entirely different things but are trying to measure the same condition of the meat. This appears to be most fortunate: a double test could be done - one on the glucose and one on the pH - and a methodology could be developed which might be more reliable than other methods to identify the DFD condition.

D.B. Lindsay *(UK)*

You can buy strips which will measure, simultaneously, both pH and glucose as well as one or two other things; they are used for diabetics. They are very expensive however.

E. Puolanne *(Finland)*

I prefer direct pH measurement; this is not so expensive. An instrument costs around £200. However, does anyone think that there is a microbiological risk when the pH value is measured by electrode?

J.T. Patterson

I would not have thought so. On the other hand, if you started off with a carcass which was heavily contaminated with Salmonella all over the surface (which is unlikely) it would undoubtedly be transferred to a number of carcasses thereafter. In a normal situation there should not be much of a problem.

TRANSLUCENCY AND COLOUR DEFECTS OF DARK-CUTTING MEAT AND THEIR DETECTION

D.B. MacDougall and S.J. Jones
Meat Research Institute, Langford, Bristol, BS18 7DY, UK.

ABSTRACT

The colour, lightness, hue and saturation, and the light scattering coefficient, Sγ, of high pH_u *dark-cutting beef were compared with the characteristics in beef of normal* pH_u. *Dark-cutting beef had lower lightness values, a more purple hue and considerably reduced saturation. Sγ doubled in value from pH 6.8 to 5.7. The response of a prototype fibre-optic probe to measure back scatter of light transmitted into meat was related to Sγ. In abattoir trials this instrument effectively detected dark-cutting meat without damaging carcasses. Instrument values of 20 or lower indicate high* pH_u *meat. A more robust and stable instrument, designed for industrial use in the abattoir, has been manufactured.*

INTRODUCTION

The environmental and physiological factors involved in the dark-cutting condition in beef have been fully examined in this seminar. Young bulls are particularly prone to dark-cutting if stressed by transport to the abattoir or excited by mixing with strangers prior to slaughter (MacDougall and Rhodes, 1972; Duchesne, 1978). The occurrence increases in late autumn when cold nights after warm days cause the animals to shiver in lairage. The dark appearance of the meat is a direct consequence of depletion of muscle glycogen by exhausting activity in unfamiliar surroundings. *Post mortem* glycolysis terminates before sufficient lactic acid is produced for the ultimate pH (pH_u) to fall to the normal value of approximately 5.5. Dark-cutting beef remains above pH_u 6.0 and in severe cases may exceed pH_u 6.5.

Comparison of the optical properties of dark-cutting meat with normal meat indicates that the major difference between them is in their opacity. This provides a basis for a technique to detect safely and conveniently the dark-cutting condition without damaging the carcass.

MUSCLE OPACITY AND pH_u

Muscle that is cut soon after an animal has been slaughtered is translucent and sticky to touch. Its dark jelly-like appearance alters during *rigor mortis* and if sufficient glycogen was initially present, it becomes progressively more opaque until pH_u is reached, at which stage its appearance on cutting and oxygenation is moist bright red. The transition from translucent to semi-opaque is detectable at pH 5.9. In dark-cutting meat this transition does not occur. In normal meat, opacity development is related to temperature as well as pH_u. If chilling conditions are such that muscle temperature is high when the pH is low, the meat will be light in colour, opaque and will exude drip. This condition obtains in muscle adjacent to the femur in beef hindquarter, chilled by traditional regimes that avoid cold shortening (Taylor et al., 1980 - 81). Opaque beef is similar in its light scattering properties to pale, soft, exudative (PSE) pork, which results from excessively fast *post mortem* glycolysis while the carcass is warm.

MUSCLE COLOUR AND pH_u

The colour terms used in this paper, lightness, hue and saturation, are the psychological concepts of colour perception, in the present situation interpreted from measurements made in Hunter colour-space. The Hunter space defined by L (lightness), a_L (green-red), b_L (blue-yellow) is a visually uniform transformation of the CIE tristimulus values X, Y, Z (Wyszecki and Stiles, 1967). Luminous reflectance Y, a measure of the eye's sensitivity to light throughout the visible spectrum is converted to uniform lightness by $10\ Y^{\frac{1}{2}} = L$.

In a study on the colour of meat from young bulls lightness was related to both haem pigment concentration and pH_u, but the relationships were different for normal and dark-cutting meat (MacDougall and Rhodes, 1972). In normal pH_u meat, lightness decreased with increase in myoglobin concentration whereas in high pH_u meat, lightness decreased with increase in pH_u but not significantly with pigment concentration. This indicates that for the 2 to 5 mg/g range of myoglobin concentration, found in meat from young bulls, variation in opacity with $pH_u > 5.7$ had a greater effect on lightness than differences in pigment absorption.

The darkest meat was least saturated initially and its hue was purple. Subjective assessment of lightness described meat after one hour's exposure to air with $pH_u > 5.9$ as moderately-to-very dark. On storage the saturation and hue slowly became identical to normal meat but the lightness did not increase.

MEASUREMENT OF OPACITY

The optical properties of light-scattering materials can be expressed in terms of two parameters, an absorption coefficient (K) and a scattering coefficient (S). The Kubelka-Munk analysis is based on the fact that reflectivity (R_∞), the reflectance of an infinitely thick layer, depends upon the ratio of the absorbing and scattering coefficients as follows:

$$\frac{K}{S} = \frac{(1 - R_\infty)^2}{2R_\infty}$$

where R_∞ is from 0 to 1. Strictly, the analysis is precise only for monochromatic light and if used for determination of absolute values, correction factors have to be included to take account of various optical effects at the medium/air interface. For most purposes relative values are adequate, provided dimensions and optical geometry are defined. The method is fully described by Judd and Wyeszecki (1975), its application to tristimulus values in foodstuffs by Francis and Clydesdale (1975) and to meat by MacDougall (1970). The scatter coefficient calculated from Y (S_Y) is adequate to describe the light-scattering properties of raw meat.

MUSCLE COLOUR, pH_u AND S_Y

The inter-relationships of light-scatter to colour and pH_u are reported for a range of meat samples selected from typically dark-cutting to pale and exudative. The samples were:

Twenty five *M. longissimus dorsi* from young bulls, whose pigment concentration ranged from 2.1 to 4.3 mg/g myoglobin, 15 of which were dark-cutting ($pH_u \geq 6.0$), and

twenty five *M. semimembranosus* from steers whose pigment concentration ranged from 4.7 to 7.9 mg/g myoglobin all with $pH_u \leq 5.6$, 9 of which were opaque, pale and wet.

Colour was measured on a Hunter D25 colour-difference meter after cutting, wrapping in oxygen permeable film and holding the meat for 1 h at +2°C. $K\gamma$ and $S\gamma$ were calculated from the reflectance of 2 mm sections of meat, in optical contact on black and white plastic, measured on a Gardner colour difference meter. Unit thickness is defined as 1 mm.

$S\gamma$ ranged from 0.06 to 0.29 (Figure 1). The dark-cutting group ($pH_u \geq 6.0$) had $S\gamma$ values < 0.11 and the pale group (normal pH_u) had $S\gamma$ values from 0.19 to 0.29. The difference in saturation between dark-cutting and normal meat was greater than the difference in lightness. The less saturated purple colour is attributable to two factors: the higher oxygen consumption rate (Hall et al., 1944; Bendall and Taylor, 1972) and the lower rate of inward diffusion of oxygen (Lawrie, 1958) which considerably increase the time for formation of a sufficiently thick layer of oxymyoglobin on the surface to appear red. Because of the greater translucence from diminished $S\gamma$, light penetrates further into the meat, more is absorbed by the pigment which makes it appear darker and that which is reflected has the absorption characteristics of myoglobin.

FIBRE OPTIC PROBE

Measurement of $S\gamma$ requires careful mounting of accurately sectioned discs of meat and cannot be contemplated as a routine method for large numbers of samples. Other techniques are available for measuring light scatter, for example the intensity of directional scatter by a light beam incident upon the scattering particles in the material. A prototype instrument was constructed to detect dark-cutting and PSE meat and its response to back scatter is linear to $S\gamma$ (MacDougall and Jones, 1975). A more robust instrument based on the same principle will be available commercially (Figure 2). It consists of a gun-handle with a sharp probe, 8 cm long, for insertion into the meat, for example from the abdominal cavity betwean the ribs to a fixed depth into *M. longissimus dorsi*. Power is supplied by rechargeable batteries and the amplified response presented on a digital

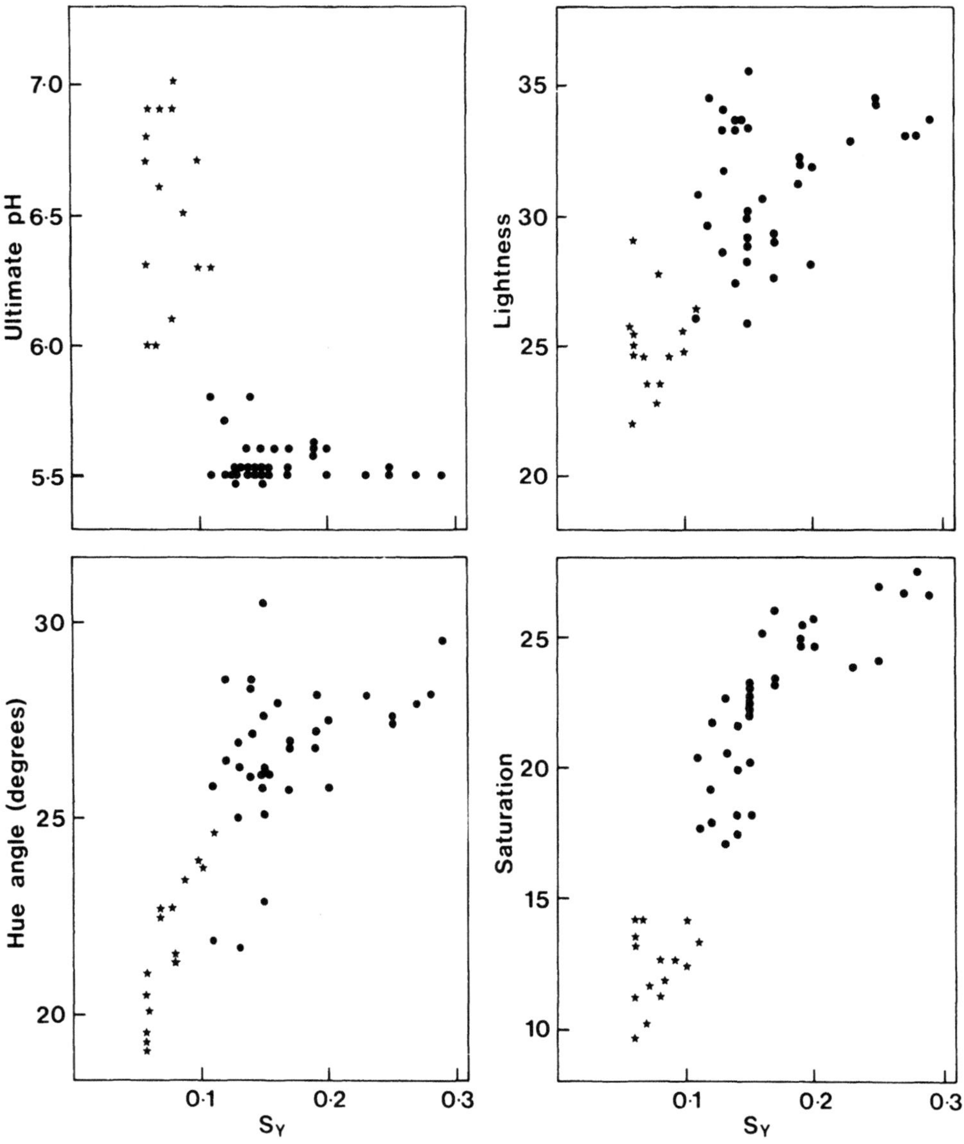

Fig. 1. Relationship of the luminous scatter coefficient, Sγ, to ultimate pH and the colour concepts lightness, hue and saturation for fresh dark-cutting, normal and pale beef exposed to air for 1 h at 2°C.

● $pH_u \leq 5.9$, ★ $pH_u \geq 6.0$

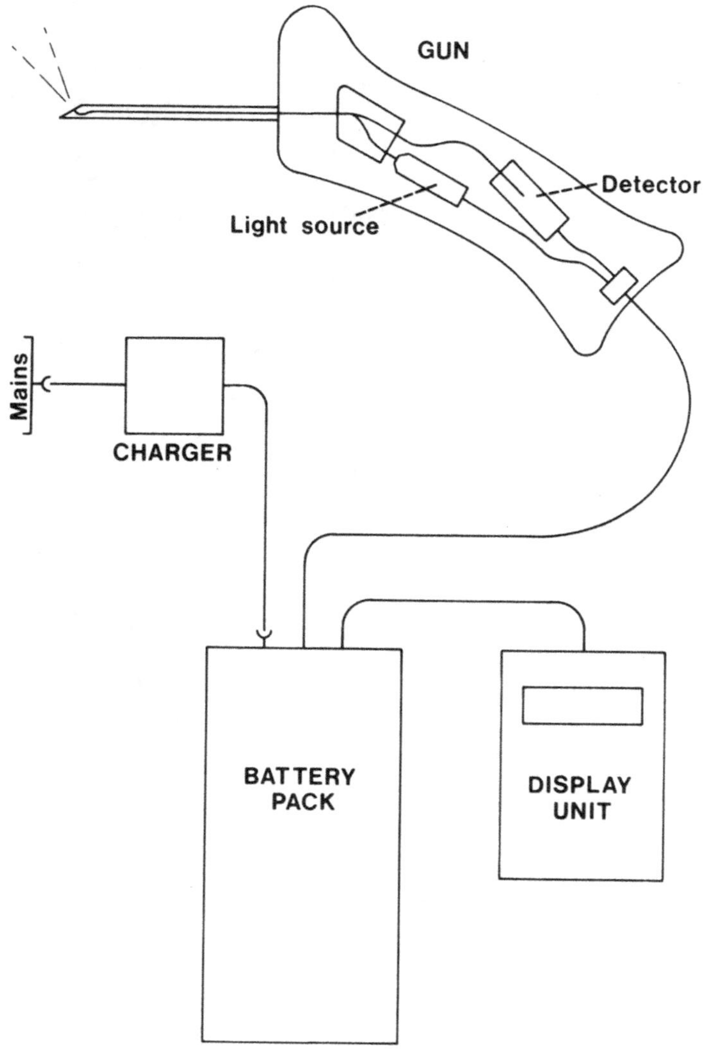

Fig. 2. Diagram of MRI fibre optic probe.

display. Calibration is by standardised blocks of translucent and semi-opaque white plastic. Light transmitted by a fibre-optic bundle illuminates the meat from the side of the tip and the intensity of returned light is a measure of scatter. Probe values were linearly related to $S\gamma$ for beef from dark-cutting through normal to pale and exudative (r = 0.93) (Figure 3). Eighty per cent of the dark-cutting samples with $S\gamma < 0.11$ had probe values of 20 or below. $K\gamma$ was not related to probe value but was related to pigment concentration (r = 0.74).

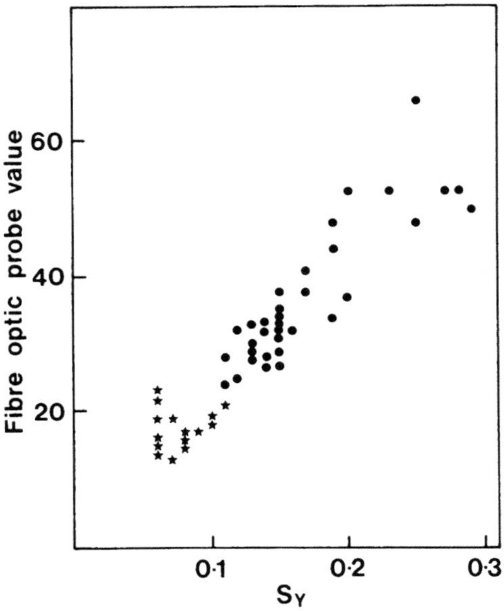

Fig. 3. Relationship of MRI fibre optic probe value to the luminous scatter coefficient, $S\gamma$, for fresh dark-cutting ($S\gamma < 0.11$), normal ($S\gamma$ 0.11 - 0.18) and pale ($S\gamma \geq 0.2$) beef.

● $pH_u \leq 5.9$, ★ $pH_u \geq 6.0$

Trials were conducted in commercial abattoirs to assess the potential of prototype instruments for detecting dark cutting meat. Approximately 1 000 carcasses of young bulls were measured over several months. Chilled sides were measured early on the morning of the day after slaughter, i.e. 16 to 22 h post-slaughter, which is insufficient time for attainment of pH_u but is the most likely time that carcasses would be assessed in a commercial operation. About 20 sides were measured on each visit. After measurement with the probe, the pH was measured using the same incision in each side. Per-cent frequency of probe-values for three pH ranges are shown in Figure 4. More than 80 per cent of those with pH of 6.1 and above had values of 20 or lower, less than 3 per cent with pH above 5.8 also had values of 20 or lower. Only one measurement had been taken on each side. The results indicate that this might be sufficient to designate carcasses with probe values below 18 as dark-cutting. However, clear decisions could not be made for carcasses with values between 18 and about 25, which is the transition stage between translucent and semi-opaque, and muscle must be measured at a second location, at least, for confirmation of the reading. Values obtained with the prototype in the survey have subsequently been shown to be less consistent than those obtained with the new model which has greatly improved electronic stability. A more effective selection of dark-cutting carcasses is possible with the new instrument, even considering the intrinsic variability in muscle of about 3 units. The extra time involved in making duplicate measurements is only a few seconds per carcass.

DISCUSSION

The most important objection to the sale of dark-cutting beef is that it is dark. Abnormal non-red colours are well known to cause rejection of pre-packaged meat if it is displayed in contrast to bright red meat (Hood and Riordan, 1973). Colour measurements of dark-cutting beef show that it is distinctly different from normal beef in all three psychological concepts of colour perception with the difference in saturation initially greater than the difference in lightness. It is not immediately apparent that the effect of a change in $S\gamma$ can be visually greater than a similar change in $K\gamma$. In the samples reported in this paper $K\gamma$ ranged from below 0.6 to above 0.7. $K\gamma$ of 0.6 is approximately equivalent to 3 mg/g myoglobin and $K\gamma$ of 0.7 to 5 mg/g. Calculated values of lightness show how relatively

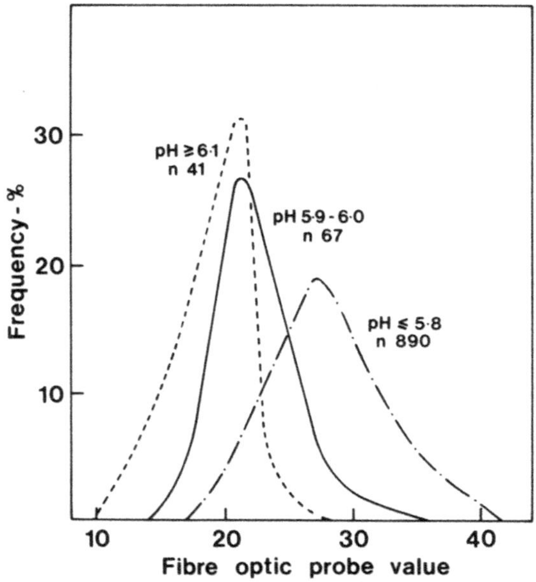

Fig. 4. Percent frequency curves of occurrence of fibre optic probe values in survey of young bull carcasses.

more important are the small changes in Sγ at the transition from translucent to opaque, compared to that produced by a large difference in pigment concentration (Table 1). A difference of 0.1 in Kγ produces a difference in L of 1.4 to 2.2 units, but a difference of only half that value in Sγ produces a difference of 7 units in L, as Sγ increases from 0.05 to 0.1 and progressively less on further increase of Sγ. In other words, the change in Sγ (0.05 to 0.1) from dark-cutting to normal has about five times the effect of a 2 mg/g change in myoglobin concentration, while the effect of the change in Sγ (< 0.2 to 0.25) from normal to pale is about twice.

TABLE 1

COMPARISON OF EFFECT OF CHANGE IN $S\gamma$ WITH CHANGE IN $K\gamma$ ON LIGHTNESS (L) IN BEEF

$S\gamma$	0.05	0.1	0.15	0.2	0.25
$K\gamma$					
0.6	19.7	26.8	31.8	35.6	38.8
0.7	18.3	25.0	30.0	33.5	36.6

Until now, selection for appropriate alternative utilisation of dark-cutting carcasses at the abattoir could be done only by visual appraisal, reflectance photometry or by using pH meters. Visual appraisal is difficult to standardise and like photometric measurements demands that the carcass be first quartered. Measurement of pH_u, although commonly used for research, cannot be condoned in commerce because of the risk of electrode breakage and contamination of the carcass with broken glass. The MRI fibre-optic probe obviates these difficulties and since it is a direct measure of the cause of darkness, or of paleness, it can be used as a quality control technique at all stages after chilling. With slight modification to make the tip flat for transmitting light through a plastic pouch, it could be used to detect vacuum-packed high pH_u meat without puncturing the pack and thus select out material that would be subject to bacterial spoilage.

ACKNOWLEDGEMENTS

The authors wish to thank Mr. R.W.R. York, Mr. M.W. Donnelly and the staff of the company specialising in fibre optics for their roles in the manufacture of the probe, Mr. J.M. Akers for conducting the survey and Mrs. A.B. Crossman for technical assistance.

REFERENCES

Bendall, J.R. and Taylor, A.A., 1972. Consumption of oxygen by the muscles of beef animals and related species II. Consumption of oxygen by *post-rigor* muscle. J. Sci. Fd. Agric., 23, 707-719.

Duchesne, H.E., 1978. The aetiology of dark-cutting beef. Ph. D. Thesis, University of Bristol.

Francis, F.J. and Clydesdale, F.M., 1975. Food colorimetry: theory and applications. AVI Publishing Company, Inc. Westport, Conneticut.

Hall, J.L., Latschar, C.E. and Mackintosh, D.L., 1944. Characteristics of dark-cutting beef. Survey and preliminary investigations. Kansas Agric. Exp. Stat. Tech. Bull., 58.

Hood, D.E. and Riordan, E.B., 1973. Discolouration in pre-packaged beef: measurement by reflectance spectrophotometry and shopper discrimination. J. Fd. Technol., 8, 333-343.

Judd, D.B. and Wyszecki, G., 1975. Color in business, science and industry. John Wiley and Sons, Inc. New York.

Lawrie, R.A., 1958. Physiological stress in relation to dark-cutting beef. J. Sci. Fd. Agric., 9, 721-727.

MacDougall, D.B., 1970. Characteristics of the appearance of meat I. The luminous absorption, scatter and internal transmittance of the lean of bacon manufactured from normal and pale pork. J. Sci. Fd. Agric., 21, 568-571.

MacDougall, D.B. and Rhodes, D.N., 1972. Characteristics of the appearance of meat III. Studies on the colour of meat from young bulls. J. Sci. Fd. Agric., 23, 637-647.

MacDougall, D.B. and Jones, S.J., 1975. The use of a fibre optic probe for the detection of pale pork. 21st European meeting of meat research workers, Berne, 113-115.

Taylor, A.A., Shaw, B.G. and MacDougall, D.B., 1980 - 81. Hot deboning beef with and without electrical stimulation. Meat Sci., 5, 109-123.

Wyszecki, G. and Stiles, W.S., 1967. Color science: concepts and methods, quantitative data and formulas. John Wiley and Sons, Inc., New York.

DISCUSSION

H. Ruderus *(Sweden)*

Have you tried to use laser light to measure the scattering effect?

D.B. MacDougall *(UK)*

I have not, but we use laser for measuring sarcomere length, but that is in very small samples. I cannot see it as a practical instrument for the abattoir but it is a very interesting point. There is literature from the States on measuring the scattering coefficient by laser light which came about 10 years after I had found the scatter values using monochromatic light within the normal spectral range. However, I have not tried it on meat.

H. Ruderus

Do you think it would be useful in the laboratory? I did not mean in the abattoir.

D.B. MacDougall

I am certain that the high intensity of the laser beam might well be helpful. It would give a measure of the direct transmittance if you set up the cell holder right and measured its divergence from direct linearity through the other side.

P.V. Tarrant *(Ireland)*

Dr. MacDougall, we are very interested indeed in the practical use of the instrument which you have developed. Can you make a comment on the effect of chilling rate on the result of a fibre optic probe measurement, particularly in relation to a hot deboning procedure?

D.B. MacDougall

We have reported on fibre optic profiles from hot deboning procedures. I gave an illustration earlier about the difference between the pale outer part of the adductor muscle and the dark inner part. The differences between these two are readily detected by the instrument, although they are at the pale end of the distribution rather than the dark one. Carcasses with low pH and high temperature are very readily distinguished by the probe. The original intention of making the probe was to detect differences in PSE but there has been more interest in the economic and practical aspects of detecting dark cutting meat. My interest is directed towards the last paper today. A meat processor may use the probe as a means of detecting a fault that cannot easily be seen. He then has the economic and moral responsibility of acting responsibly on that information. At the moment it is only the person who finally cuts up the carcass that has the problem. This does not apply to the United States' situation where the carcass is already quartered, but many carcasses in the UK or Europe are sold as complete carcasses or sides. It is only the person at the end of the chain - the supermarket or the retailer - who has to break it up and who discovers the fault. If this is put into the abattoir, then someone at the abattoir end will discover the fault and there may have to be some rearrangement of the logic of costing.

Patricia McGloughlin *(Ireland)*

I would like to ask a general question. Is there any agreed measurement of DFD in cattle, or in beef, that could be taken as a bench-mark against which all other instruments and techniques can be measured?

D.B. MacDougall

Earlier in the proceedings I was very happy to hear from Dr. Tarrant the break down and the logic of ultimate pH from more than 6.3, 6.0 - 6.3, 5.8 - 6.0 and less than 5.8 as an arbitrator. This is also the case with the probe. If you had to make an ultimate decision on it, it would be done by a second method: either the pH to the probe, or the probe to pH. Far better to use two methods, whose agreement you know, than to use one twice.

D.E. Hood *(Ireland)*

It also depends on the category of beef that you are dealing with. This is the difficulty; a pH of 6.2 is perhaps not particularly significant with cows, but it would be with steers or bulls.

D.B. MacDougall

I forgot to mention this, but I could see a similar instrument with a flat head being used for detecting low light scatter beef inside a vacuum pack, provided that you put the end against a portion of the muscle that had no fat interface between it and the film. The only thing that is required is to recalibrate the instrument, taking account of the extra distance between the tip and the sample because of the film. This could become a rapid way of screening out those high ultimate pH samples from vacuum packed meat, particularly if hot deboning and vacuum packing becomes a normal practice so that the material is in the pack before any pH measurement is made on it. It would be a way of screening out all those that are suspect without damaging the package.

D.E. Hood

Would you increase the size of the tip?

D.B. MacDougall

Yes, it should not be too difficult to redesign a handle with a wider tip.

Before we finish, I would like to make one plea. There has been a great deal of interest expressed by several people here over a period of time. The company who made the original fibre part in conjunction with the MRI is no longer in operation. However, the personnel who were involved with the operation have now formed their own small company to make fibre optic instruments. They will start making the instrument if there is enough genuine interest in it. Now I am not here to ask you to buy - I am not trying to sell it - but if you would like to write to me perhaps that would give some indication of the interest in this project. It may get off the ground - otherwise it has got to a stage where I might abandon it. By the way, the price is estimated at about £1 000. That is very cheap considering the optical components that are in optical instruments (I don't have any shares in the company)!

EATING QUALITY OF DFD BEEF

E. Dransfield
Meat Research Institute, Langford, Bristol, BS18 7DY, UK.

ABSTRACT

Eating quality of DFD beef has been studied using chemical, instrumental, sensory and consumer tests.

Laboratory tests have shown that DFD beef is markedly more tender than beef of normal pH. The relationship between tenderness and pH depends upon the muscle, the cooking conditions and the method of assessment.

DFD beef had less beef flavour and consequently was less preferred and less acceptable than meat of normal pH. It was found that pH had little influence on juiciness.

Eating quality of beef is notoriously variable, resulting from a wide range of production factors. In general, therefore, the use of ultimate pH alone would be a poor indicator of eating quality.

INTRODUCTION

Overall quality of beef comprises a complex judgement based on its appearance, cooking and eating characteristics. Eating quality, judged as tenderness, juiciness and flavour, is affected by many production factors and by variations in rigor development and proteolysis of the meat. Factors affecting eating quality have been well reviewed (Lawrie, 1979; Patterson, 1974).

After slaughter, ATP is consumed in an attempt to maintain cellular integrity and, for a while, is regenerated by anaerobic glycolysis with the accompanying production of lactic acid, ultimately from glycogen. The rate of *post mortem* glycolysis increases below 15°C as the muscle is stimulated to contract. Such contraction, known as cold shortening, has a major influence on toughness. When the glycogen reserve is reduced prior to slaughter, little or no lactate can be produced resulting in high ultimate pH. Variations in pH affect protein hydration and water holding capacity of the meat which could affect toughness and juiciness. Endogenous enzymes damage the myofibrillar proteins in the early *post mortem* period. Proteolysis in the region of the Z disc is thought to be mainly responsible for tenderising during *post mortem* storage and general proteolysis for flavour development in the lean. Enzyme activity is dependent mainly on pH and temperature.

In this paper, the relationships between tenderness, juiciness and flavour and ultimate pH are described and examined, where possible in terms of water binding, proteolysis and the generation of flavour precursors.

TENDERNESS

Tenderness of meat depends mainly on variations in myofibrillar proteins, connective tissue proteins and water and their interactions with cooking conditions. In studying tenderness, in particular, various methods have been employed to alter pH and hence water binding capacity. Altering pH by *post mortem* injections of lactic acid or ammonia into meat (Winkler, 1939) gave minimum tenderness at pH 6 and pre-slaughter injections of epinephrine and/or iodoacetate (Penny et al., 1963) increased ultimate pH and tenderness. More recently, increases in tenderness associated with high ultimate pH have been shown in beef (Fredeen et al., 1974), venison (MacDougall et al., 1979), rabbit (Miles and Lawrie, 1970) and mutton (Bouton et al., 1971). In beef and venison *M. semitendinosus* heated to 80° and in venison *M. semimembranosus* (MacDougall et al., 1979) heated to 75°C, toughness decreased linearly with increasing pH (Figure 1). However, the relationship varies between muscles and the cooking conditions. In mutton, minimum tenderness values were found at pH 5.6, 5.9 and 6.1 for *M. biceps femoris*, *M. semitendinosus* and *M. longissimus dorsi*, respectively (Bouton and Shorthose, 1969) and for beef, topside roast, sirloin roast and grilled rump, minimum tenderness occurred in the pH range 5.8 to 6.1 (Bouton et al., 1957). Cooking mutton at 65°C produced minimum tenderness at pH 5.9 in *M. semimembranosus* and *M. biceps femoris* but a linear relation when cooked at 90°. Within muscle, toughness was highly correlated with cooking losses and water holding capacity determined by centrifugation (Bouton et al., 1971). In DFD meat, the moisture content after cooking produces a more open structure and more tender meat, although the shear strength of raw DFD meat is unaffected by pH (Figure 1).

The extent of tenderising in high pH meat is also dependent on the degree of muscle shortening and ageing. At high pH, pre-*rigor* stretching or *post mortem* ageing have no effect on tenderness (Bouton et al., 1973).

Enzyme inactivation in beef after slaughter will arrest glycolysis and also result in high pH meat. High pH may be obtained in this way by cooking meat rapidly soon after stunning, but this also causes contraction and toughness. After removing the contribution due to shortening, the remaining toughness is related to pH, with maximum toughness occurring at pH 5.9 in *M. semitendinosus* as in DFD meat (Dransfield and Rhodes, 1975). The toughness due to muscle shortening, therefore, may be offset by high pH.

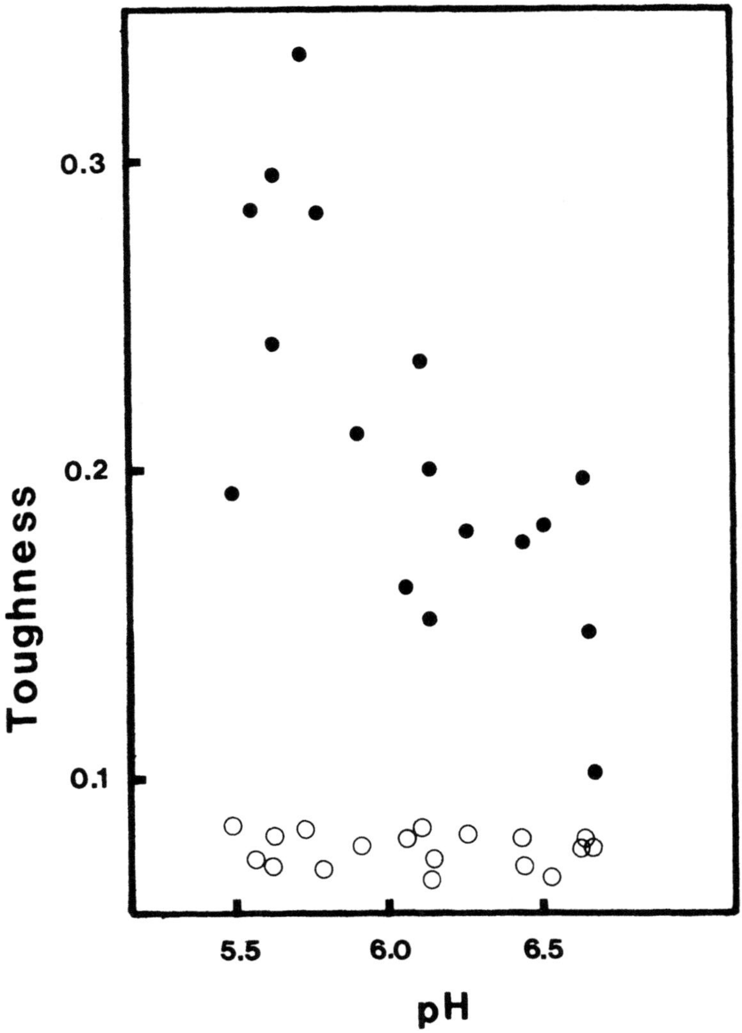

Fig.1. Relationship between toughness and pH.
Toughness was measured instrumentally raw (open circles) and cooked (closed circles) on *M. semitendinosus* from bulls.
pH values are those of the raw muscle.

Many factors other than pH affect tenderness. Chilling pre-*rigor* meat below 10°C within 10 h of slaughter induces muscle shortening and severe toughness (called 'cold shortening' toughness) and, in the carcass, *M. longissimus dorsi* is particularly susceptible. Storage (ageing) of beef causes a progressive tenderising over 3 weeks at chill temperatures. However, even under slow cooling conditions followed by storage for 7 days, wide variations in tenderness of LD occur (Figure 2). With wider variations in cooling and storage conditioning pertaining to commerce, pH alone would be a poor indicator of tenderness.

Most laboratory studies, like those discussed above, are confined to a few muscles and to direct 'side-by-side' comparisons using experienced tasters. To assess consumer reactions, meat from grilling, frying, roasting and casserole cuts were given to consumers to eat as part of their normal meal. Half of the consumers were given DFD and half control beef, and about one week later the tests were repeated using control and DFD beef respectively. The results of such trials (expressed as differences between treatments) are given in Table 1. Normal pH steer beef was assessed equal in tenderness to DFD bull beef (1st trial) and marginally (0.2 points on a 14 point scale) tougher than normal pH bull beef (2nd trial) suggesting that DFD meat is, on average, only marginally more tender than normal pH.

Tenderising during storage (ageing) is related to proteolysis (Penny and Dransfield, 1979). Overall proteolytic activity, measured by the production of amino nitrogen, in beef homogenates was highest at pH 3.5 and showed little activity about pH 7.0 (Drabikowski et al., 1977). It might be anticipated, therefore, that the rate of tenderising during storage in DFD beef would be less than in normal pH beef, but no such observations have been reported.

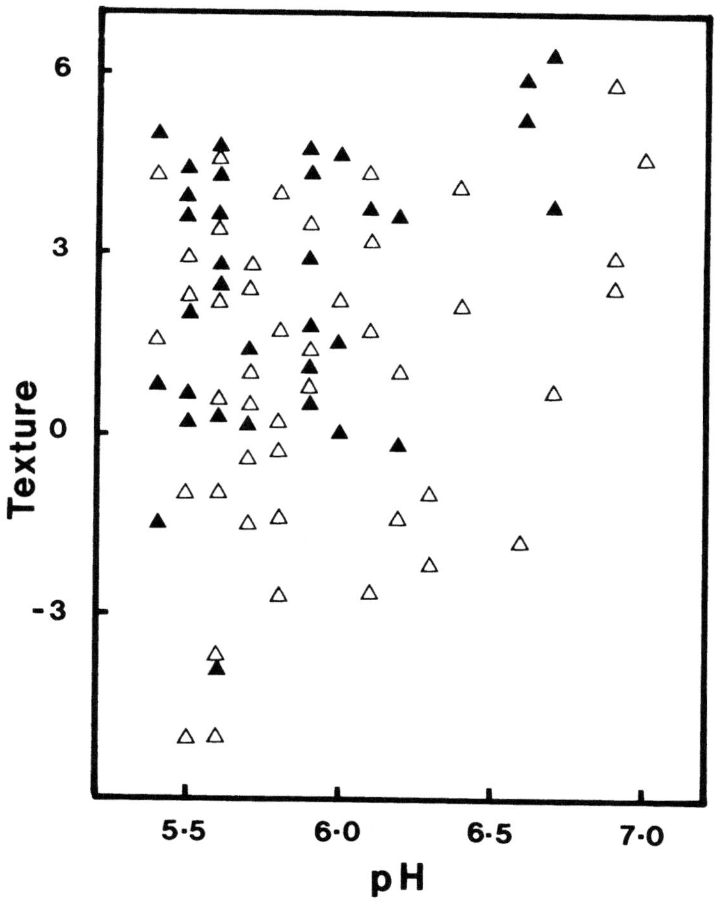

Fig.2. Relationship between tenderness and pH.
Tenderness of roast *M. longissimus dorsi* was assessed by experienced staff of the institute on a scale: extremely tough (-7) to extremely tender (7). Shaded triangles are results for steer beef and open triangles those of bull beef. pH values are those of raw muscle.

TABLE 1

CONSUMER ASSESSMENTS OF EATING QUALITY OF DARK-CUTTING BEEF

Cooking method	Number of tasters	Flavour	Juiciness	Texture
Dark-cutting trial				
Grill/fry	153	-0.2*	-0.0	-0.0
Roast	218	-0.1	-0.2*	-0.4
Casserole	27	-0.1	-0.0	1.0
All	398	-0.1**	-0.1	-0.2
Normal pH trial				
Grill/fry	91	0.1	0.0	-0.3
Roast	439	-0.1	0.0	-0.3
Casserole	55	-0.1	-0.2	-0.2
Stew	21	0.4	0.4	1.0
All	606	-0.0	0.0	-0.2**

Consumers in SW England were asked to cook joints and steaks in their usual way and assess them for flavour on a scale: not satisfactory (1), poor (2), good (3), and excellent (4); juiciness on a scale: dry (1), slightly juicy (2), moderately juicy (3) and very juicy (4); texture on a scale: very tough (-5), moderately tough (-3), slightly tough (-1), slightly tender (1), moderately tender (3) and very tender (5). Values are average differences (bull-steer) for 16 animals in dark-cutting trial (pH 5.5 - 6.8) and 8 animals in normal pH trial (5.5 - 5.7).

* $P \nless 0.05$; ** $P < 0.01$

JUICINESS

Although juiciness may be described as two organoleptic components - an initial impression of wetness during the first few chews and sustained juiciness appreciated during mastication and salivation - such a distinction has not been made in studying DFD beef.

Studies at MRI showed that juiciness of roast *M. longissimus dorsi* tended to increase with increase in pH in steer beef but not in bull beef (Figure 3). In steer beef, juiciness is increased, on average, 1 point (of a 5 point scale) from pH 5.5 to 7.0, whilst the variation between animals of similar pH was 1 - 2 points (Figure 3).

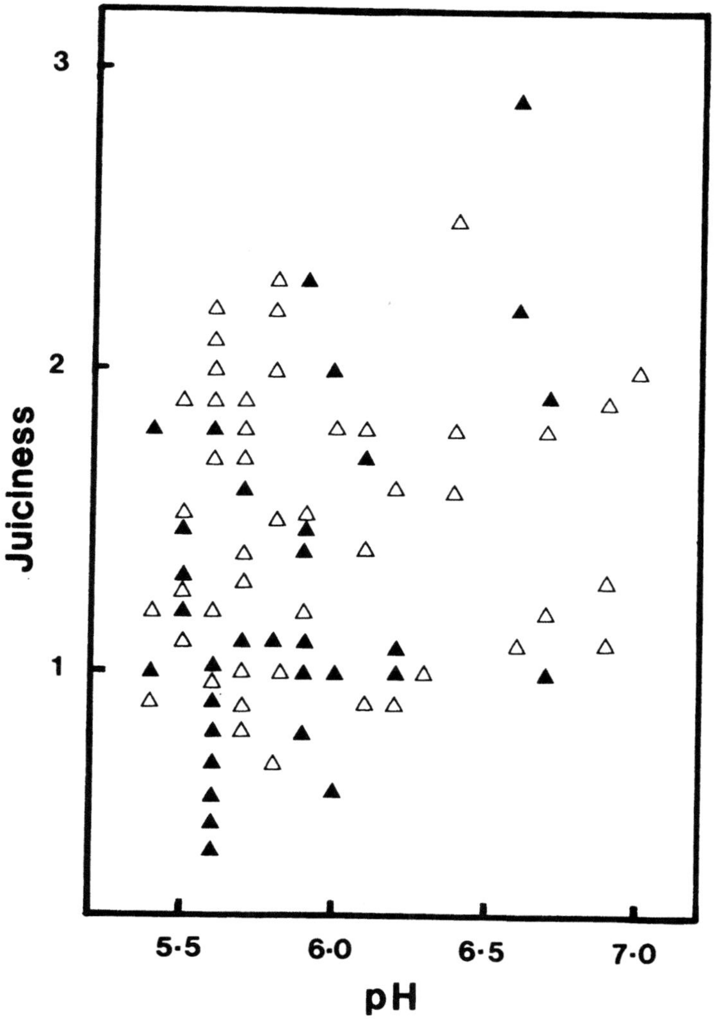

Fig.3. Relationship between juiciness and pH.
Juiciness of roast *M. longissimus dorsi* was assessed by experienced staff of the institute on a scale: dry (0) to extremely juicy (4). Shaded triangles are the results of steer beef and open triangles those of bull beef. pH values are those of raw muscle.

As part of the EEC beef co-ordination programme, quality assessments have been compared between 5 institutes, each using their standard methods for grilled sirloin steaks. Part of these results are reported here in relation to pH (Table 2). Juiciness of steaks was not significantly related to pH in any of the five laboratories (Table 2).

TABLE 2

RELATIONSHIP BETWEEN pH AND FLAVOUR AND JUICINESS IN STEAKS GRILLED ACCORDING TO REGIONAL PREFERENCE

Cooking	Number of tasters	Institute	Correlation coefficients: pH against	
			Flavour intensity	Juiciness
75° centre	14	Langford	- 0.6**	- 0.0
70° centre	10	Dublin	- 0.4	- 0.1
170° for 10 min	9	Roskilde	- 0.2	- 0.1
Contact grill 6 min	6	Kulmbach	0.1	0.0
50° centre	12	Theix	- 0.6**	0.3

Steaks of *M. longissimus dorsi* from 20 animals whose pH ranged from 5.8 to 6.8 were assessed using standard methods at five institutes. The work formed part of an eating quality co-ordination programme with the EEC and was funded by the Commission of the European Communities. A full report will be published

** $P < 0.01$

In consumer trials (Table 1) in England, bull beef of normal pH was equal in juiciness to steer beef of normal pH (2nd trial) and, overall, DFD bull beef and normal pH steer beef were equally juicy (1st trial). In roasting joints only, DFD bull beef was slightly drier than steer beef of normal pH (2nd trial).

The pH did not affect juiciness in roast and grilled beef joints (Bouton et al., 1957), in beef muscles (Bouton et al., 1973), nor in roast venison (MacDougall et al., 1979). However, in thawed beef, Penny et al. (1963) showed that fresh and dehydrated high pH beef were ranked more juicy than normal pH beef

FLAVOUR

With the lack of intrumentation to measure flavour, studies are confined to subjective assessments which are more open to interpretation. Flavour of cooked beef, referred to here, is a general term combining taste and odour, assessed by using hedonic, intensity and acceptability scales. In contrast to studies on tenderness, little work has been reported on the influence of pH on flavour.

Flavour of roast *M. longissimus dorsi* tended to be disliked more as pH increased in steer beef, although there was no noticeable effect in bull beef (Figure 4). There were wide variations in flavour scores at all pHs and, on average, flavour scores fell only 3 points of the 14 point scale when the pH was raised from pH 5.5 to 7.0. Similar tests on roast venison *M. semimembranosus* showed no significant relationship between pH and panel mean hedonic flavour scores (MacDougall et al., 1979).

However, averaging hedonic scores may obscure differing trends between panellists because of their individual preferences. Panellists who tested normal and DFD beef were therefore considered individually. Of the nine panellists (who tasted between 22 and 44 samples) eight tended to dislike the flavour of DFD meat, although only four showed significant trends (Table 3). At best (panellist 1) variations in pH accounted for half the variation in flavour scores. The dislike for flavour of DFD meat was not associated with the sex or age of the panellist. Using flavour intensity scales on grilled beef at MRI showed that there was less beef flavour in DFD meat (Table 2) and undoubtedly explains its general dislike. Bouton et al. (1957) also found a similar trend, although only five values above pH 6 were reported.

Comparison of results in five laboratories (Table 2) showed that the relationship between pH and flavour intensity was similar in Theix and Langford despite wide differences in their normal cooking methods. Relationship of pH and flavour intensity were

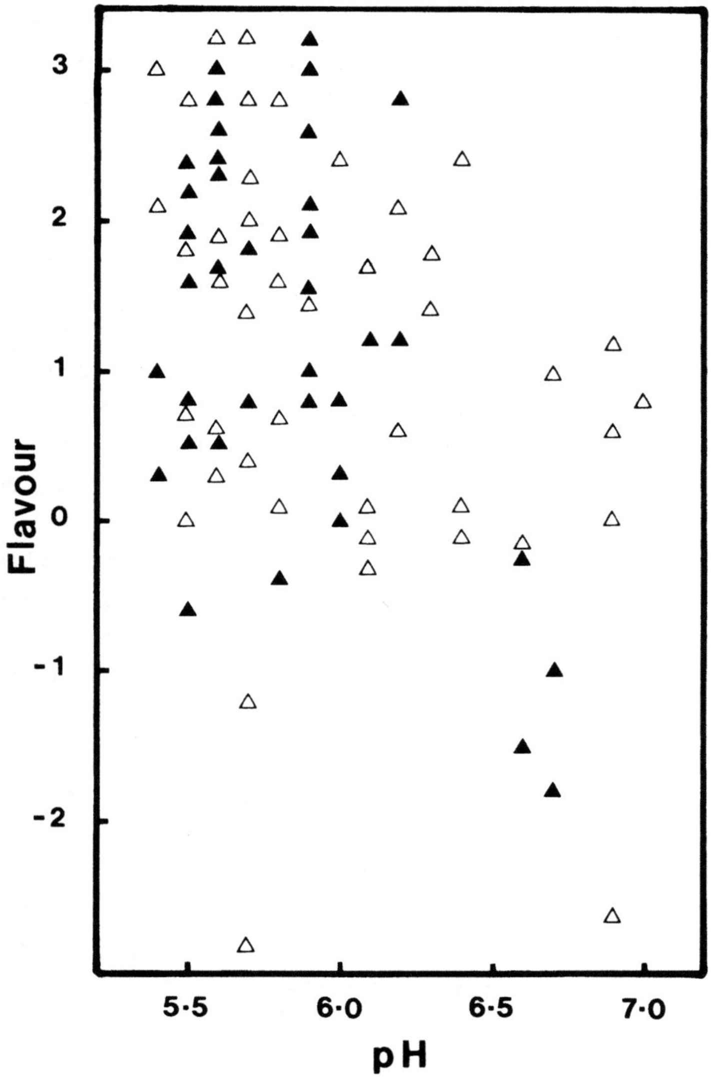

Fig.4. Relationship between flavour and pH.
Flavour of roast *M. longissimus dorsi* was assessed by experienced staff of the institute on a scale: dislike extremely (-7) to like extremely (7). Shaded triangles are results of steer beef and open triangles those of bull beef. pH values are those of raw muscle.

not signficantly related when assessed in Dublin and Roskilde but correlation coefficients were again negative. The results suggest that regional differences exist and more comparisons of this type would be valuable.

TABLE 3

INTERACTION BETWEEN FLAVOUR ACCEPTABILITY AND pH OF BEEF

Panellist	n	Range of flavour score	Correlation coefficient
1	28	-7 to 5	-0.75***
2(F)	40	-3 to 5	-0.49**
3	32	-3 to 5	-0.46**
4	44	-3 to 5	-0.36*
5(F)	26	-3 to 3	-0.21
6	22	-3 to 3	-0.18
7	28	-1 to 3	-0.04
8	38	-5 to 5	-0.01
9(F)	26	-5 to 3	0.17

Samples of loin in which *M. longissimus dorsi* ranged from pH 5.4 to 6.7 were roasted and flavour assessed on a scale: dislike extremely (subsequently scored -7), dislike very much (-5), dislike moderately (-3), dislike slightly (-1), like slightly (1), like moderately (3), like very much (5), like extremely (7). Panellists' assessments were correlated with pH of the raw meat.
(F) - female; * $P < 0.05$; ** $P < 0.01$; *** $P < 0.001$

The acceptability of flavour of DFD beef was assessed from consumer trials carried out in England (Table 1). The first trial compared DFD bull beef with steer beef of normal pH and estimated the effect of pH alone; the results of a second trial, comparing bull and steer beef of normal pH, are included. With normal pH (2nd trial), flavour was equally acceptable in bull and steer beef, but DFD bull beef (1st trial) had a poorer flavour. The overall effect of pH was small - only 0.1 points on a 4 point scale.

Summarising: beef of normal pH was more acceptable than DFD beef because people, in general, preferred stronger beef flavour.

Lawrie (1979) suggested that the lower flavour might result from the swollen structures of high pH beef interfering with the access of the palate to flavour substances. A similar phenomenon had been noted in bacon (Ingram, 1949) where normal pH muscles had more 'free' (unbound) saline available for taste than at high pH where the water was bound and the salt unavailable for taste. However, although this phenomenon may play some role in reducing the flavour of DFD beef, it is not the complete cause since steam volatiles from lamb and beef at pH 6.0 are different from those at pH 5.5 - 5.8 (Park and Murray, 1975).

It seems likely that weak flavour results from the lack (or very low level) of carbohydrate expected in meat of high ultimate pH, producing little interaction with amino acids or proteins. In meat of normal pH, those interactions are mostly responsible for the development of odour and flavour (Patterson, 1974). Sugar and sugar phosphates, isolated from meat at normal pH, include fructose, fructose-6-phosphate, fructose-1, 6-diphosphate, glucose-6-phosphate, ribose and ribose-5-phosphate (Jarboe and Mabrouk, 1974). Levels of carbohydrate in meat are reduced on heating, and heating *in vitro* produces meaty odour by Maillard reactions with amino acids which form the base of some patents for meat flavour.

REFERENCES

Bouton, P.E., Carroll, F.D., Fisher, A.L., Harris, P.V. and Shorthose, W.R., 1973. Effect of altering ultimate pH on bovine muscle tenderness. J. Fd. Sci., 38, 816-820.

Bouton, P.E., Harris, P.V. and Shorthose, W.R., 1971. Effect of ultimate pH upon the water holding capacity and tenderness of mutton. J. Fd. Sci., 36, 435-439.

Bouton, P.E., Howard, A. and Lawrie, R.A., 1957. Studies on beef quality: Part VI: Effects on weight losses and eating quality of further pre-slaughter treatments. Spec. Rept. Fd. Invest. Bd. Lond., No. 66.

Bouton, P.E. and Shorthose, W.R., 1969. Correlations between ultimate pH and some quality traits of sheep meat. Proc. 15th European Meeting of Meat Research Workers, Helsinki, 78-83.

Drabikowski, W., Gorecka, A. and Jakubeic-Puka, A., 1977. Endogenous proteinases in vertebrate skeletal muscle. Inst. J. Biochem., 8, 61-71.

Dransfield, E. and Rhodes, D.N., 1975. Texture of beef *M. semitendinosus* heated before, during and after development of rigor mortis. J. Sci. Fd. Agric., 26, 483-491.

Fredeen, H.T., Martin, A.H. and Weiss, G.M., 1974. Changes in tenderness of beef *M. longissimus dorsi* as related to muscle colour and pH. J. Fd. Sci., 39, 532-536.

Ingram, M., 1949. Salt flavour in bacon. J. Soc. Chem. Ind., 68, 356-359.

Jarboe, J.K. and Mabrouk, A.F., 1974. Free amino acids, sugars and organic acids in aqueous beef extracts. J. Agric. Fd. Chem., 22, 787-791.

Lawrie, R.A., 1979. In: Mean Science, Pergamon Press, Oxford, 3rd Ed. p.359.

MacDougall, D.B., Shaw, B.G., Nute, G.R. and Rhodes, D.N., 1979. Effect of pre-slaughter handling on the quality and microbiology of venison from farmed young red deer. J. Sci. Fd. Agric., 30, 1160-1167.

Miles, C.L. and Lawrie, R.A., 1970. Relation between pH and tenderness in cooked muscle. J. Fd. Technol., 5, 325-330.

Park, R.J. and Murray, K.E., 1975. Meat Res. in CSIRO, p22.

Patterson, R.S.L., 1974. The flavour of meat. Meat: Proc. Univ. Nottingham, 21st Easter School in Agricultural Science. D.J.A. Cole and R.A. Lawrie, Eds., London, Butterworths, 1975 p.359-379.

Penny, I.F. and Dransfield, E., 1979. Relationship between toughness and troponin T in conditioned beef. Meat Sci., 3, 135-141.

Penny, I.F., Voyle, C.A. and Lawrie, R.A., 1963. A comparison of freeze-dried beef muscles of high or low ultimate pH. J. Sci. Fd. Agric., 14, 535-543.

Winkler, C.A., 1939. Tenderness of meat. I: A recording apparatus for its estimation and relationship between pH and tenderness. Can. J. Res., 17D:8.

DISCUSSION

E. Puolanne *(Finland)*

At what time after slaughter did you make these experiments? We found different results one day after slaughter and one week and so on.

E. Dransfield *(UK)*

Normally at 7 days, which is an average of British practice. Meat was stored for 7 days and then tasted in the laboratory and in the consumer trials.

G. Monin *(France)*

What was the range of pH in the experiment between different institutes in the EEC?

E. Dransfield

It was 5.5 to 6.8 in *M. longissimus dorsi*.

C.L. Davey *(New Zealand)*

I was always under the impression that if you trim meat it is very difficult to distinguish between species as far as flavour is concerned. In fact it is very difficult to identify any flavour at all. In other words, most of the flavour comes from the fat. Under those circumstances you would not expect any flavour variation with meat ultimate pH because this is not affecting the pH in the fat.

E. Dransfield

I think that both the lean and the fat are recognised as contributing to the flavour. Fat is said to be mainly responsible for species differences and the lean for quantitative differences within species. When I say flavour, all of these experiments refer to the normal eating situation. Experiments have been done to distinguish between odour and taste. Most of the flavour differences, due to dark-cutting, would also affect odour as well.

H. Ruderus *(Sweden)*

I think it is surprising that you found so little difference in flavour. Were the samples prepared so that they had a 'frying crust', or were they just 'heated meat'?

E. Dransfield

Normal laboratory data refers to roast *M. longissimus dorsi*. The EEC studies were done on grilled steaks. The consumer trials were done on a whole range of muscles cooked to the requirements of the consumer - therefore we know little about the cooking in those situations.

H. Ruderus

You get very little Maillard reaction in this DFD meat, which I suppose should influence the flavour scores.

E. Dransfield

If the Maillard reaction is involved then it is coming from the high temperatures in the outside of the meat.

G. van Logtestijn *(The Netherlands)*

I wonder if we are justified in speaking of the tenderness of DFD meat in total, because we have to distinguish between the role of collagen and contractile proteins.

E. Dransfield

In all the subjective trials it is an overall tenderness assessment. I presented two illustrations: one showed that if you use the same muscle, under exactly the same conditions, there is a large effect of pH. It is about the equivalent of age in beef - unaged and aged beef, it is that size. However, if you let all the other production factors come into the experiment, then there is very little relationship between a pH measurement and tenderness. All the other factors, rapid chilling, variations in ageing and connective tissue then override the effect due to pH.

PRACTICAL ASPECTS OF THE USE OF DARK FIRM DRY (DFD) MEAT

J. Sornay[1], B.L. Dumont[2] and Jeanne Fournaud[2]

[1] Institut Technique d'Elevage Bovin (ITEB), 149 Rue de Bercy, 75579 Paris Cedex 12

[2] Laboratoire de Recherches sur la Viande de l'INRA, CNRZ, 78350 Jouy-en-Josas, France

ABSTRACT

From a practical point of view DFD carcasses cause problems for the packer, on the one hand through financial loss and on the other by causing serious difficulties in day-to-day management of the company. The expression 'DFD' covers a wide range of meats with variable characteristics. For the user different questions are not yet fully answered:

- *the choice of an adequately discriminating criterion which will allow the detection of DFD carcasses as soon as possible after slaughter*
- *the choice of an adequate method of measurement or visual assessment*
- *the choice of location on the carcass where measurement or observation should be applied.*

To answer these questions and to have a better understanding of the biochemical mechanisms involved in the DFD condition, a number of fundamental studies remain to be done.

In general, packers do not take adequate account of the risk of encountering DFD in normal management practice so that on the one hand preventive measures can be adopted and on the other adequate outlets can be provided for DFD carcasses. The paper considers what these outlets might be and examines the problems of utilisation of DFD beef.

INTRODUCTION

In this article we consider the characteristics of DFD meat from the point of view of the meat packer, drawing attention to its major defects which lead on the one hand to serious financial loss and on the other to difficulties in processing.

A COSTLY PROBLEM IN THE BEEF CHAIN

The term DFD is relatively new but the phenomenon itself has been known in many countries for a long time. In the last few years the problem has become more acute and this is probably linked, at least in Europe, to changes which have taken place in rearing systems for beef (particularly the production of young bulls by intensive systems) and in economic and technical structures, particularly those concerned with packing and distribution (concentration of slaughterhouses, development of supermarkets, packaging of fresh meat etc.).

The phenomenon of DFD is worrying to meat packers because of the unacceptably high percentage of affected carcasses. In France many slaughterers acknowledge that the incidence of DFD carcasses is on average 3 - 4 per cent of their cattle throughput. These rates may go up to about 10 per cent where the cattle slaughtered are young bulls and in any case there is considerable variation from one abattoir to another (see Figure 1). The observed rate also depends on the criteria used to define DFD meat. The incidence of carcasses classified as DFD may differ significantly depending on whether assessment is based on visual judgement or on pH measurement.

A DFD carcass will be depreciated more or less depending on the particular conditions of a company, but we estimate that the financial loss is on average from 25 - 30 per cent of the value of a normal carcass.

Finally the problem has further economic consequences, the effects of which depend on who bears the major part of the financial responsibility i.e. the feeder, the slaughterer or the packer.

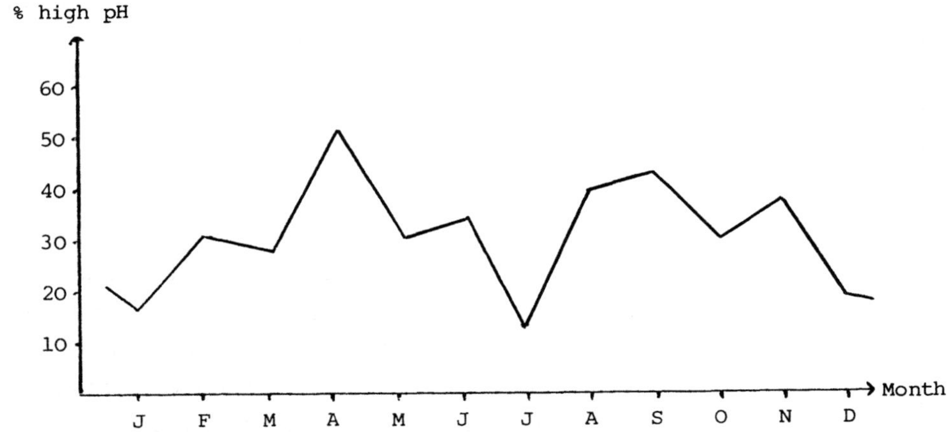

Fig. 1. Percentage of high pH carcasses (pH > 5.9) for a sample of 1 480 young bulls in a French abattoir during 1977.

Average per cent of carcasses with high pH for the total year: 31.5%

(ITEB)

DFD MEAT HAS A RANGE OF CHARACTERISTICS

The designation 'DFD' cannot be applied to a specific product with precisely defined characteristics which distinguish it clearly from normal meat. From a practical point of view, meat is considered to be DFD when certain abnormal characteristics occur which can be seen or easily measured, or both.

Between meat which is obviously DFD (very dark colour, firm consistency and a sticky surface on the cut muscle) and so-called normal meat, there is a wide range of intermediate stages of the condition. Under certain circumstances meat which is considered to be DFD may even have a normal colour.

The characteristics which distinguish DFD meat are themselves due to abnormal values of certain physico-chemical parameters whose biochemical mechanisms are now beginning to be understood. These are high ultimate pH, low glucose concentration and high water-holding capacity.

DIFFICULTY OF USING DFD MEAT

The abnormal characteristics of DFD meat make it more difficult to use than normal meat.

The dark colour of DFD meat makes it less attractive to the consumer who is apt to confuse the colour with that of very old animals or with meat which has been badly stored.

The sticky character of DFD meat, for which an objective method of measurement remains to be found, not only makes it less acceptable but also makes the preparation of the muscles more difficult i.e. cutting, trimming, preparation into portions for retail sale etc.

The high water-holding capacity of DFD meat results from its high ultimate pH; this can be an advantage at the practical level. As fresh meat it is subject to less weight loss during storage and cooking. In the case of processing i.e. curing and cooked meat products, high water-holding capacity is a particular advantage. In this respect DFD meat is similar to freshly slaughtered meat. This advantage disappears when DFD meat is used for dry sausage.

ABNORMAL BACTERIAL CHARACTERISTICS

During the storage of fresh DFD meat, undesirable odours and green discolourations may develop very rapidly. Bacterial growth is enhanced and the metabolism altered in such a way that there is a more direct attack on muscle proteins with the development of unpleasant odours. In the case of vacuum-packaging all bacterial flora develop at the same time, without the usual inhibition of specific types. It should be noted that there is a lack of comparative work on oxygen utilisation between DFD and normal meat under vacuum; were oxygen more readily available in vacuum-packaged DFD meat it could lead to abnormal development of aerobic bacteria, such as *Pseudomonas*. Similarly there has been little work done on the migration of micro-organisms in the deep tissues of muscle during storage.

It should also be stressed that the DFD characteristic in itself presents no danger to the consumer.

PRACTICAL LIMITATIONS OF STORAGE

As long as it remains whole or quartered, a DFD carcass does not present any particular problems during storage since under these conditions there should be few micro-organisms in the deep tissues. It is, therefore, recommended that DFD carcasses should not be jointed too quickly. Removal of the subcutaneous fat during preparation of the carcasses in the abattoir should be avoided since it constitutes a natural protection for the underlying muscle tissues.

After de-boning, the DFD muscle exposed to the air will not keep more than one day at most and even less if it is cut. When vacuum-packed in a highly impermeable bag and kept at a strict temperature of 0 to +2°C the meat will keep for a week at most, provided the initial contamination is low.

PROBLEMS OF CENTRAL PACKAGING

Modern meat trading (packaging industry/supermarkets) is much less suitable than the traditional butcher's shop for disposing of DFD meat because of the new techniques involved (early de-boning after slaughtering, packaging for long-term storage, prepackaging for retail sale etc.).

THE PROBLEM OF DIAGNOSIS

A major problem for the wholesaler is the ability to determine DFD carcasses with reliability soon after slaughter.

Although there is general agreement about the definition of DFD meat, in practice the parameters which characterise it are far from homogeneous.

In order to diagnose the DFD condition it is necessary to use one or more of the parameters which together characterise the condition: colour, pH, water-holding capacity, glucose concentration, sticky surface, bacterial growth, microfloral composition and consistency of the meat.

The inter-relationships which exist between some of these characteristics, notably between pH, colour and water-holding capacity, have already been extensively studied. In practice it is possible to say that correlation coefficients are not high. Correlations of -0.52 and -0.44 illustrate the poor relationship observed respectively between pH and loose water, and between pH and reflectance on a sample of 20 young bulls slaughtered under similar conditions (Sornay, unpublished results).

Inter-relationships between other characteristics are not well known. With regard to bacterial growth and storage potential it is not known how long is required to reach a contamination of 10^7 or 10^8 micro-organisms/cm^2 over a range of pH's and low temperatures. Observations have been made using artificial media in model systems but results on meat *per se* are lacking.

Similarly, little is known about the relationship between glucose concentration and the DFD condition. Newton and Gill (1980) have observed that glucose is always absent from 'suspected DFD' meat when the pH is greater than pH 6.4 and, to a lesser extent, even down to pH 6.0. The question then arises as to whether glucose concentration is the significant parameter to be measured in order to define DFD meat. If so, what is the critical threshold and the distribution of glucose among the important beef muscles? These questions have not been answered at the present time.

It seems worthwhile and a matter of some urgency to study further these inter-relationships, particularly those between glucose concentration, storage life and pH. However, until more information is available the wholesaler is likely to choose the descriptive criterion for DFD meat which will fit his particular working conditions. Thus the traditional butcher will continue to pay particular attention to the colour of the meat whilst others who are more concerned with long-term storage will measure pH.

From a practical point of view, measurement of pH is an appropriate method in most cases. Although relatively simple, it has the disadvantage that it only gives an answer to the wholesaler at 20 - 24 hours *post mortem*, which is the time necessary to reach the ultimate pH in beef. However, it must be remembered that any pH chosen to define DFD, such as pH > 6.0, is an arbitrary index which does not give absolute security. Mistakes can still be made which have serious economic consequences, such as accepting carcasses with close to normal pH which are in fact DFD. Another difficulty is that pH measurements may be unreliable because they are taken by non-specialised staff in the slaughterhouses.

Whatever descriptive criteria are chosen by the wholesaler, problems still remain as to where to measure pH or to observe colour. Distribution patterns of pH and colour are required for all muscles in the carcass to establish both inter- and intra-muscle incidence of the DFD condition. Some information is available on the distribution of pH throughout the carcass and more studies are in progress on this topic but as far as other parameters are concerned, such as glucose, much remains to be done. To avoid making mistakes about colour, ideally it is necessary to observe a number of cut muscles in the carcass, but this involves jointing which is precisely what must be avoided in the case of DFD carcasses.

It would be valuable to the wholesaler to have quicker methods at his disposal. On this point some slaughterers say that DFD carcasses tend to produce a more pronounced *rigor* at bleeding, but this needs to be checked experimentally.

THE USE OF DFD MEAT

The priority for the slaughterer is to know as quickly as possible that a carcass is likely to produce DFD meat. If the meat is returned to him by an angry retailer de-boned ten days after dispatch his only recourse at this stage is to divert it to pet-food manufacture. A wholesaler who is faced with this problem will try to find a way of reducing his economic loss to a minimum. He may have the opportunity to divert DFD carcasses to intervention (EEC countries) but this may not always be possible and in any case could not be regarded as a permanent solution to the problem. He may also be able to export to markets where customers are less discriminating.

The use of DFD meat in the fresh meat market can be contemplated only under special circumstances which correspond more to the traditional butcher's trade in which ageing is carried out on half carcasses, the meat being prepared at the point of sale. Here, the butcher has the opportunity to explain to the customer that the potential for storage is limited. If DFD meat is not shown side by side with normal meat, it is possible that under these circumstances the customer has a higher tolerance towards dark-cutting beef, especially if the carcass is rather fat. Provided it is not too dark, the colour anomaly may be offset by a degree of marbling.

In the exceptional case when a wholesaler manages to sell a DFD carcass to a traditional butcher he will get 30 per cent less than the normal price, unless of course the butcher does not notice that the carcass is DFD. This may happen with forequarters in which the DFD character is less apparent than in hindquarters.

As far as supermarkets are concerned, all the difficulties mentioned above are compounded. The storage of meat is inevitably short-term with the result that ageing may be insufficient, thereby limiting the use to which the meat can be put; the storage temperature at which retail prepackaged cuts are held is often badly regulated (5°C or more); DFD meat is shown side by side with normal beef on the counter. For these reasons the sale of DFD meat through modern distribution channels is practically ruled out.

Concerning chilled, vacuum-packaged beef, recent studies permit some interesting speculation about the possibility of controlling the DFD condition. Newton and Gill (1980) have used citrate to increase the preservative effect of vacuum-packaging; it was possible to keep DFD muscles up to 12 weeks at -1°C. This treatment allows only a partial solution to the problem, however, since it reappears once the bags are opened. The regulatory aspects of this method are also stressed by these authors, particularly the continued use of the term 'fresh meat' to describe a product thus treated.

Concerning processed products, problems due to DFD meat are more or less similar in both beef and pork. The solution for using beef would be similar to that for pork, but processed products which use beef are less numerous. The fundamental case for using DFD meat in curing processes is its high water-holding capacity and this is of particular interest when meats are finally comminuted for use in meat emulsions. However, one cannot recommend the use of DFD beef in dry-sausage manufacture even though bacteriological considerations are unimportant in this case. Similarly, for ready-to-eat dishes and canned beef there should be no problem from this point of view.

The decision to use a carcass for processing rather than for sale as fresh meat necessarily implies an important financial loss, when the difference in price between processing and fresh meat is taken into account. The loss will vary depending on whether or not the company has its own processing department. A wholesaler who is carrying on processing operations will be able, on de-boning a carcass, to save certain muscles or parts which are not affected by DFD for use as fresh meat. On the other hand, some packers who do not themselves process, debone the carcass and keep the less affected joints as fresh meat, freezing the rest to sell it to a processor.

CONCLUSION

The first point which we would make is that the economic and practical consequences of the DFD problem will vary from one country to another (types of animal, consumption habits etc.) and from one company to another (conditions under which animals are collected, processing operations, export policy, etc.).

It appears that there is a lack of fundamental knowledge on a number of points which indicates where more study is required These include the importance of glucose concentration, certain bacteriological aspects, variation of pH and other physical and chemical parameters between and within muscles.

Apart from possible ways of avoiding DFD meat, certain treatments such as the use of citrate could result, in the near future, in a partial solution to the problem, particularly the extension in storage life for DFD muscles which would give time to the packer to search for suitable outlets.

It nevertheless seems to us that DFD carcasses remain as an inevitable problem for the slaughterer, one that he tries to overcome in various ways, ultimately passing on the cost to the consumer.

Packers need to become more aware of the phenomenon and its consequences. On the one hand they should try to remedy the problem or to reduce its effect by taking a number of preventive measures such as correct design of cattle trucks, care in loading and unloading, choice of routes and reduction in transportation time before slaughter, design of lairage at the abattoir (individual boxes etc.). On the other hand, he needs to be aware of the risk of encountering DFD meat and through good management reduce the effect to a minimum both by providing an adequate supply of cattle and also finding suitable outlets.

Finally, let us emphasise the urgency of solving the problem of DFD carcasses for we will have to contend with a far more serious evil if solutions are not found, i.e. 'the stress of the packer'!

REFERENCES

Newton, K.G. and Gill, C.O., 1978. Storage quality of Dark, Firm, Dry meat. Appl. Environ. Microbiol., 36: 375-376.

Newton, K.G. and Gill, C.O., 1980. Control of spoilage in vacuum packaged Dark, Firm, Dry (DFD) meat. J. Food Tech., 15: 227-234.

Sornay, J. and Legras, P., 1978. Cartographie du pH dans les carcasses de gros bovins. Industries Agricoles et Alimentaires, 4: 392-397.

Wirth, F., 1978. pH-Wert und Fleischwaren herstellung. Die Fleischwirtschaft, 9: 1458-1468.

DISCUSSION

E. Puolanne *(Finland)*

I was surprised to hear that the economic loss is so high in your country. We calculate it to be somewhere between 5 and 10 per cent. We recommend that DFD meat is used by restaurants etc., and it can be used a few days after slaughter because it is tender. The alternative is to freeze it, because the cooking loss, freezing and thawing loss of DFD meat is low. When DFD meat is used in large kitchens it is not dangerous because the pH value decreases during the cooking. As for cured meat, we have developed new products to use DFD meat. Perhaps this is why we have such a low economic loss.

M.J. Sornay *(France)*

In France, the processing and the fresh meat trades are completely separate. The difference in price between the two types of carcass is very high - about 30 per cent. Contrary to your experience the restaurant trade in France will not buy DFD carcasses. Of course when carcasses are sold to intervention there is no loss at all and the actual economic loss will depend on specific circumstances. Regarding your argument for the freezing of DFD carcasses I agree completely. It is the best way at present to find an outlet for this type of meat.

E. Puolanne

I am not speaking of the DFD carcass when I speak of DFD meat. When a DFD carcass is found, it is cut so that the meat that is not DFD is used as usual, and the affected parts - sirloins and rounds - are used as DFD meat. The only complaint that the consumer has is that it is red after cooking; and suspects that there may be nitrite there, even in fresh products.

M.J. Sornay

Is the meat red after cooking?

E. Puolanne

Yes, it is, even without nitrite.

H. Ruderus *(Sweden)*

That may depend on a very slow rate of heat transfer in DFD meat as compared with ordinary meat.

E. Puolanne

No, the heating rate is higher in DFD meat than in normal meat, at least at the beginning. It may be that the water flow goes in the opposite direction to the heat flow. Also, the surface of normal meat is very wet.

D.B. MacDougall *(UK)*

Is there any country that has a positive demand for DFD meat as part of its normal production? If DFD meat was available in a regulated supply, even though it came in through the intervention system, is there a process or a product? Its increased worth in binding capacity for the manufacturer of all types of sausages might well only need the link-up of a continual supply.

J.J. Sheridan *(Ireland)*

There is a microbiological difficulty in using it in sausages and other comminuted meats - it does not keep.

G. Eikelenboom *(The Netherlands)*

You mentioned in your paper that some slaughterhouses observed that potential DFD carcasses are already stiff when they are bled.

M.J. Sornay

Yes, we heard that on different occasions.

G. Eikelenboom

In Germany they have observed that there is a high temperature in DFD meat, *post mortem*. It is approximately 1°C. Do you think that this temperature exists prior to slaughter?

Chr. Augustini *(FRG)*

I think it is an effect of the stress before slaughter. However, if you fast the animals before slaughter there is a DFD effect but not a temperature effect.

E. Kallweit *(FRG)*

I would like to comment on a question that we have had before about the water binding capacity of DFD meat in sausage production. As soon as there is legal limitation on the amount of water to be added, then it is no help, even if the water binding capacity of the meat is really high. The amount of water allowed for sausage making is so low that even beef with a lower water holding capacity will do the job quite well. This is one reason why hot boning is of less interest than before, because then one wanted to use the high water binding capacity of pre-*rigor* meat. However, this is now of less interest in view of the limitations by law.

D.E. Hood *(Ireland)*

Would it not also be an advantage, from the point of view of preventing excessive cooking losses of cooked meat products?

E. Kallweit

I am not in meat processing so I cannot say.

E. Puolanne

The firmness of the sausage will decrease if you use DFD meat which has a pH value higher than 6.2. This is very important if the sausage is to be sliced afterwards.

POSTER PRESENTATIONS

Chairman: J. Wismer-Pedersen

INFLUENCE OF HOLDING ANIMALS BEFORE SLAUGHTER

Chr. Augustini
Bundesanstalt für Fleischforschung, E.-C.-Baumann-Strasse 20, D 8650 Kulmbach, Federal Republic of Germany.

ABSTRACT

The effect of different waiting times and group compositions of loose-yard bulls in the lairage was investigated. The great excitability and often heavier physical stress of bulls managed in this way are considered to contribute to the development of dark-cutting beef.

It was found that lengthening the waiting time on the day of arrival and also prolonging the time in lairage till the next morning was closely associated with an increase of dark-cutting beef in M. semimembranosus. Only if the animals were slaughtered immediately after arrival was dark-cutting avoided. When bulls were mixed together, i.e. when they were not kept in the same group at the lairage as they had been on the farm, waiting times of up to 90 min resulted in some incidence of high ultimate pH values. The frequency of dark-cutting in beef was lower in groups which were not mixed together. In these groups a prolonged waiting time (at least 1.5 to 3 h) was necessary to produce this quality fault. The pH value at 48 h post mortem was closely correlated with glycogen concentration and meat temperature (both measured in M. semimembranosus at 30 min post mortem) but not with the concentrations of creatine phosphate, ATP and lactate.

INTRODUCTION

Previous experiments have shown that young bulls are more frequently affected by dark-cutting than cows or heifers. Bulls housed untethered are particularly prone to this condition. The greater excitability of bulls managed in this way, combined with the heavier physical stress during transport and at the slaughterhouse, could be of major importance. These factors cause a depletion of the glycogen stores in the muscles of the living animal, resulting in a low muscle lactate concentration *post mortem* and a high ultimate pH.

An experiment with bulls out of loose yards was carried out to examine the effect of a systematic prolongation of lairage time to a maximum of overnight lairage; in addition the effect of grouping was studied.

METHODS

The experiment was carried out on well finished Simmental bulls. An average carcass weight of 374.5 ± 39.0 kg was registered. Generally, the animals were fed for the last time the evening before slaughter. All bulls came out of loose yards and remained untethered during transport as well as in the lairage. Relatively high environmental temperatures and relative humidity of the air were recorded during the course of the experiment (20 and 25°C, 80 and 90 per cent average day values in lairage).

On arrival at the factory the bulls were allocated to groups according to required holding time before slaughter: 0 - 30 min, 31 - 90 min, 91 - 180 min, 181 - 300 min, 301 - 480 min and overnight lairage. Each time-group was further subdivided; the first sub-group was mixed with bulls ('strangers') from different fattening pens (mixed group) and the second with familiar bulls from the same fattening pen (unmixed group) until slaughter. In total there were 11 groups, i.e. 5 parallel groups and one consisting of bulls slaughtered immediately after arrival. The following parameters were measured in *M. semimembranosus* :

pH value at 48 h *post mortem* (pH_u), meat temperature (30 min *post mortem*), concentration of glycogen, lactate, ATP and creatine phosphate (all at 30 min *post mortem*).

RESULTS

Lengthening the waiting time was closely associated with an increase of dark-cutting beef in *M. semimembranosus*. Figure 1 shows group mean pH values at 48 h *post mortem*. Normally the lowest ultimate pH values were found in animals which were slaughtered immediately after arrival; here no dark-cutting was registered. For bulls mixed with strangers during lairage at the slaughterhouse, a lairage time of 90 min or less was sufficient to produce some animals with high ultimate pH values.

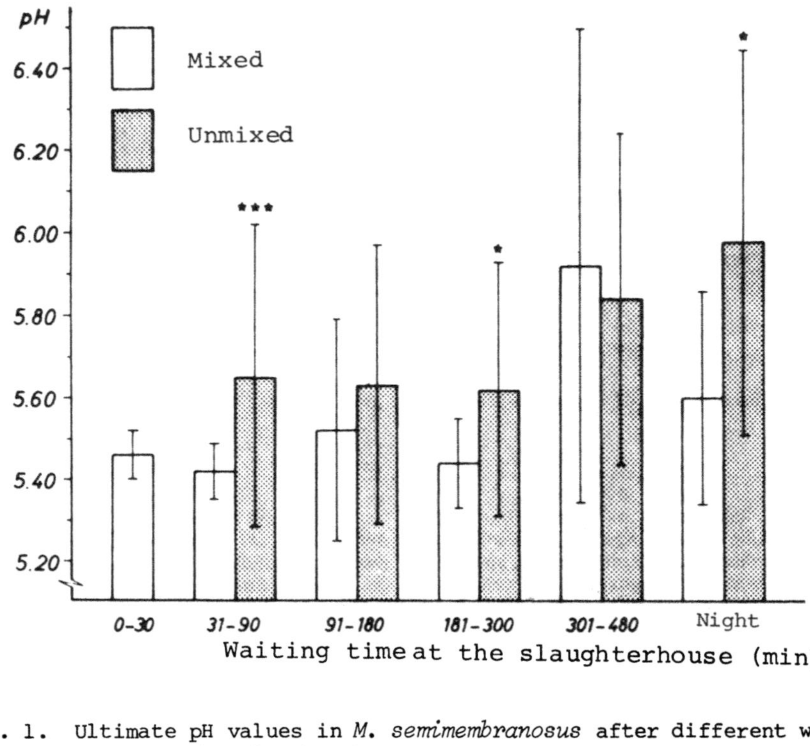

Fig. 1. Ultimate pH values in *M. semimembranosus* after different waiting times at the slaughterhouse.

The percentage of dark-cutting beef (pH_u > 6.1 in *M. semimembranosus*) in groups mixed with strangers for 31 - 90 min was 11.1 per cent, after 91 - 180 min 21.6 per cent, after 181 - 300 min 10.5 per cent, after 301 - 480 min 23.5 per cent and in the case of overnight lairage 55.5 per cent. In the groups which were not mixed the dark cutting percentage was in most cases significantly lower (31 - 90 min 0 per cent, 91 - 180 min 12.5 per cent, 181 - 300 min 5 per cent, 301 - 480 min 33.2 per cent, and overnight 8.3 per cent).

The distribution of pH_u values at the different waiting times is shown in Figure 2. In this case the group composition was not taken into account.

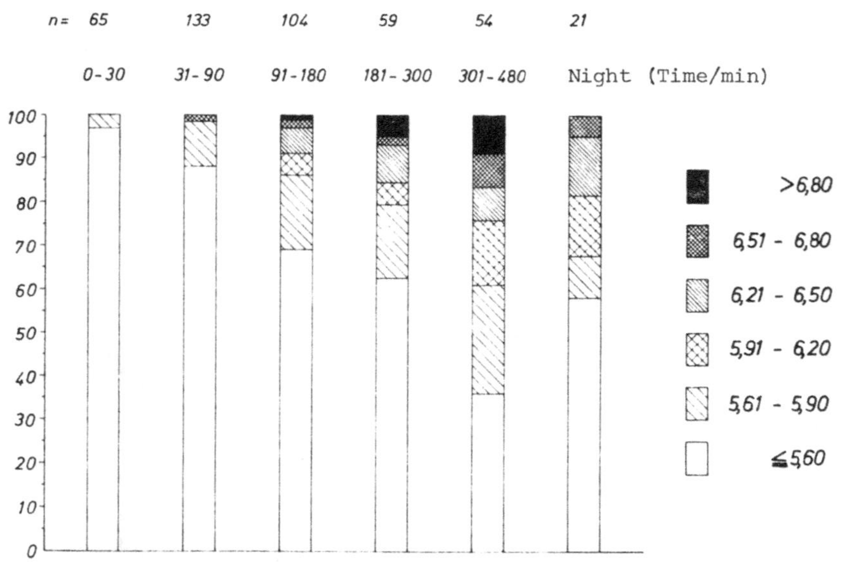

Fig. 2. Percentage distribution of final pH stages (*M. semimembranosus*) after different waiting times at the slaughterhouse.

It is evident that with the prolongation of lairage time the percentage of normal meat was reduced. Thus, after a lairage of 5 to 8 h, only 60 per cent of pH_u values were below 5.9 and only 37 per cent were below 5.6.

The result of excitement before slaughter can be seen very clearly in the meat temperatures 30 min *post mortem* (Figure 3). Differences between bulls in mixed groups and unmixed groups are apparent and, in spite of considerable individual differences, they are partly statistically significant.

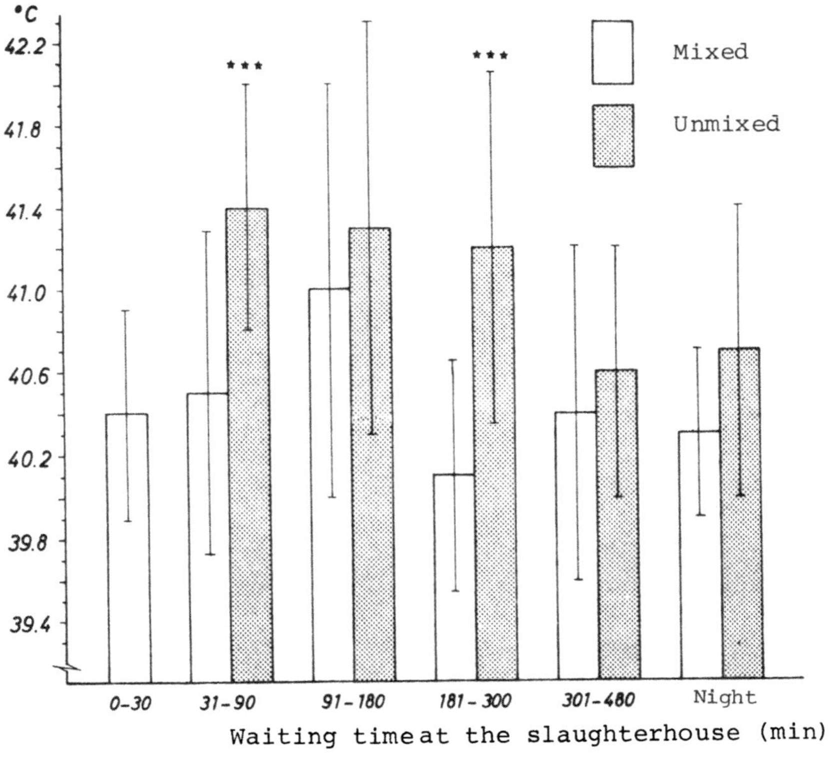

Fig. 3. The meat temperature 30 min *post mortem* in *M. semimembranosus* after different waiting times at the slaughterhouse.

Comparison of meat temperatures (*M. semimembranosus*) in muscles with ultimate pH values above 6.0 and those with ultimate pH values of 5.6 or lower, showed highly significant differences ($pH_u > 6.0$, $41.35 \pm 0.88^{\circ}C$; $pH_u \leqslant 5.6$, $40.43 \pm 0.72^{\circ}C$).

The concentration of glycogen is a good parameter for judging the degree of pre-slaughter stress of the animal. In Figure 4 there is a marked decline in glycogen concentration with increase in lairage time. The mixed group normally had lower concentrations.

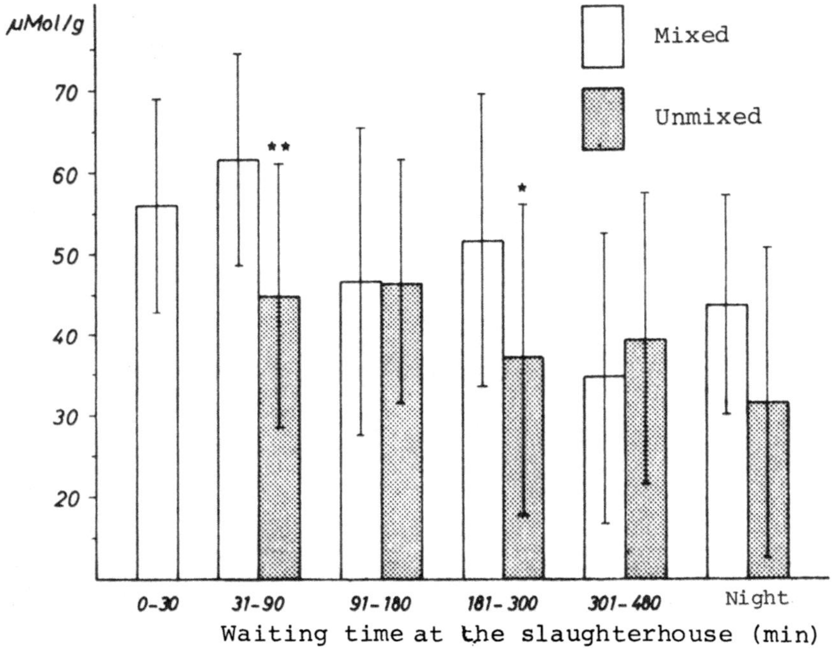

Fig. 4. Glycogen concentration 30 min *post mortem* in *M. semimembranosus* after different waiting times at the slaughterhouse.

Compared with results in pigs, lactate concentrations found in *M. semimembranosus* of bulls at 30 min *post mortem* were relatively low (Table 1). The low lactate concentrations after short lairage times were associated with high muscle glycogen concentrations. On the other hand, the low lactate values after longer waiting times were associated with low muscle glycogen content and indicate the final stage of glycolysis.

TABLE 1

LACTATE CONCENTRATION (µmol/g) 30 MIN *post mortem* IN *M. semimembranosus* AFTER DIFFERENT WAITING TIMES AND DIFFERENT STABLING AT THE SLAUGHTERHOUSE (LOOSE STABLING BULLS).

Holding time (min)	Unmixed group			Mixed group		
	n	$\bar{x}$	s	n	$\bar{x}$	s
M. semimembranosus						
0 - 30	10	17.44	6.52	(slaughtered immediately)		
31 - 90	12	12.95	7.93	11	18.24	11.59
91 -180	34	25.00	16.52	42	24.67	15.31
181 -300	18	32.71	26.99	16	27.56	20.48
301 -480	11	14.67	9.58	37	18.12	13.31
overnight	12	18.57	8.47	9	12.03	5.60

TABLE 2

CREATINE PHOSPHATE AND ATP (µmol/g) IN *M. semimembranosus* AFTER DIFFERENT WAITING TIMES AND DIFFERENT STABLING AT THE SLAUGHTERHOUSE (LOOSE STABLING BULLS).

Holding time (min)	Unmixed group			Mixed group		
	n	$\bar{x}$	s	n	$\bar{x}$	s
Creatine phosphate						
0 - 30	10	5.51	2.39	(slaughtered immediately)		
31 - 90	12	7.72	2.74	11	4.73	2.65
91 - 180	34	3.93	2.57	42	3.41	1.87
181 -300	18	3.67	2.43	16	3.87	2.54
301 -480	11	6.25	2.48	37	5.07	3.57
overnight	12	5.40	2.21	9	5.37	3.15
ATP						
0 - 30	10	5.99	1.33	(slaughtered immediately)		
31 - 90	12	7.74	0.85	11	4.92	1.43
91 -180	34	5.02	1.27	42	4.95	1.66
181 -300	18	4.07	1.70	16	4.91	1.71
301 -480	11	3.96	0.83	37	4.36	1.81
overnight	12	6.00	1.36	9	5.63	0.61

The concentrations of the energy-rich phosphates (ATP and creatine phosphate) tended to decline with length of waiting time in the slaughterhouse (Table 2). However, the concentrations were still relatively high in groups with high incidences of dark-cutting beef.

CONCLUSIONS

Taking the conditions of the experiment into consideration, results show that for bulls from loose-yards the situation in the slaughterhouse could be of major importance in determining the incidence of dark-cutting beef. It is therefore concluded that bulls from loose-yards which remain loose on transport and lairage should be slaughtered as quickly as possible after arrival in the slaughterhouse. Mixing of bulls out of different fattening pens or farms should be especially avoided.

POST-MORTEM MUSCLE BIOCHEMISTRY AND BEEF QUALITY

Chr. Fischer and R. Hamm
Bundesanstalt für Fleischforschung,
D-8650 Kulmbach,
Federal Republic of Germany.

ABSTRACT

Samples of M. semimembranosus from 50 carcasses of young bulls were taken 30 min after slaughter. The pH value was measured and the concentration of ATP, glycogen, lactate and the metabolites of glycogenolysis were determined. The ultimate pH value, water-holding capacity, plasticity and colour brightness were measured 48 h post mortem. Samples with higher ultimate pH showed a higher water-holding capacity and plasticity and a darker colour. Compared with normal muscle, dark-cutting beef with extremely high ultimate pH (pH_u > 6.81) had remarkably lower concentrations of glycogen, glucose, hexose-phosphates and the following metabolites of glycogenolysis: DAP, GAP, 3-PG, 2-PG, PEP and lactate. Only the pyruvate concentration was at the same level as in normal muscle. On the other hand in moderately dark-cutting beef with pH_u of 5.81 - 6.20, a low glycogen concentration was combined with high levels of hexose-monophosphates similar to that found in fast glycolysing bovine muscle 30 min after slaughter. The concentration of lactate was approximately the same as in normal bovine muscle. Low concentration of glycogen in combination with an accumulation of hexose-monophosphates indicate a stimulation of the phosphorylase system in the moderate dark-cutting beef, possibly induced by a secretion of epinephrine before slaughter.

INTRODUCTION

Dark-cutting beef is characterised by a high water-holding capacity and a closed structure combined with a dark colour which are due to its high ultimate pH. The reason for the incomplete pH fall *post mortem* is a much reduced glycogen concentration immediately before slaughter. The purpose of this investigation was to get some information on *post mortem* glycolysis and breakdown of ATP in dark-cutting beef in comparison to normal bovine muscle. In addition to the ultimate pH (pH 48 h *post mortem*) the water-holding capacity, colour brightness and plasticity were used as indices of meat quality.

MATERIAL AND METHODS

The experiments were carried out with 50 young bulls of the German Simmental breed at a slaughter-weight of about 320 kg. Thirty minutes after slaughter the pH value was measured in *M. semimembranosus*. Perchloric acid extracts were prepared and the concentration of glycogen was determined in an aliquot after Dalrymple and Hamm (1973). In the extract the levels of free glucose, glucose-1-phosphate (G-1-P), glucose-6-phosphate (G-6-P) and fructose-6-phosphate (F-6-P) were determined by the enzymic methods of Bergmeyer et al. (1970). For fructose-1, 6-diphosphate (FDP), dihydroxyacetone-phosphate (DAP) and glyceraldehyde-3-phosphate (GAP) the method of Bücher and Hohorst (1970) was used. 2-phosphoglycerate (2-PG), 3-phosphoglycerate (3-PG), phosphoenol pyruvate (PEP) and pyruvate were determined by the method of Czok and Lamprecht (1970). The concentration of ATP was determined after Jaworek et al. (1970). The assay of lactate was carried out according to the procedure of Hohorst (1970).

At 48 h *post mortem* the ultimate pH (pH_u) value and the wateriness (cm^2 liquid area/300 mg tissue on filter-paper) and plasticity (cm^2 meat area/300 mg tissue) was measured by a filter-paper press-method (Grau and Hamm, 1957). The colour brightness was measured after Mirna (1965); in this method the

the sample is visually compared with a combination of a coloured glass filter with 20 different grey tones. A very light colour is expressed as 'step one', a very dark one as 'step twenty'.

RESULTS

For a better understanding of the results the 50 muscle samples were classified into 9 groups according to the pH value 48 h *post mortem* (pH_u) with intervals of 0.2 pH units. For each pH_u group the mean values and standard deviations of the characteristics of meat quality and of the metabolite concentrations of glycogenolysis were calculated as presented in Figure 1 and 2.

As Figure 1 shows, with increasing pH_u the wateriness was decreased i.e. dark-cutting beef had a better water-holding capacity. Higher pH_u values corresponded with a higher plasticity, a darker colour and also with a higher pH_1 (pH 30 min after slaughter).

In Figure 2 the concentrations of glycolytic metabolites and of ATP at 30 min *post mortem* for the different pH_u groups are presented.

With increasing pH_u the concentration of glycogen, FDP and of the following metabolites of glycogenolysis, DAP, GAP, 3-PG, 2-PG, PEP and lactate were lowered. On the other hand, the concentrations of hexose-monophosphates and pyruvate showed a maximum between pH_u groups 3 and 6. Mean values for ATP concentration 30 min *post mortem* were decreased at $pH_u > 6.01$, but the standard deviation was relatively high. For a better interpretation of the metabolism of dark-cutting beef a 'crossover plot' was used (Figure 3). In dark-cutting beef with extremely high pH_u compared with normal bovine muscle all levels of glycolytic metabolites were decreased. Only the pyruvate concentration was normal. Presumably due to an extremely low glycogen concentration at the time of slaughter, the following metabolites of glycogenolysis were correspondingly lowered.

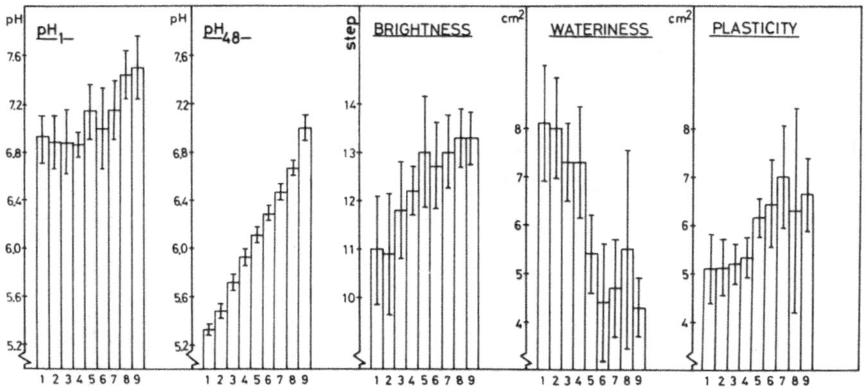

Fig. 1. Meat quality characteristics: pH_1, colour brightness (low brightness stage, light; high brightness stage, dark), wateriness (cm^2 liquid area) and plasticity (cm^2 meat area) in *M. semimembranosus* for the following pH_u groups:

pH_u group	pH_u range	n
1	5.21 - 5.40	8
2	5.41 - 5.60	8
3	5.61 - 5.80	5
4	5.81 - 6.00	4
5	6.01 - 6.20	5
6	6.21 - 6.40	7
7	6.41 - 6.60	4
8	6.61 - 6.80	3
9	> 6.81	6

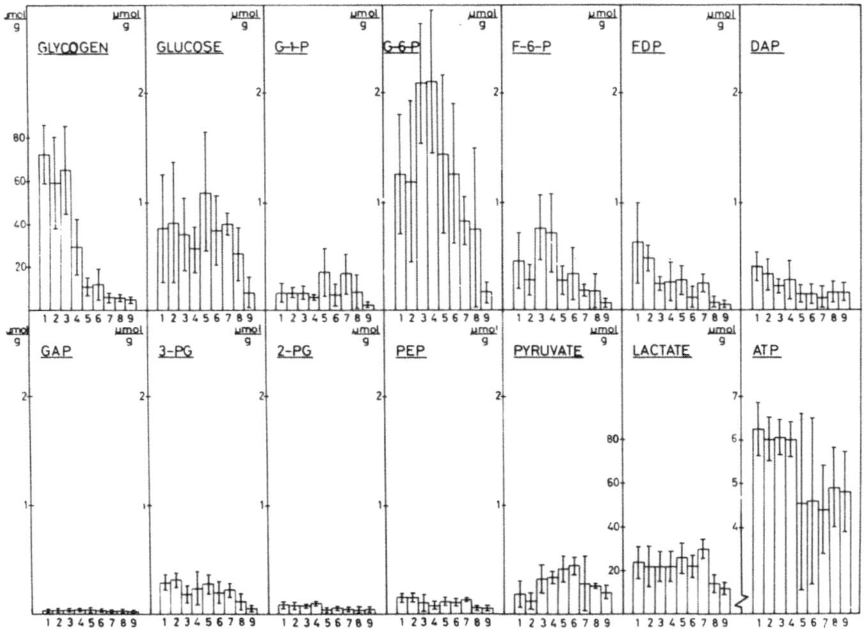

Fig. 2. Concentration of metabolites of glycogenolysis and of ATP 30 min *post mortem* for different pH_u groups (see Figure 1). The glycogen concentration is expressed as μmol glucose units/g tissue.

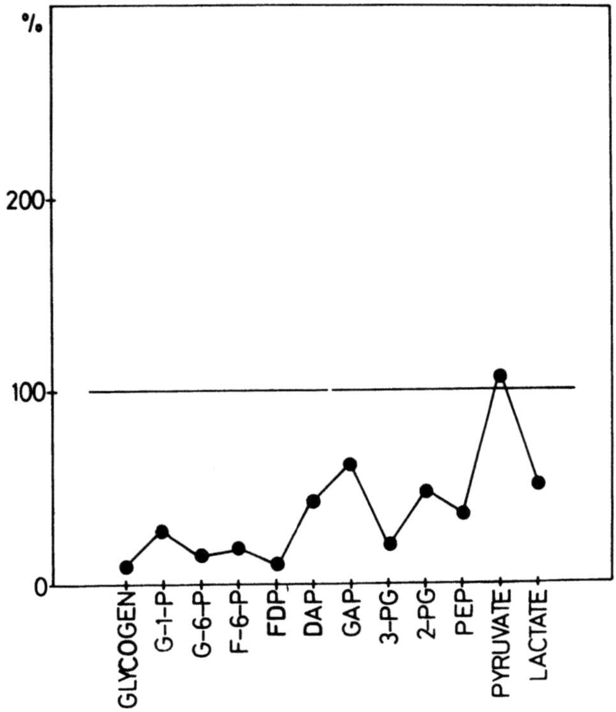

Fig. 3. Crossover plot of metabolite concentrations of glycogenolysis 30 min *post mortem* in dark-cutting beef with an extremely high final pH value (pH_u group 9) related to concentrations in normal musculature (100 per cent).

On the other hand, dark-cutting beef with slightly increased ultimate pH in relation to normal muscle (Figure 4) showed an accumulation of the hexose-monophosphates which indicates a stimulation of the phosphorylase system. We found a similar crossover plot in fast glycolysing bovine musculature compared with normal muscle at the same time after slaughter (30 min *post mortem*) (Fischer and Hamm, 1980).

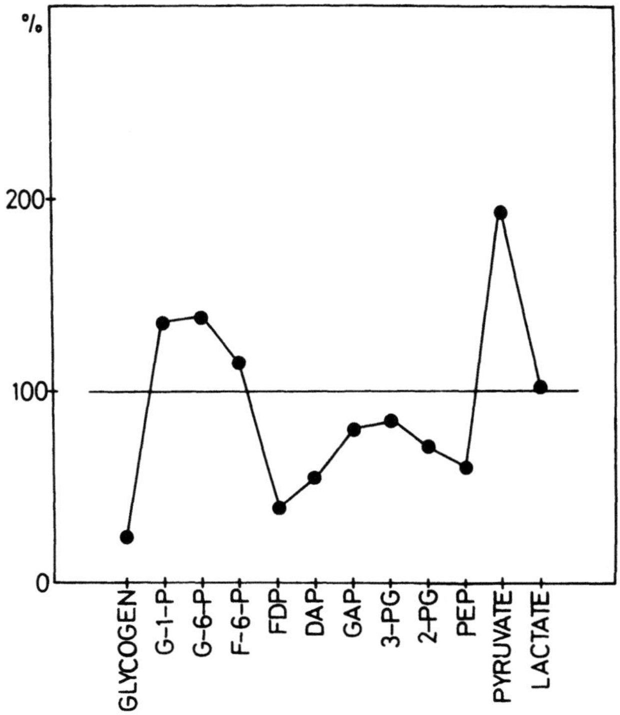

Fig. 4. Crossover plot of metabolite concentrations of glycogenolysis 30 min *post mortem* in dark-cutting beef with slightly increased final pH value (pH_u groups 4 and 5) related to concentrations in normal musculature (100 per cent).

CONCLUSIONS

The high concentration of hexose-monophosphates combined with a low glycogen concentration at 30 min *post mortem*, observed in dark-cutting beef with slightly increased pH_u, indicates an increased activity of the phosphorylase system. This could result from a stress reaction and an accelerated epinephrine secretion immediately before slaughter. In dark-cutting beef with extremely high pH_u values the glycogen level at slaughter is so low that a possible influence of epinephrine on the phosphorylase system could not be demonstrated.

REFERENCES

Bergmeyer, H.U., Bernt, E., Schmidt, F. and Stork, H., 1970. In: Methoden der enzymatischen Analyse (Bergmeyer, H.U. ed.); Verlag Chemie, Weinheim/Bergstrasse, 1163.

Bucher, T. and Hohorst, H.-J., 1970. In: Methoden der enzymatischen Analyse (Bergmeyer, H.U. ed.); Verlag Chemie, Weinheim/Bergstrasse, 1282.

Czok, R. and Lamprecht, W., 1970. In: Methoden der enzymatischen Analyse (Bermeyer, H.U. ed.); Verlag Chemie, Weinheim/Bergstrasse, 1407.

Dalrymple, R.H. and Hamm, R., 1973. A method for the extraction of glycogen and metabolites from a single muscle sample. J. Fd. Technol. 8, 439.

Fischer, C. and Hamm, R., 1980. Biochemical studies on fast glycolysing bovine muscles. Meat Sci. 4, 41.

Grau, R. and Hamm, R., 1957. Uber das Wasserbindungsvermogen des Säugetiermuskels. Z. Lebensm. Untersuch.-Forsch. 105, 446.

Hohorst, H.-J., 1970. In: Methoden der enzymatischen Analyse (Bergmeyer, H.U. ed.); Verlag Chemie, Weinheim/Bergstrasse, 1425.

Jaworek, D., Gruber, W. and Bergmeyer, H.U., 1970. In: Methoden der enzymatischen Analyse (Bergmayer, H.U. ed.); Verlag Chemie, Weinheim/Bergstrasse, 2020.

Mirna, A., 1965. Über ein vereinfachtes Verfahren zur Farbbeurteilung von Fleisch und Fleischwaren. Fleischwirtschaft 45, 332.

INFLUENCE OF TEMPERATURE, FASTING AND TRANSPORTATION

K. Fischer
Bundesanstalt für Fleischforschung, E.-C.-Baumann-Strasse 20,
D 8650 Kulmbach, Federal Republic of Germany.

ABSTRACT

The influences of different temperatures during transport (+2°C, +12°C, +36°C), and an additional fasting period of 48 h before slaughter were investigated in relation to characteristics of meat quality and post mortem glycogenolysis in 48 young bulls of the German Simmental breed. Feeding of animals was discontinued 22 h before transportation to the slaughterhouse. The duration of transport lasted four hours and the RH in the air-conditioned truck was 65 per cent. Final pH values 48 h post mortem in M. semimembranosus, M. semitendinosus, M. longissimus dorsi, M. psoas major and M. biceps femoris were determined. Water-binding capacity (Grau/Hamm), and essential metabolites of glycogen metabolism at 45 min post mortem were also measured.

Different temperatures during transport, followed by immediate slaughter did not lead in any case to dark-cutting beef; only at the highest temperature were lower glycogen contents and higher lactate and glucose concentrations found, especially in M. semitendinosus. The additional fasting led in all muscles examined to a drastic decline in glycogen concentration, particularly in M. longissimus dorsi, M. semitendinosus and M. semimembranosus. Highly significant differences were also found in ultimate pH values and in the water-binding capacity, compared with unfasted animals. Glucose, ATP and creatine phosphate levels were almost unaffected by the experimental treatments.

INTRODUCTION

In considering the causes of dark-cutting beef, the factors that require particular attention are those that bring about a drop in the glycogen level in living muscle. The stresses that frequently occur during marketing of animals, such as bad transport conditions or fasting of animals for a long time, are of practical importance. In two experiments described in this paper the effects of various transport temperatures and of an additional 48 h fasting period were investigated.

METHODS

Forty-eight young bulls (German Simmental) were used in the experiments. In order to judge the effects of temperature, 8 animals were transported for 4 h in an air-conditioned truck at +2°C, +12°C or +36°C, with constant RH of 65 per cent, and slaughtered immediately on arrival at the slaughterhouse (experiment I). A further 24 young bulls were transported in the same way but were not slaughtered until after an additional fasting period of 48 h, during which time the animals were held in loose pens containing 2 animals each, with free access to water (experiment II). All animals were last fed 22 h before transportation. A summary of treatments is given in the following review:

	n	Fasting period before transport (h)	Transport temperature (°C)	Transport duration (h)	Fasting period after transport (h)
Experiment I	8	22	+ 2	4	0
	8	22	+12	4	0
	8	22	+36	4	0
Experiment II	8	22	+ 2	4	48
	8	22	+12	4	48
	8	22	+36	4	48

Characteristics of *post mortem* glycogen metabolism (45 min *post mortem*) and of meat quality (48 h *post mortem*) were determined in *M. semimembranosus, M. semitendinosus, M. longissimus dorsi, M. psoas major* and *M. biceps femoris*.

RESULTS

Experiment I

Heart rate was continuously recorded during the journey and was not affected by alterations in temperature on the truck (Figure 1). On the other hand at the highest ambient temperature during transport rectal temperatures at the end of the journey were statistically significantly above starting values (Figure 2).

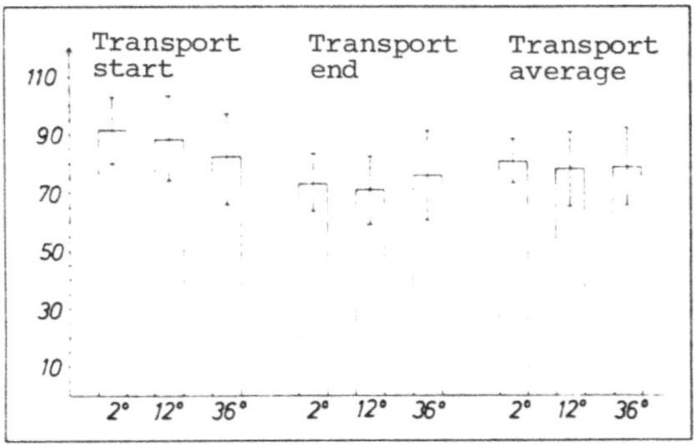

Fig. 1. Heart frequency values during transport at different temperatures (°C) - mean values ± standard deviations.

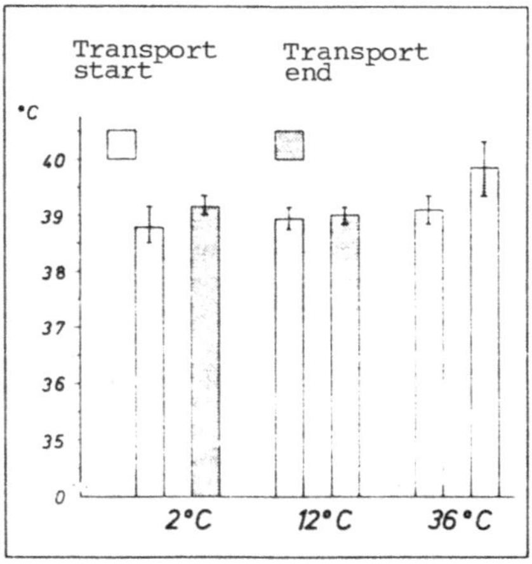

Fig. 2. Rectal temperatures before and after transport at different temperatures (°C) - mean values ± standard deviations.

In recent work no differences in final pH values and water-binding capacity were found between treatments based on various temperature levels - moreover, there was no indication of quality faults with respect to dark-cutting (Figure 3).

After journeys at the highest temperature level there was a tendency towards lower glycogen contents and higher lactate and glucose contents, particularly in *M. semitendinosus* and *M. semimembranosus* (Table 1, Figure 4).

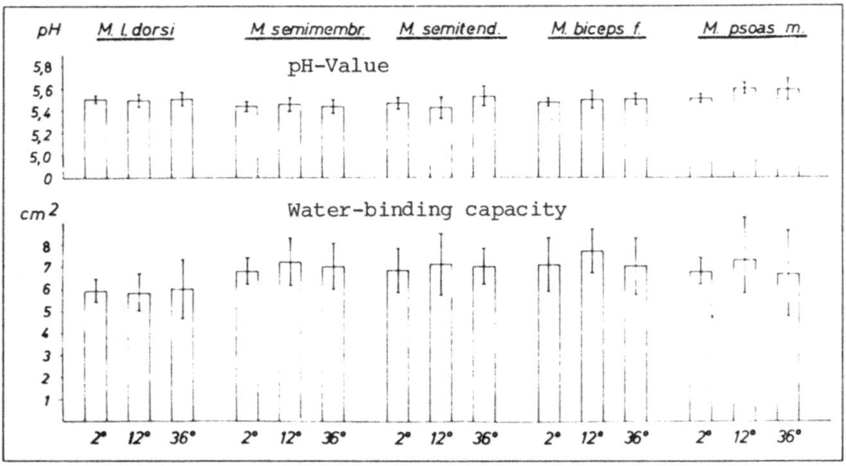

Fig. 3. pH value and water-binding capacity (liquid area - method of Grau/Hamm) 48 h *post mortem* after transport at different temperatures (°C) and immediate slaughter - mean values ± standard deviations.

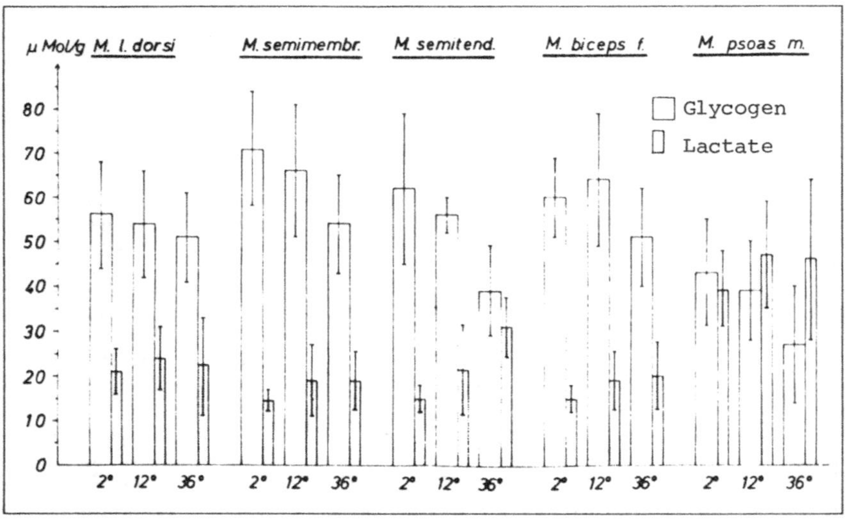

Fig. 4. Concentrations (µmol/g) of glycogen (Glucose units) and lactate 45 min *post mortem* after transport at different temperatures (°C) and immediate slaughter - mean values ± standard deviations.

TABLE 1

GLUCOSE CONCENTRATION 45 MIN *post mortem* (μmol/g) IN DIFFERENT MUSCLES AFTER SUBJECTING THE ANIMALS TO DIFFERENT TRANSPORT TEMPERATURES - MEAN VALUES AND STANDARD DEVIATIONS

Muscle		Transport temperature (°C)			t-Test		
		2°C	12°C	36°C	2°:12°	12°:36°	2°:36°
M. semimembranosus	$\bar{x}$	0.76	0.62	1.70		++	++
	s	0.36	0.33	0.69			
M. semitendinosus	$\bar{x}$	0.81	1.00	1.50			+
	s	0.22	0.37	0.68			
M. longissimus dorsi	$\bar{x}$	1.02	0.73	0.96			
	s	0.65	0.17	0.74			
M. psoas major	$\bar{x}$	2.47	2.28	2.68			
	s	1.20	0.92	1.27			
M. biceps femoris	$\bar{x}$	1.08	1.04	1.21			
	s	0.89	0.91	0.47			

Experiment II

In the second experiment it was found that about 50 per cent of the fasted animals had final pH values higher than 6.2 in *M. longissimus dorsi* (Figure 5). Highly significant differences were also found in the final pH values and in the water-binding properties (Grau/Hamm) of the other muscles, compared with the muscles of animals that had not been fasted (Table 2).

Compared with experiment I the glycogen contents of all the muscles examined had dropped on average by half (Figure 6). On the other hand there were no clear signs of the treatment affecting concentrations of lactate, glucose, ATP or creatine phosphate (Table 3).

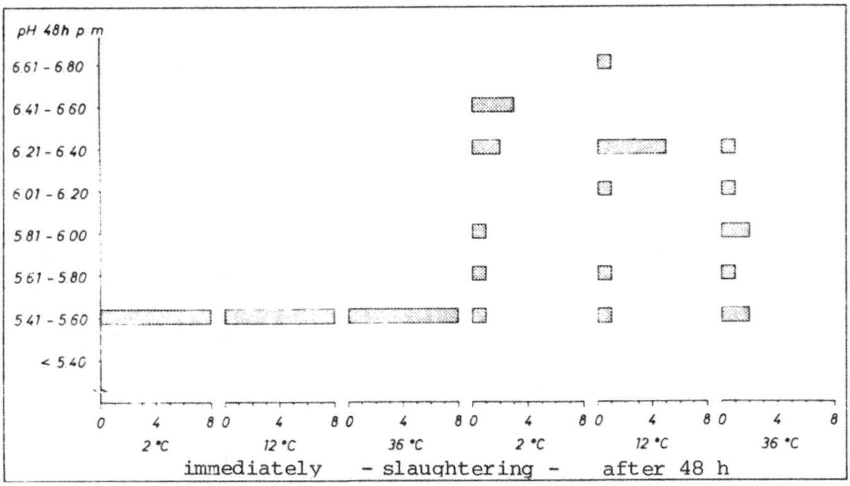

Fig. 5. Absolute distribution of pH 48 h *post mortem* in *M. longissimus dorsi* after different transport temperatures and slaughtering times.

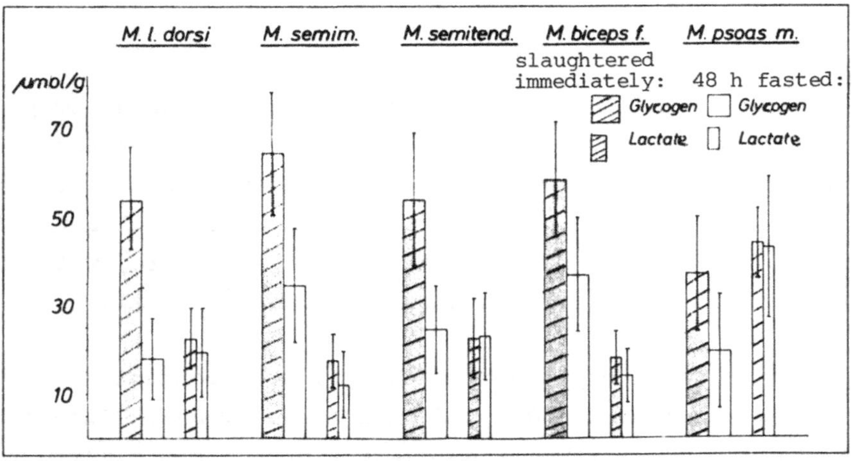

Fig. 6. Concentrations (µmol/g) of glycogen (glucose units) and lactate 45 min *post mortem* in the treatment groups 'immediate slaughter' and 'additional fasting' (mean values ± standard deviation, n = 24)

TABLE 2

MEAT QUALITY CHARACTERISTICS 48 h *post mortem* FOR THE 'IMMEDIATE SLAUGHTER' PART OF THE EXPERIMENT (S) AND FOR THE 'ADDITIONAL FASTING' GROUP (N) - MEAN VALUES, STANDARD DEVIATIONS, T-TEST.

Muscle		Final pH value			Juice area (cm^2)			Meat area (cm^2)		
		S	N	t-Test	S	N	t-Test	S	N	t-Test
M. semimembranosus	$\bar{x}$	5.44	5.77	+++	7.00	5.93	+	5.55	6.06	
	s	0.05	0.32		0.91	1.74		0.74	1.11	
M. semitendinosus	$\bar{x}$	5.47	5.81	+++	6.97	5.35	+++	5.84	6.53	+
	s	0.09	0.23		0.99	1.62		0.63	1.12	
M. longissimus dorsi	$\bar{x}$	5.50	6.07	+++	5.83	4.51	++	6.05	7.09	+++
	s	0.05	0.35		0.96	1.29		0.69	0.96	
M. psoas major	$\bar{x}$	5.55	5.62	+	6.96	5.78	++	5.86	6.55	+
	s	0.08	0.11		1.29	1.47		0.80	0.98	
M. biceps femoris	$\bar{x}$	5.48	5.71	+++	7.10	6.36		5.63	5.92	
	s	0.05	0.28		1.19	1.36		0.63	1.19	

TABLE 3

CONCENTRATIONS (µmol/g) 45 MIN *post mortem* OF GLUCOSE, ATP AND CREATINE PHOSPHATE (CP) IN THE MUSCLES EXAMINED FOR THE 'IMMEDIATE SLAUGHTER' (S) AND 'ADDITIONAL FASTING' (N) GROUPS - MEAN VALUES, STANDARD DEVIATIONS, T-TEST

Muscle		Glucose			ATP			CP		
		S	N	t-Test	S	N	t-Test	S	N	t-Test
M. semimembranosus	$\bar{x}$	0.97	0.79		5.63	5.58		11.33	11.02	
	s	0.64	0.62		0.96	0.40		3.73	3.99	
M. semitendinosus	$\bar{x}$	1.04	1.33		5.52	5.19		7.36	7.97	
	s	0.48	0.87		0.84	0.53		3.94	3.90	
M. longissimus dorsi	$\bar{x}$	0.98	1.15		5.18	4.85		8.01	6.02	+
	s	0.53	0.87		1.01	0.55		3.75	2.62	
M. psoas major	$\bar{x}$	2.46	2.51		4.64	4.30		2.08	2.38	
	s	1.08	1.07		1.77	1.42		1.59	1.59	
M. biceps femoris	$\bar{x}$	1.00	1.02		5.47	5.26		8.68	8.87	
	s	0.63	0.61		1.16	0.53		4.39	2.53	

CONCLUSIONS

Young bulls do not seem to be as sensitive to climatic stress as fattening pigs.

Even under high environmental temperature the muscle metabolism of young bulls shows no serious malfunction.

A prolonged fasting time (more than 2 days) before slaughter seems to have an important effect on the aetiology of dark-cutting beef.

The incidence of dark-cutting meat in young bulls is not initiated by an accelerated breakdown of ATP as frequently found in pigs.

EFFECTS OF TRANSPORTATION AND PRE-SLAUGHTER HOLDING ON SOME BLOOD PARAMETERS AND ON MEAT QUALITY IN FATTENING BULLS

E. Kallweit, J. Unshelm, K. Wemken and D. Smidt
Institut für Tierzucht und Tierverhalten Mariensee (FAL),
3057 Neustadt 1, Federal Republic of Germany

ABSTRACT

Dark-cutting beef seems to be a management problem; it is particularly dependent on the way animals are held during the time shortly before slaughter. In the present experiment the influence of stress on some blood metabolites, hormones and enzymes and on meat quality traits was investigated, as indicators of stress. Fattening bulls were kept in groups, during the last 12 - 14 h prior to slaughter, either under tied-up or loose housing conditions.

Higher physical activity of the loosely-housed groups caused increased plasma contents of hormones and enzymes.

Meat quality traits indicated a tendency in this group towards dark-cutting characteristics.

MATERIALS AND METHODS

The experiment was carried out with 23 fattening bulls, 10 Holstein-Friesian and 13 German Fleckvieh bulls at 18 months of age. They were equipped with Silastic catheters in the external jugular vein and well acquainted with the blood sampling procedure 12 weeks prior to the experiment. All animals were kept in groups on straw bedding. Groups of equal size from each breed were slaughtered on three different days. One day before slaughter they were transported by truck over a distance of approximately 200 km. After arrival at the slaughterhouse the bulls were divided into two holding groups for the remaining time until slaughter. They were kept either under tied-up or loose-housing conditions in groups of 3 - 4 animals.

Blood samples were taken before transportation, after arrival at the slaughterhouse and the next morning before slaughter. On each of these occasions a sequence of three samples at time intervals of 15 min were collected, individually analysed and the results pooled for the calculation of one mean value.

Blood plasma concentrations of cortisol, aldosterone, lactate, creatine kinase (CK), lactate dehydrogenase (LDH) and LDH-isoenzyme 5 were determined. The pH value in *M. longissimus dorsi* (8th/9th rib) was measured at 1, 24 and 48 h *post mortem*. On muscle samples from the rib (48 h *post mortem*) the following traits were evaluated: dry matter, fat content, cooking loss, juice and meat area on filter-paper; the Volodkevich tenderometer and the Göfo reflectance meter were used to measure tenderness and colour brightness respectively.

RESULTS AND CONCLUSIONS

Changes due to transport and holding before slaughter are illustrated in Figure 1 for blood lactate, cortisol and aldosterone, and in Figure 2 for CK, LDH and LDH-isoenzyme 5. Cortisol increased due to the stress of transport and remained at a high level until slaughter. This hormone is therefore an indicator

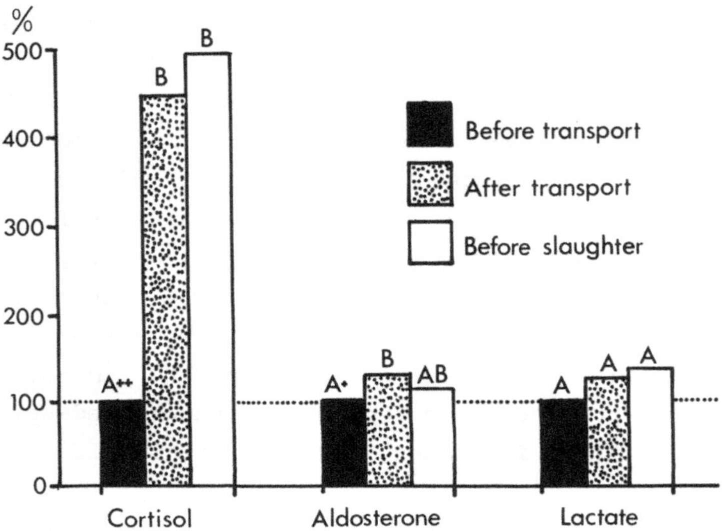

Fig. 1. Changes in cortisol, aldosterone and lactate due to transport and holding before slaughter.

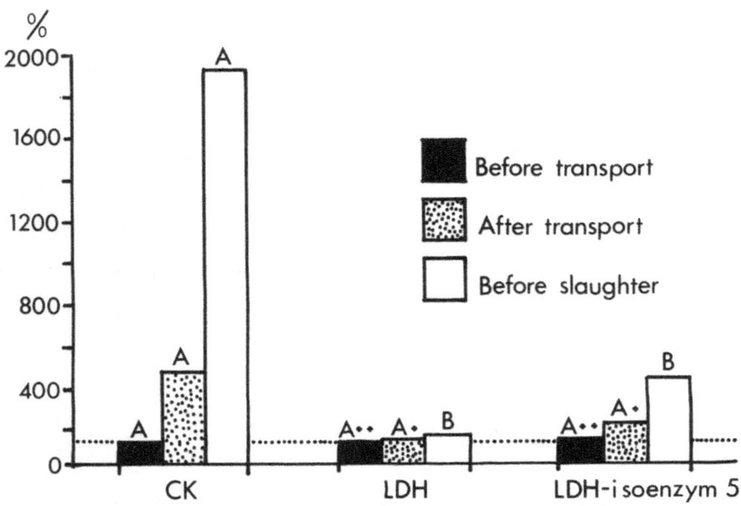

Fig. 2. Changes in creatine kinase, lactate dehydrogenase and lactate dehydrogenase isoenzyme 5 due to transport and holding before slaughter.

TABLE 1

INFLUENCE OF THE METHOD OF HOLDING YOUNG BULLS BEFORE SLAUGHTER ON SOME BLOOD CONSTITUENTS AND MEAT QUALITY CHARACTERISTICS. LEAST SQUARES ANALYSIS WAS CARRIED OUT, VALUES FOR DIFFERENT BREEDS AND DAYS (OF EXPERIMENT) WERE INCLUDED IN THE REGRESSION EQUATION ALTHOUGH THESE FACTORS DID NOT SIGNIFICANTLY INFLUENCE THE TRAITS INVESTIGATED.

	N	Before transport		After transport		Before slaughter	
		$\hat{C}$	$s\hat{C}$	$\hat{C}$	$s\hat{C}$	$\hat{C}$	$s\hat{C}$
Cortisol (log ng/ml)							
Individually tied	11	-0.013	0.049	-0.160*	0.056	-0.081*	0.039
Loose group	12	0.013	0.049	0.160*	0.056	0.081*	0.039
$\hat{\mu}$	23	0.717	0.049	1.31	0.056	1.40	0.039
Blood lactate (mg/100 ml)							
Tied	11	0.99	0.83	0.23	0.56	-2.13**	0.61
Loose group	12	-0.99	0.83	-0.23	0.56	2.13**	0.61
$\hat{\mu}$	23	7.27	0.83	8.54	0.56	9.24	0.61
LDH-isoenzyme 5 (%)							
Tied	9	-0.30	0.29	0.14	0.55	-4.07*	1.89
Loose group	8	0.30	0.29	-0.14	0.55	4.07*	1.89
$\hat{\mu}$	17	2.73	0.30	3.80	0.58	8.42	1.98

($\hat{C}$, regression coefficient; $s\hat{C}$, standard error of coefficient; *, $P \leq 0.05$; **, $P \leq 0.01$).

TABLE 1, cont.

	N	Before transport $\hat{C}$	$S\hat{C}$	After transport $\hat{C}$	$S\hat{C}$	Before slaughter $\hat{C}$	$S\hat{C}$
pH in *M. longissimus dorsi*		pH 60 min		pH 24 h		pH 48 h	
Tied	12	-0.099*	0.028	-0.328*	0.086	-0.254*	0.076
Loose group	12	0.099*	0.028	0.328*	0.086	0.254*	0.076
$\hat{\mu}$	24	6.795	0.028	5.802	0.086	5.716	0.076
Meat quality		Göfo		Cooking loss		Juice area (filter press)	
Tied	12	-3.44*	0.90	2.728*	1.066	1.32*	0.44
Loose group	12	3.44*	0.90	-2.728*	1.066	-1.32*	0.44
$\hat{\mu}$	24	87.4	0.90	40.25	1.07	11.9	0.44
Meat quality		Meat area (filter press)		Volodkevich (kg)			
Tied	12	-1.24*	0.46	1.243	1.279		
Loose group	12	1.24*	0.46	-1.243	1.279		
$\hat{\mu}$	24	10.9	0.46	18.65	1.28		

($\hat{C}$, regression coefficient; $S\hat{C}$, standard error of coefficient; *, $P \leq 0.05$; **, $P \leq 0.01$)

for long-term stress. Aldosterone increased during transport but did not continue to rise during the holding period before slaughter. It may therefore be an indicator of short-term stress. Blood lactate and the blood enzymes increased almost continuously throughout the transport and holding period.

Breed of cattle or day of experiment did not substantially influence the blood parameters or meat quality traits investigated.

The holding system (tied-up or loose in a group) significantly influenced some blood parameters and meat quality traits (Table 1). Tied-up animals were lower in cortisol, lactate and LDH-isoenzyme 5, probably due to less physical activity of these animals during this period.

Differences between tied and loose animals in CK, aldosterone and LDH were not statistically significant.

Water and fat content of muscle tissues were not influenced by holding conditions.

A high level of physical activity among the loosely-housed bulls caused differences in meat quality with a tendency towards dark-cutting beef in this group (Table 1). This was indicated by significantly higher pH values, darker meat colour, a higher water-holding capacity, as well as improved tenderness.

DEVELOPMENT OF SPECIAL FEEDS FOR YOUNG BULLS KEPT IN OVERNIGHT LAIRAGES

K. Kousgaard
Danish Meat Research Institute, Maglegaardsvej 2,
DK-4000 Roskilde, Denmark

ABSTRACT

By carefully transporting and then slaughtering animals the same day they leave the farm, it is almost possible to avoid high ultimate pH in the meat of young bulls.

However, overnight lairage at the abattoir cannot be totally avoided at the moment and the possible use of highly digestible feed to reduce the occurrence of high pH has been investigated.

An experiment with a special mixture of concentrates showed that the occurrence of high pH meat can be appreciably reduced. However, to be effective the animals must be kept in lairage for 2 nights, which means that practical interest in this method is limited.

In order to obtain muscle glycogen deposition as quickly as possible the following experiments are in progress:

1. *Feeding with a mixture of concentrates containing sodium propionate, which is glucogenic and is assumed to pass through the rumen very quickly.*
2. *Feeding with liquid dairy products, which by utilisation of the oesophageal groove closure may bypass the rumen and enter the abomasum directly.*
3. *Encapsulation of glucose in order to avoid microbiological degradation in the rumen.*

INTRODUCTION

Almost all Danish male calves (500 000 per year) are fattened intensively and slaughtered as young bulls at a live-weight of 400 kg. Over half of the animals are delivered directly to the abattoir, and the remainder are sold through live cattle markets. Although distances in Denmark are small, and overnight lairage is avoided as far as possible, it still takes place to some extent.

Normally animals kept in overnight lairage are fed only water and straw. An experiment with a total of 68 young bulls, from a cattle market, which were exhausted at slaughter (Kousgaard, 1975), showed that this feeding did not improve the condition of these animals. After overnight lairage 18 per cent of the animals had pH values higher than 6.0, 24 h after slaughtering, and after two nights lairage 23 per cent had pH values higher than 6.0.

The next approach was to make a highly digestible feed which might make it possible to raise the content of muscle glycogen quickly to a normal level, and possibly in this way reduce the occurrence of high pH meat.

EXPERIMENT 1

For this experiment (Sørensen, 1978), with a total of 60 young bulls bought at market, an experimental feed was made with the following composition:

Dried sugarbeet pulp	43 per cent
Molasses	13 per cent
Barley	35 per cent
Soyabean meal	8 per cent
Fat with flavours	1 per cent

At arrival, the young bulls weighing from 280 to 425 kg live-weight were divided into four groups of 15 animals each.

These were tied separately and treated in the following way in the lairage before slaughter:

Group	Feeding	Number of nights in lairage
1	Straw + water	1
2	Straw + water + 2.5 kg experimental feed	1
3	Straw + water	2
4	Straw + water + 3 x 2.5 kg experimental feed	2

At slaughter liver samples were removed for determination of glycogen and glucose contents. Forty-eight hours after slaughter the pH value was measured in various muscles, and a sample of *M. longissimus dorsi* was removed for colour measurement (Hunterlab L-values). The results are shown in Table 1.

From the experiment the following can be concluded:

1. Prolonged transport results to a great extent in increased pH value.
2. One night lairage gave no difference in the pH value between fed and unfed animals.
3. After two nights lairage only one animal among the fed group had an increased pH value, whereas an obvious deterioration and a lower content of liver glycogen were observed among the unfed animals.
4. The variation in pH values could only partly be explained from the content of liver glycogen, which might indicate psychological as well as physical stress (Duchesne, 1978).

The occurence of high pH values in young bulls kept in overnight lairages can be reduced by feeding, but as the effect requires two nights in lairage the practical value of the experiment is limited. The results are in accordance with an experiment using molasses (Wichlach et al., 1979).

TABLE 1

INFLUENCE OF EXPERIMENTAL FEED AND TIME IN LAIRAGE ON ULTIMATE pH VALUES, LIVER GLYCOGEN PLUS GLUCOSE CONTENT AND COLOUR OF *M. longissimus dorsi* IN YOUNG BULLS.

	Experi-mental feed	Number of animals	pH *M. longimissimus dorsi*			Aver-age pH	Glucose + glycogen mg/g liver	Hunterlab L-values
			<5.8	5.8-6.2	>6.2			
1 night)	-	15	10	3	2	5.82	34.6	33.0
lairage)	+	15	11	1	3	5.81	41.8	32.5
2 nights)	-	15	7	6	2	5.82	21.6	33.3
lairage)	+	15	14	1	0	5.53	38.4	35.4

EXPERIMENT 2

In order to accelerate the desired effect, an experimental feed was prepared containing varying quantities of sodium propionate (4, 8, 12 and 16 per cent). The advantages of using sodium propionate should be that the propionate directly enters the glycogenic pathway, so that the time for fermentation is saved, and quite a large quantity could give a substantial and rapid increase in glycogen level.

An experimental feeding was carried out (Klastrup, 1979) with sodium propionate added to a ground mixture of concentrates for young bulls. Large individual differences between the animals' appetites were found, and not more than 12 per cent sodium propionate should be added. As the feed was very dusty it was decided to use the same pelletised mixture as in experiment 1, but adding 4, 8 or 12 per cent sodium propionate.

Further experimental feeding showed that the animals preferred the mixture with the smallest amount of sodium propionate, and a consumption of 5 kg feed per animal was not reached until after one night in lairage. Addition of sodium propionate may have the physiological effect of causing rapid satiation.

Experimental feeding of sodium propionate to 12 month old bulls will be continued. Also the following subjects will be investigated:

1. Rumen bypass of liquid dairy products through oesophageal groove closure.
2. Feeding with encapsulated glucose.

CONCLUSION

The best way to prevent development of DFD meat in young bulls is a short and careful transport with slaughter as soon as possible after arrival.

At present beef animals have to be tethered individually during transport and in lairages at market places and slaughterhouses. How appropriate this will be in future is an open question, because an increasing number of beef animals are now placed in pens with slatted floors in groups of eight to ten animals.

Use of a highly digestible mixture for young bulls kept in lairages overnight has not yet given the desired effect, proably because it takes time to build up glycogen depots and also because of psychological as well as physical stress factors when the animals are held in new environments.

REFERENCES

Butcher, L., 1980. Development of procedures for identification and minimisation of DFD in young bulls under Danish conditions. Proc. EEC Seminar - The problem of dark-cutting in beef. October 7-8, Brussels.

Duchesne, H.E., 1978. The aetiology of dark-cutting beef. Ph.D. Thesis, University of Bristol.

Klastrup, S., 1979. Fodring af ungtyre med varierende maengder Na-propionat. Personlig meddelelse. Slagteriernes Forskningsinstitut, Roskilde.

Kousgaard, K., 1975. Oplysninger af 3. februar. KALVE - KØDKVALITET. Slagteriernes Forskningsinstitut, Roskilde.

Sørensen, S.E., 1978. Fodring af ungtyre, der opstaldes på slagteri. Arbejde nr. 17.152 - Rapport. Slagteriernes Forskningsinstitut, Roskilde.

Wichlach, H., Grzeskowiak, E. and Krzywicki, K., 1979. The reduction of dark-cutting beef incidence through administration of molasses solution to young bulls before slaughtering. Proc. 25th European Meeting of Meat Research Workers, Budapest, Hungary, 11-13.

SELECTIVE GLYCOGEN DEPLETION AND RECOVERY IN SKELETAL MUSCLES FIBRE TYPES OF YOUNG BULLS SUBJECTED TO A BEHAVIOURAL STRESS

A. Lacourt[1] and P.V. Tarrant

[1]INRA, Station de Recherches sur la Viande, Theix 63110 Beaumont, France

Meat Research Department, Agricultural Institute, Dunsinea Research Centre, Castleknock, Co. Dublin, Ireland.

ABSTRACT

The response of the three major fibre types in beef M. longissimus dorsi during stress and recovery was examined with respect to cellular glycogen content. Stress was induced by mixing experimental animals (eight 15 month old Friesian bulls) with strangers for a period of 5 h. This treatment resulted in significant increases ($P < 0.001$) in heart rate, rectal temperature and plasma CPK activity. The glycogen concentration of M. longissimus dorsi fell to 45 per cent of the resting concentration during the 5 h period of stress ($P < 0.001$). Muscle glycogen concentration returned to 111 per cent of the resting value during a three-day recovery period. Statistically significant differences were observed during stress between the SO fibre type and the FG and FOG fibre types for percent glycogen positive fibres ($P < 0.05$) and percent glycogen negative fibres ($P < 0.001$). Glycogen was lost rapidly during stress from FG and FOG fibre types while SO fibres showed much slower glycogen loss during stress. On the first day of recovery, FG and FOG fibres showed an increase in glycogen content whereas SO fibres continued to lose glycogen. On the third day of recovery all fibre types displayed glycogen contents similar to resting muscle.

INTRODUCTION

Beef skeletal muscle, like that of most animals, contains three major fibre types. These may be classified as slow twitch, oxidative fibres (SO), fast twitch, glycolytic fibres (FG) and fast twitch fibres with both oxidative and glycolytic capacity (FOG). The muscle is also rich in glycogen, an essential requirement for normal meat quality.

Selective glycogen depletion in different muscle fibre types during muscular contraction has been observed in a number of species including man (Gollnick et al., 1973). The response of the different muscle fibre types is largely determined by the intensity and duration of the work performed. Differences between fibre types in beef muscle are of particular interest because they may indicate the mechanism of muscle glycogen depletion in a specific stress situation, for example the mixing stress imposed on the present experimental animals. The relative importance of endocrine (mainly adrenaline) mediated glycogenolysis as opposed to glycogenolysis mediated by contractile events in the muscle cell has not been established.

There is also evidence that glycogen depletion before slaughter occurs in specific muscles, resulting in dark-cutting beef in the corresponding parts of the carcass (Tarrant and Sherington, 1980). As the fibre type composition varies considerably between individual muscles it is of interest to examine the response of the three main fibre types to a typical stress situation.

The object of the experiment was therefore to determine the pattern of glycogen breakdown and recovery in the different fibre types and to establish if the response is significantly different between fibre types.

EXPERIMENTAL PROCEDURE

Animals

Eight Friesian bulls, 14 - 15 months old and 350 - 400 kg liveweight, were tied in stalls and fed a concentrate diet containing rolled barley.

Stress

The experimental bulls were subjected to a social stress by mixing them, two at a time, with a group of ten unfamiliar bulls of the same age and breed. The period of stress was 5 h and recovery was monitored until 72 h. During recovery the experimental animals were returned to their individual stalls and fed *ad libitum*.

Sampling

Muscle samples were taken from *M. longissimus dorsi* using a Bergstrom biopsy needle with an internal diameter of 5 mm. Blood samples were taken from the jugular vein by venepuncture. Resting samples were obtained 3 - 4 days before stress. Samples were taken during stress (+ 3 h), at termination of stress (+ 5 h) and during recovery (+ 24 h and + 72 h).

Treatment

Four of the eight experimental animals were given a treatment designed to elevate blood glucose levels and to stimulate glucose uptake by muscle. This consisted of a subcutaneous injection of 30 mg (15 ml) of a glucocorticoid (Dexadreson, Intervet Laboratories Ltd., Cambridge, England) administered 16 h before the start of stress and an intravenous infusion of 250 g (500 ml) of glucose (Dextrose Injection B.P., 50% w/v, Travenol Laboratories, Norfolk, England) after stress and an intramuscular injection of 240 units (3 ml) of insulin (Protamine Zinc Insulin Injection, B.P. Wellcome Foundation, England). The effect of this treatment on blood and muscle constituents is the subject of a

Fig. 1 A-H. Histochemical analysis of needle biopsy samples of beef *M. longissimus dorsi*. Micrographs A - D are transverse serial sections of a sample taken 3 h after the start of the stress. A, succinic dehydrogenase activity; B, α-glycerophosphate dehydrogenase activity; C, ATPase activity after preincubation at pH 10.2; D, PAS-coloured glycogen. This procedure allowed individual fibres to be identified (A - C) and their glycogen content estimated (D).

Micrographs E - H show muscle glycogen content at the remaining sampling times for the same animal. The complete sequence of muscle glycogen depletion and recovery is: E control sample, ABCD after 3 h of stress, F after 5 h of stress, G recovery after 24 h, H recovery after 72 h. Magnification factor: x 60.

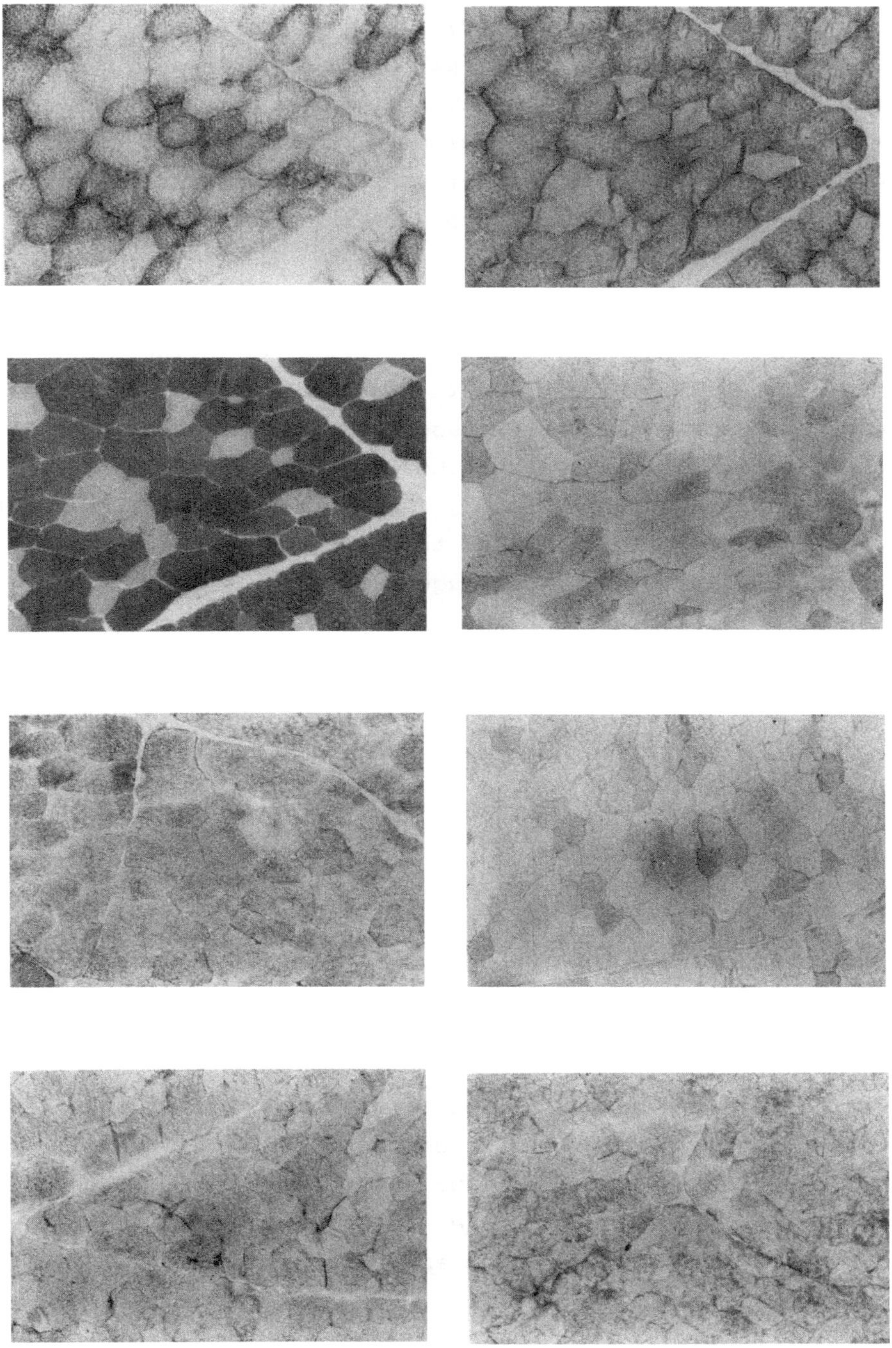

A B C D E F G H

separate report (in preparation). The treatment had no obvious effect on the response of the muscle fibre types to stress nor had it a marked effect on muscle glycogen concentration. Therefore, for the purposes of the present histochemical report, the results for the eight experimental animals were pooled and analysed as a single group.

Biochemical analyses

Muscle glycogen was hydrolysed using amyloglucosidase from *Aspergillus niger* (Boehringer, Mannheim) and determined as free glucose using glucose oxidase (type 5) and peroxidase (type 2, Sigma Chemical Co., St Louis). Creatine kinase activity was measured in fresh plasma as the rate of reduction of $NADP^+$ in the reaction linked to hexokinase and glucose-6-phosphate dehydrogenase (Boehringer).

Histochemical analysis

Transverse serial sections of muscle tissue were prepared. Fibres were classified and typed according to the following scheme:

	FG	FOG	SO
ATPase at pH 9.4 after preincubation at pH 10.2	+	+	-
α-Glycerophosphate dehydrogenase	+	+	-
Succinic dehydrogenase	-	+	+

The relative concentration of glycogen in each fibre was determined by subjective assessment on periodic acid schiff (PAS) stained sections and reported as glycogen positive, glycogen intermediate or glycogen negative in each case. The present analysis is based on an examination of thirty fibres in each muscle sample.

Figure 1 shows fibre typing (A, B, C) and glycogen content (D) for a specimen of muscle taken after 3 h of mixing stress. The sequence of glycogen depletion and recovery for a single animal is shown in micrographs E, D, F, G, H.

Statistical analysis

The percentage glycogen positive, glycogen intermediate and glycogen negative fibres were analysed using factorial analysis of variance, with animals, fibre type and time (after start of stress) as factors. The arcsin transformation of the percentages was used.

RESULTS

Mixing the experimental bulls with strangers resulted in a high level of physical activity and a strong response was observed in the physiological measurements. Significant increases were recorded in heart rate and body temperature (Table 1). These persisted throughout the 5 h period of stress. Plasma creatine kinase activity (Figure 2) was significantly higher at 3 h ($P < 0.01$), 5 h ($P < 0.001$) and again at 24 h ($P < 0.001$) compared with the control value. Quantitative analysis for muscle glycogen (Figure 2) showed a decline to 53 per cent of the control value (87 µmol glucose units/g wet tissue) after 3h of stress ($P < 0.001$) and to 45 per cent of the control value after 5h of stress ($P < 0.001$).

TABLE 1

EFFECT OF MIXING TOGETHER OF UNFAMILIAR FRIESIAN BULLS (FROM 0 h TO 5 h) ON HEART RATE AND BODY TEMPERATURE

Time	Heart rate	Rectal temperature
Control	106 ± 3.5	102.7 ± 0.14
0 h	108 ± 4.6 NS	
+ 3 h	135 ± 3.6***	104.3 ± 0.29**
+ 5 h	133 ± 3.3***	103.9 ± 0.15***
+ 24 h	102 ± 3.2 NS	102.6 ± 0.17 NS
+ 72 h	100 ± 4.9 NS	102.6 ± 0.18 NS

Values are presented as means ± SEM for eight animals. Deviation of results from the mean control value was tested by student's t test for paired values: ***$P < 0.001$, **$P < 0.01$, NS = No statistical significance.

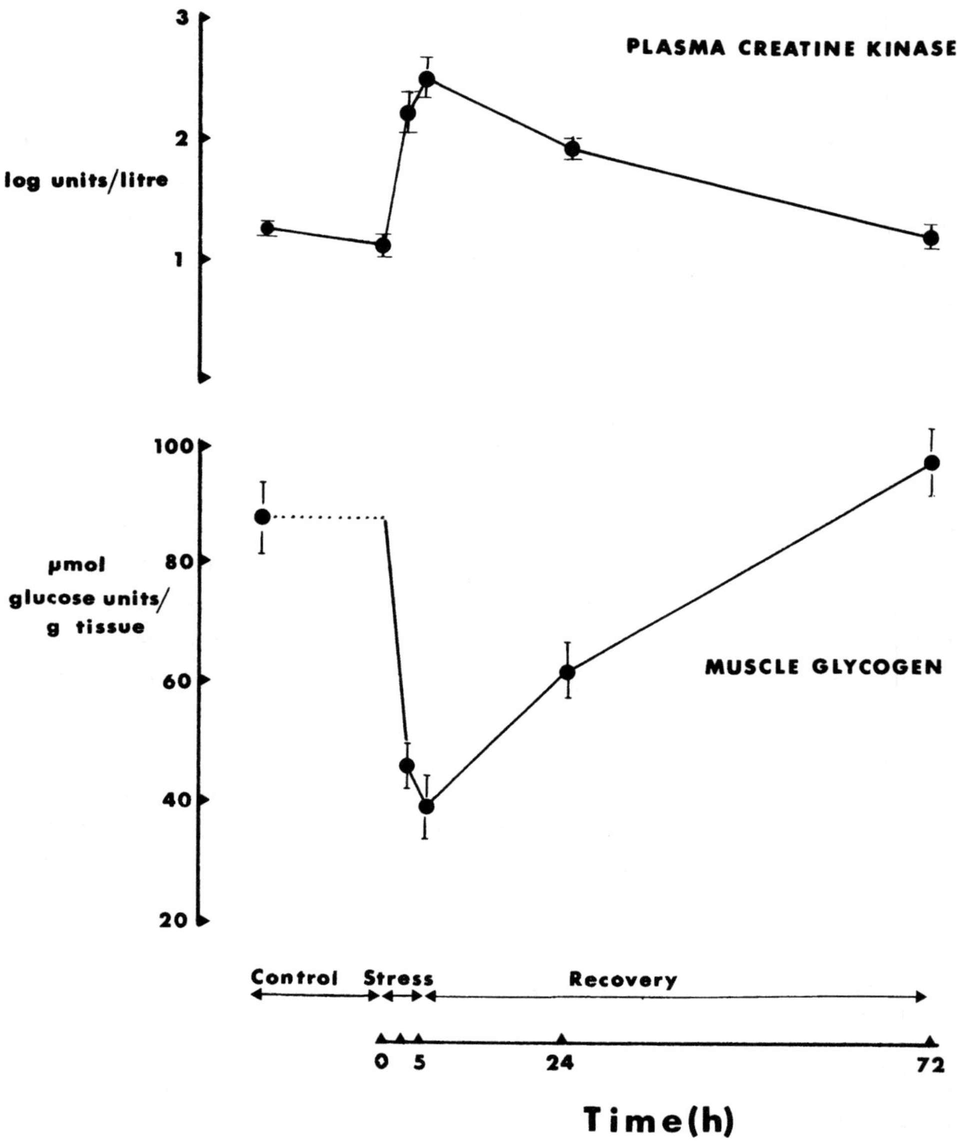

Fig. 2. Plasma creatine kinase activity and muscle (*M. longissimus dorsi*) glycogen concentration in Friesian bulls at rest and during mixing and recovery. Mean values and standard errors are shown for eight animals.

During recovery the concentration of muscle glycogen increased to 71 per cent after one day and to 111 per cent after three days.

The percentage of fibres judged positive, intermediate and negative for glycogen for each of the three beef muscle fibre types (FG, FOG and SO) are shown in Figure 3. Major differences are apparent between the response of SO fibres compared with the FG and FOG fibre types. Statistical analysis of the data (Table 2) confirmed a significant interaction between fibre type and glycogen content, with respect to the percent of fibres positive ($P < 0.05$) and negative ($P < 0.01$) for glycogen.

TABLE 2

FACTORIAL ANALYSIS OF VARIANCE USING THE ARCSIN TRANSFORMATION OF THE PERCENTAGES OF GLYCOGEN POSITIVE (+), INTERMEDIATE (±) AND NEGATIVE (-) FIBRES, WITH ANIMALS (A) TIME AFTER START OF STRESS (T) AND FIBRE TYPE (F) AS FACTORS

Source of variation	Degrees of freedom	Means squared		
		Glycogen +	Glycogen ±	Glycogen -
A	7	0.3165 **	0.5135 **	0.2041 **
T	4	6.4836 ***	4.1573 ***	0.9094 ***
F	2	0.3914 *	0.0070	0.596 ***
AT	28	0.4539 ***	0.3936 ***	0.1058 *
AF	14	0.2412 **	0.1094	0.1785 ***
TF	8	0.6078 ***	0.1914	0.3231 ***
Residual	56	0.0929	0.1394	0.0624

During the first three hours of stress the FG and FOG fibre types showed a large decrease in percent glycogen positive and a corresponding increase in percent glycogen intermediate and glycogen negative fibres (Figure 3). On the contrary SO fibres showed essentially no change in glycogen content during the first three hours of mixing. During the final two hours (3 ⟶ 5 h) a further loss of glycogen was observed and this was mainly associated with the SO fibre type.

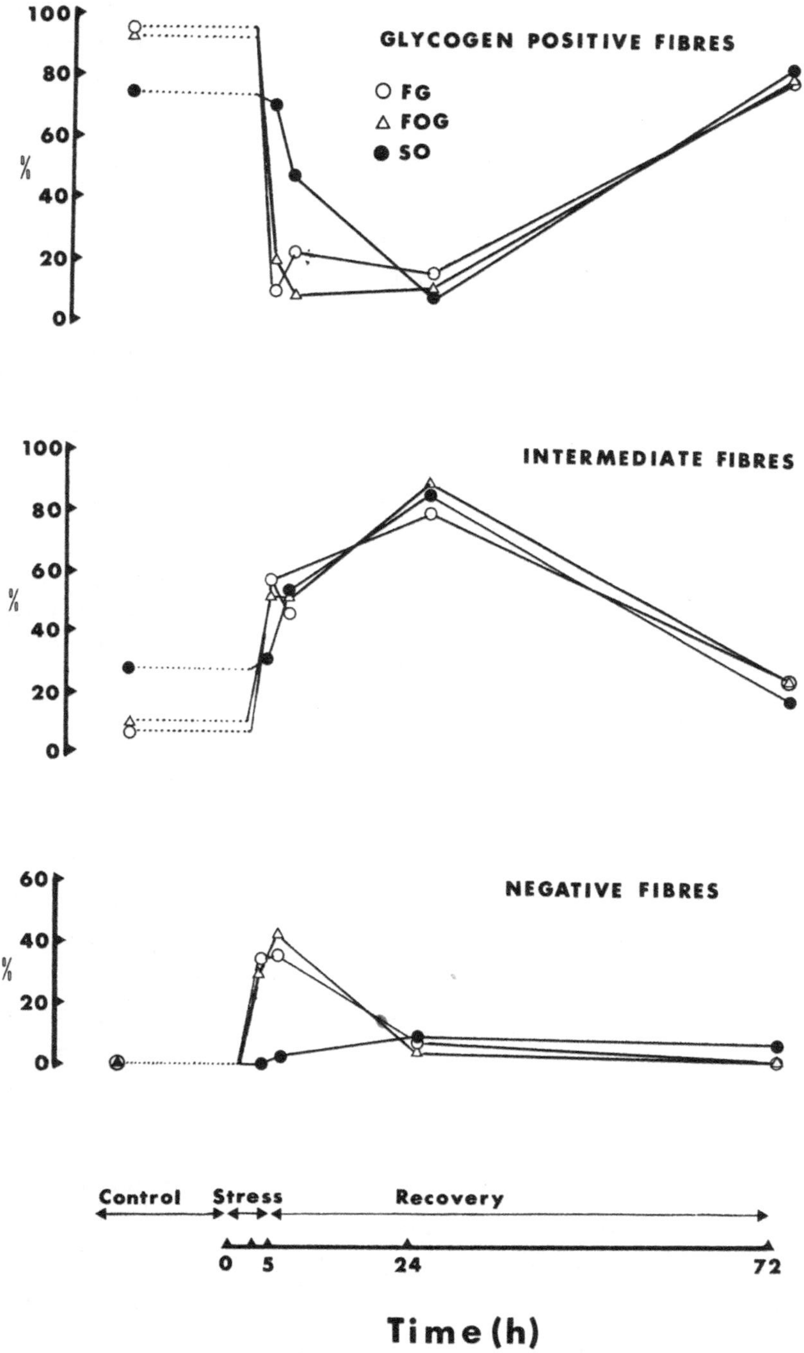

Fig. 3. Percent glycogen positive, intermediate and negative fibres (subjective rating) in Friesian bulls at rest and during mixing and recovery. Results are shown for the three main fibre types in beef *M. longissimus dorsi*. Each point represents the mean value for eight animals.

The glycogen positive fibres declined by 23 per cent and the glycogen intermediate increased by 21 per cent. A notable feature at the termination of the stress period (at 5 h) was the almost total absence of SO fibres negative for glycogen (Figure 3).

During the initial phase of recovery (24 h) FG and FOG fibre types showed an increase in glycogen. This was due to a decrease in percent glycogen negative and a corresponding increase in percent glycogen intermediate fibres. In contrast, the SO fibre type showed further loss of glycogen at 24 h. This was due to a substantial decline in percent glycogen positive and an increase in percent glycogen intermediate fibres.

During the final phase of recovery (24 ⟶ 72 h) the three fibre types showed equally substantial increases in glycogen content. This was manifested by large increases in the percent glycogen positive and corresponding decreases in the percent glycogen intermediate fibres for the three fibre types (Figure 3).

CONCLUSIONS

The three principal fibre types in beef skeletal muscle undergo changes in glycogen content during behavioural stress and recovery. Selective glycogen depletion occurs between SO fibres and the other two fibre types (FG and FOG). Glycogen losses from FG and FOG fibre types are more rapid and more extensive than those occurring in SO fibres. The results suggest that a heavy recruitment of the former two fibre types occurs during the behavioural stress, which is associated with a high level of physical activity. As the glycogen content of the FG and FOG fibres becomes exhausted, SO fibres are gradually recruited. This pattern resembles that observed in man during muscular work of high intensity (Edgerton et al., 1973) and is in contrast to that seen during prolonged, moderately intense exercise when SO fibres are the first to become depleted of their glycogen reserves. The continuing loss of glycogen from SO fibres during the early stages of recovery (5 $\longrightarrow$ 24 h) is of particular interest and the mechanism of this is presently unexplained.

ACKNOWLEDGEMENT

The statistical analysis was performed by J. Sherington, An Foras Taluntais, Sandymount Avenue, Dublin 4.

REFERENCES

Edgerton, V.R., Essén, Birgitta, Saltin, B and Simpson, D.R., 1973. Glycogen depletion in specific types of human skeletal muscle fibres in intermittent and continuous exercise. In: Metabolic Adaptation to Prolonged Physical Exercise. Proc. Second International Symposium on Biochemistry of Exercise, Magglingen. Eds. H. Howald and J.R. Poortmans. Birkhäuser Verlag Basle.

Gollnick, P.D., Armstrong, R.B., Sembrowich, W.L., Shepherd, R.E. and Saltin, B., 1973. Glycogen depletion pattern in human skeletal muscle fibres after heavy exercise. J. appl. Physiol. 34 (5), 615-618.

Tarrant, P.V. and Sherington, J., 1980. An investigation of ultimate pH in the muscles of commercial beef carcasses. Meat Science 4, 287-297.

THE BREAKDOWN OF MUSCLE GLYCOGEN DURING BEHAVIOURAL STRESS IN NORMAL AND BETA-ADRENORECEPTOR BLOCKED YOUNG BULLS

J.M. McVeigh and P.V. Tarrant

Meat Research Department, Agricultural Institute,
Dunsinea Research Centre, Castleknock, Co. Dublin, Ireland.

ABSTRACT

Barley-fed Friesian bulls were stressed by mixing with other bulls for a period of five hours. Afterwards the experimental animals were returned to individual stalls for recovery. At intervals during stress and during recovery, needle biopsy samples were taken from M. longissimus dorsi for glycogen determination. One half of the experimental animals were given propranolol, to study the effect of blockade of beta-adrenergic receptors on muscle glycogen breakdown.

During stress in young bulls, highly significant increases ($P < 0.001$) above resting levels were observed in body temperature, heart rate, serum NEFA and plasma CPK. Muscle glycogen concentration fell to 37 per cent of the value at rest ($P < 0.001$). During a three-day recovery period the glycogen concentration increased to 85 per cent of the value at rest. In the propranolol-treated animals, the muscle glycogen concentration fell to 45 per cent of the resting value at the end of stress ($P < 0.01$) and increased to 91 per cent of the resting value after a three-day recovery period.

The results show that glycogen breakdown occurred continuously during a period of behavioural stress in young bulls. Recovery was a relatively slow process. Propranolol had a small protective effect during the initial part of the stress period ($P < 0.02$) but subsequently was totally ineffective in preventing muscle glycogen depletion. The result suggests that muscle glycogen depletion in cattle during mixing stress is not predominantly mediated by catecholamines.

INTRODUCTION

Muscle glycogen depletion results from physiological stress, including heavy muscular work, during which muscle glycogenolysis is activated. Several factors may be responsible for this activation, including adrenaline release and biochemical changes associated with muscle contraction. In this study the involvement of adrenaline in muscle glycogenolysis during a behavioural stress was examined.

Adrenaline is released *in vivo* in stressful situations and may be a causative agent in the development of dark cutting in beef (Hedrick et al., 1959). Subcutaneous adrenaline administration caused muscle glycogen depletion in steers and this response was successfully inhibited by prior administration of propranolol (Ashmore et al., 1973). Consequently, propranolol was proposed to be an effective agent for the prevention of dark-cutting in beef. Its capacity to prevent muscle glycogen breakdown during stress induced by mixing unfamiliar cattle was examined in the present experiment.

EXPERIMENTAL PROCEDURE

Animals

Twelve Friesian bulls aged 12 - 17 months and weighing 381 - 450 (mean 410) kg were used in the study. They were fed a concentrate ration containing rolled barley *ad libidum* and were kept tied in individual stalls from 10 months of age.

Stress

The experimental animals, in pairs, were mixed with an established group of 9 (or 10) similar bulls for five hours. Afterwards, the animals were returned to their individual stalls for recovery and fed the barley ration *ad libidum*.

Beta-blockade

One of each pair of experimental animals was given an

intravenous infusion of propranolol solution (Propranolol Hydrochloride BP, ICI Limited, England) at a dosage of 0.5 mg/kg liveweight, at one hour before mixing and again at 0, 1 h and 3 h after mixing. A preliminary trial (Table 1) established that this dosage was completely effective for preventing glycogen depletion in *M. longissimus dorsi* of adrenaline-treated (0.26 mg/kg liveweight) Friesian bulls.

TABLE 1

VARIATION IN MUSCLE GLYCOGEN IN FRIESIAN BULLS TREATED WITH PROPRANOLOL AND ADRENALINE AND SUBSEQUENTLY WITH ADRENALINE ONLY. TREATMENTS WERE GIVEN AT TIME 0. DEVIATION OF RESULTS FROM THE CONTROL VALUE AT REST WAS TESTED FOR SIGNIFICANCE BY ANALYSIS OF COVARIANCE.

	Glycogen (μmol glucose units/g wet weight of tissue)			
	Mean value	Standard error	Number of animals	Significance level
Control value	90.1	± 5.66	6	
Propranolol/Adrenaline				
+ 24 h	85.6	± 3.56	6	N.S.
+ 72 h	94.2	± 5.15	6	N.S.
Adrenaline				
+ 24 h	38.0	± 5.58	6	$P < 0.01$
+ 72 h	66.6	± 5.91	4	$P < 0.05$

Sampling times

Blood and muscle samples were taken at 3 - 4 days before mixing (control samples), at 1 h, 3 h and 5 h after the start of stress and again during recovery at 24 h and 72 h.

METHODS

Tissue samples

Muscle samples were obtained from *M. longissimus dorsi* using a Bergström needle of 5 mm internal diameter. Blood was collected by venepuncture of the jugular. Heart rate was determined by stethoscopic examination.

Biochemical analyses

Muscle glycogen was extracted and hydrolysed using amyloglucosidase and the glucose liberated was determined enzymatically.

Creatine kinase activity was measured in fresh plasma as the rate of reduction of $NADP^+$ in the reaction linked to glucose-6-phosphate dehydrogenase and hexokinase. A unit of enzyme activity is defined as 1 μmol of substrate used per min at $25^{o}C$.

Free fatty acids were extracted from serum using a two-phase system and measured in duplicate by an automated colorimetric procedure.

Statistical analysis

The data was statistically evaluated using an analysis of covariance, adjusting for resting values.

RESULTS

The mixing procedure usually resulted in a high level of physical activity, eventually leading to fatigue in both the control and propranolol-treated animals. Major changes were observed in all of the physiological parameters examined.

A. Response to stress in untreated bulls:

Significant increases above the mean resting values occurred in the heart rate ($P < 0.01$, Figure 1), rectal temperature ($P < 0.001$, Table 2) and blood glucose concentration ($P < 0.05$, Table 2). These parameters were elevated after one hour of mixing and remained elevated throughout the stress period (5 h). Serum NEFA concentration (Figure 2) and plasma CPK activity (Table 2) increased gradually and were significantly elevated at +3 h ($P < 0.05$ and $P < 0.01$ respectively). Values for NEFA and CPK showed further large increases at +5 h.

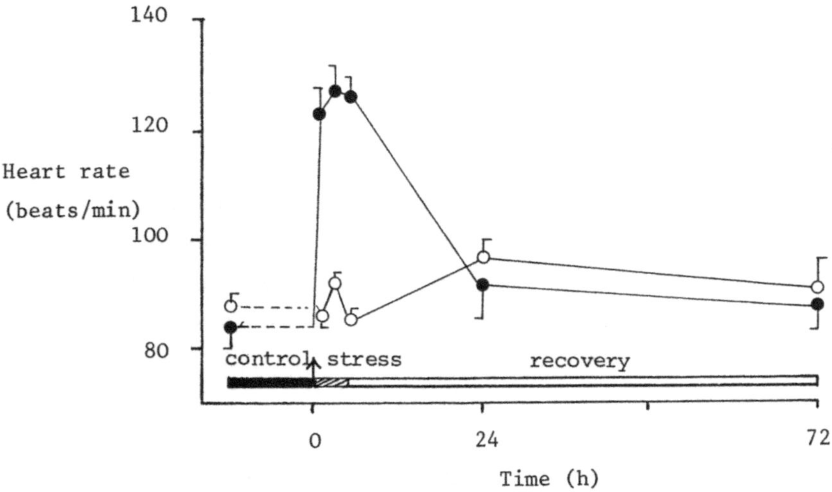

Fig. 1. Heart rate in untreated (●) and propranolol-treated (O) Friesian bulls at rest and during mixing stress and recovery. The results are presented as mean values and standard errors for six animals in each group.

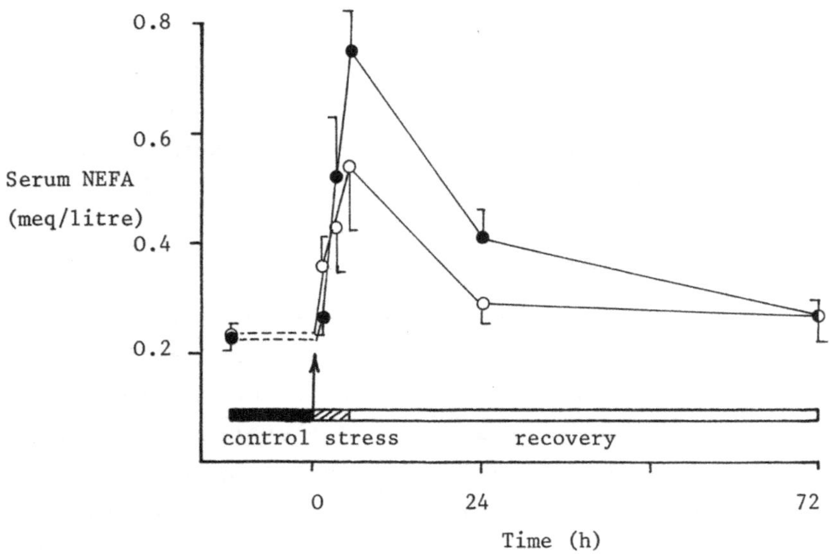

Fig. 2. Serum non-esterified fatty acids in untreated (●) and propranolol-treated (O) Friesian bulls at rest and during mixing stress and recovery. The results are presented as mean values and standard errors for six animals in each group.

TABLE 2

CHANGES IN BLOOD GLUCOSE, PLASMA CPK AND RECTAL TEMPERATURE DURING A FIVE HOUR PERIOD OF STRESS (COMMENCING AT TIME O) AND DURING RECOVERY IN FRIESIAN BULLS. RESULTS (MEAN VALUES AND STANDARD ERRORS) ARE PRESENTED FOR SIX UNTREATED AND SIX PROPRANOLOL-TREATED BULLS.

TIME		BLOOD GLUCOSE (mmol/litre)		PLASMA CPK (units/litre)		RECTAL TEMPERATURE (°C)	
		UNTREATED	PROPRANOLOL-TREATED	UNTREATED	PROPRANOLOL-TREATED	UNTREATED	PROPRANOLOL-TREATED
RESTING VALUES	-3/-4 days	3.23 ± 0.10	3.23 ± 0.12	33 ± 5	39 ± 6	39.1 ± 0.12	39.1 ± 0.12
	-1 h	3.09 ± 0.06	3.19 ± 0.09	37 ± 5	46 ± 12	38.9 ± 0.19	38.8 ± 0.11
STRESS	+1 h	3.80 ± 0.25	5.77 ± 0.86	185 ± 68	135 ± 24	40.8 ± 0.15	40.9 ± 0.25
	+3 h	3.82 ± 0.19	5.52 ± 1.37	520 ± 88	563 ± 137	40.7 ± 0.19	41.0 ± 0.39
	+5 h	3.44 ± 0.07	3.64 ± 0.09	1238 ± 190	1008 ± 192	40.7 ± 0.22	40.5 ± 0.26
RECOVERY	+1 day	3.11 ± 0.20	3.33 ± 0.16	551 ± 89	539 ± 111	38.9 ± 0.13	39.2 ± 0.18
	+3 days	3.39 ± 0.09	3.40 ± 0.18	63 ± 9	60 ± 8	39.0 ± 0.07	39.3 ± 0.18

During the recovery period all values returned gradually towards normal. On day 1 (approximately 19 h after terminating stress) the heart rate, rectal temperature and blood glucose concentration were not significantly different from mean resting values. On the third day of recovery serum NEFA concentration was close to the resting value and plasma CPK was still significantly elevated ($P < 0.05$).

B. Response to stress in propranolol-treated bulls:

Some parameters (rectal temperature and plasma CPK activity, (Table 2) showed an identical response to that observed in untreated bulls. However, the responses of heart rate, serum NEFA and blood glucose were significantly altered by propranolol. The pulse remained constant during stress and did not vary significantly from the resting value. This was in contrast to an elevation of about 50% observed in the untreated animals.

Serum NEFA concentration increased significantly during stress in the propranolol-treated bulls ($P < 0.05$ at +3 h). However, the increase was not as great as that observed in untreated bulls (Figure 2). Blood glucose concentration also increased significantly in the propranolol-treated bulls ($P < 0.05$ at +1 h, Table 2) and this response was significantly greater than that of the untreated bulls ($P < 0.05$ at +1 h). A feature of the hyperglycaemia in the propranolol-treated bulls was the large standard errors associated with the mean values, indicating the irregularity of the hyperglycaemic response.

C. Effect of stress on muscle glycogen concentration in untreated and in propranolol-treated bulls:

Muscle glycogen was significantly lower at all points of the stress period in both the untreated and treated bulls (Figure 3).

In the untreated animals, after 1 h of stress, muscle glycogen had decreased from a resting value of 86.5 μmol

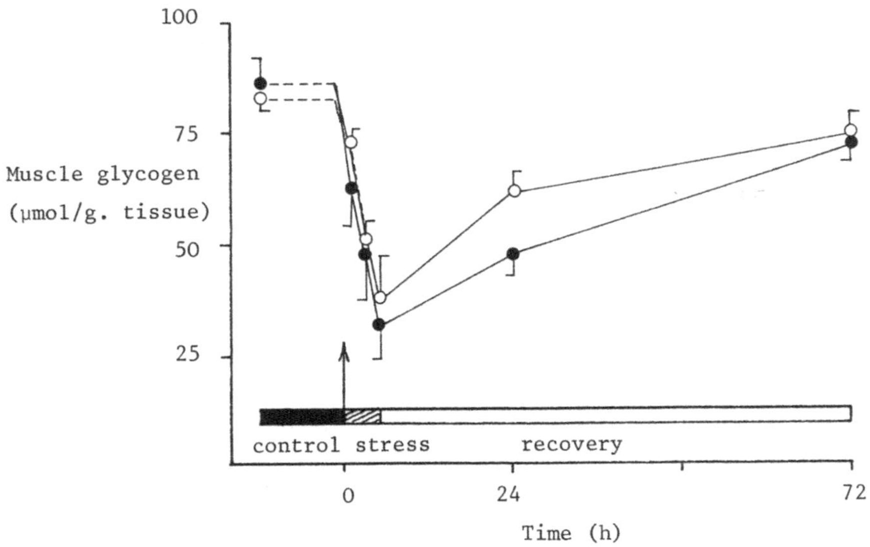

Fig. 3. Muscle glycogen concentration in untreated (●) and in propranolol-treated (O) Friesian bulls at rest and during mixing stress and recovery. The results are presented as mean values and standard errors for six animals in each group.

glucosyl unit/g wet weight of tissue to 62.8 μmol/g. It had decreased further at 3 h and by 5 h was at 32.1 μmol/g (37 per cent of the resting value).

In the propranolol-treated animals muscle glycogen decreased from a resting level of 83.5 μmol/g to 73.4 μmol/g after one hour of stress. Glycogen continued to decrease throughout the stress period and after five hours was at 37.9 μmol/g (45 per cent of the resting concentration).

Propranolol had a protective effect on muscle glycogen during the early stages of mixing. During the first hour the rate of glycogen depletion was reduced from 23.7 μmol/g per hour to 10.1 μmol/g per hour by propranolol treatment ($P < 0.02$).

Some glycogen repletion was observed on day 1 (19 h after the termination of stress). On day 3 muscle glycogen concentration was at 85 per cent and 91 per cent of the resting concentration in the untreated and propranolol-treated groups respectively. The repletion rates were similar in both groups during the 3-day recovery period and were 14.8 and 13.5 µmol/g per day in the untreated and treated animals, respectively.

CONCLUSIONS

The results of the experiment support the following conclusions:

a) The stress of mixing with unfamiliar animals produces a strong physiological response. During mixing, glycogen breakdown in *M. longissimus dorsi* is substantial and continuous. Recovery, under favourable conditions, is a comparatively slow process, requiring three days.

b) An effective blockade of beta-adrenergic receptor sites was established, as shown by:

1. Total inhibition of muscle glycogenolysis following adrenaline injection;
2. Inhibition of the increase in pulse rate during stress; and
3. Reduction in NEFA during stress.

c) Propranolol is largely ineffective in preventing muscle glycogen depletion during mixing stress.

d) Muscle glycogen depletion during mixing stress is not predominantly mediated by catecholamines. The most likely alternative controlling factors are the intracellular events associated with the performance of work, notably the breakdown of high-energy phosphates and elevated calcium ion concentrations.

REFERENCES

Ashmore, C.R., Carroll, F. and Doerr, L., 1973. Effects of propranolol on characteristics of beef carcasses. J. Anim. Sci. 37, 435-437.

Hedrick, H.B., Boillot, J.B., Brady, D.E. and Nauman, H.D., 1959. Etiology of dark-cutting beef. Missouri Agr. Exp. Sta. Res. Bull. 717.

FACTORS INFLUENCING MUSCLE GLYCOGEN SYNTHESIS AFTER ADRENALINE INDUCED DEPLETION IN BEEF HEIFERS

J.M. McVeigh and P.V. Tarrant
Meat Research Department, Agricultural Institute, Dunsinea, Castleknock, Co. Dublin, Ireland

ABSTRACT

Muscle glycogen content was reduced to one quarter of its resting value by subcutaneous injection of adrenaline in Hereford heifers. Recovery of muscle glycogen was followed in needle biopsy samples of M. longissimus dorsi, under conditions of fasting and hay feeding. Also measured were muscle glycogen synthase activity, glucose-6-phosphate, blood glucose, insulin and non-esterified fatty acid contents.

Replenishment of muscle glycogen in hay-fed heifers averaged 4.8 μmol glucose units/g wet weight of tissue/day. This is equivalent to 5.6 per cent of the resting concentration. Fasting reduced the rate of repletion to 1.5 μmol/g/day.

Fasting alone had a small but significant effect on resting muscle glycogen content, amounting to 15 per cent loss during a nine day fast.

The specific activity of beef muscle glycogen synthase (I+D) was 2.13 μmol UDPG/min/g wet weight of tissue at 30°C and pH 7.8. The per cent active form (synthase I) of the enzyme increased from values close to 40 per cent in resting muscle to 70 per cent in glycogen-depleted muscle.

Low muscle glycogen content was associated with low muscle glucose-6-phosphate (not statistically significant) and plasma immunoreactive insulin ($P < 0.01$) contents. Blood glucose content was not affected by fasting or by low muscle glycogen; the combination of fasting and low muscle glycogen caused a slight decrease ($P < 0.05$).

Serum non-esterified fatty acid concentration was not affected by glycogen depletion per se but increased to very high values (> 2.0 mmol/l) in fasted animals.

INTRODUCTION

The glycogen content of the muscles of meat animals at slaughter has an important influence on the *post mortem* biochemical reactions in the muscle and ultimately on meat quality. Dark-cutting meat is a direct result of low muscle glycogen stores at the time of slaughter leading to a high ultimate pH in the meat. Glycogen deficiency, in turn, may result from physiological stress caused by physical activity or emotional excitement. Both of these conditions are commonly encountered by meat animals in the immediate pre-slaughter period.

The rate of repletion of muscle glycogen stores depends on rest and an adequate feed intake. Much work has been done on human subjects on the effect of different diets on muscle glycogen repletion rates. Such *in vivo* work was facilitated by the development of a muscle biopsy needle capable of taking small muscle samples for biochemical and histochemical analysis. Previous studies on meat animals have relied on data obtained from animals slaughtered during the course of the experiment. However, in the present work, the muscle needle biopsy removed this constraint and permitted continuous assessment of muscle glycogen metabolism over extended periods. Muscle sampling was shown not to cause undue stress or loss of muscle glycogen in cattle (McVeigh and Tarrant, 1979).

The objective of this study was to determine the rate of repletion of skeletal muscle glycogen in fasted and hay-fed beef heifers. In addition the effect of glycogen depletion and fasting on plasma immunoreactive insulin and blood glucose concentration and on muscle glycogen synthase activity and glucose-6-phosphate content was examined.

EXPERIMENTAL PROCEDURE

Animals

Hereford heifers, 18 - 36 months old, and weighing 329 - 435 kg were tied in stalls and fed hay to appetite. A minimum of 2 weeks was allowed from tying in stalls to the start of experimental work. During this pre-experimental period the animals were familiarised with some of the experimental procedures, by removing them from their stalls and restraining them in a cattle crush on a number of occasions. Blood sampling and heart rate measurements were performed at these times.

Treatments

The animals were divided into 4 groups as follows:
Group A, fed controls (N = 4)
Group B, fed and adrenaline treated (N = 4)
Group C, fasted controls (N = 6)
Group D, fasted and adrenaline treated (N = 6)

Fasting

Fasting consisted of a 9 day period during which animals had access to water only. In group D, fasting commenced 2 days before adrenaline injection and terminated 7 days after adrenaline. Fasting animals were then returned to a full intake of hay over a 4 day period (day 7 - day 11 in Figure 1). Animal liveweights at the termination of fasting averaged 86 per cent (group D) and 89 per cent (group C) of the fed liveweight.

Sampling times

Control samples of muscle and blood were taken at 6 and 3 days before adrenaline treatment and the mean value for these 2 samples was taken as control. Further samples were taken immediately before adrenaline treatment (day 0) and at the following points of the recovery period; days 1, 2, 4, 7, 11, 14, 17 and 25.

METHODS

Tissue sampling

Muscle samples were taken from *M. longissimus dorsi* using a Bergstrom biopsy needle of 5 mm internal diameter. Blood was collected by venepuncture from the jugular vein.

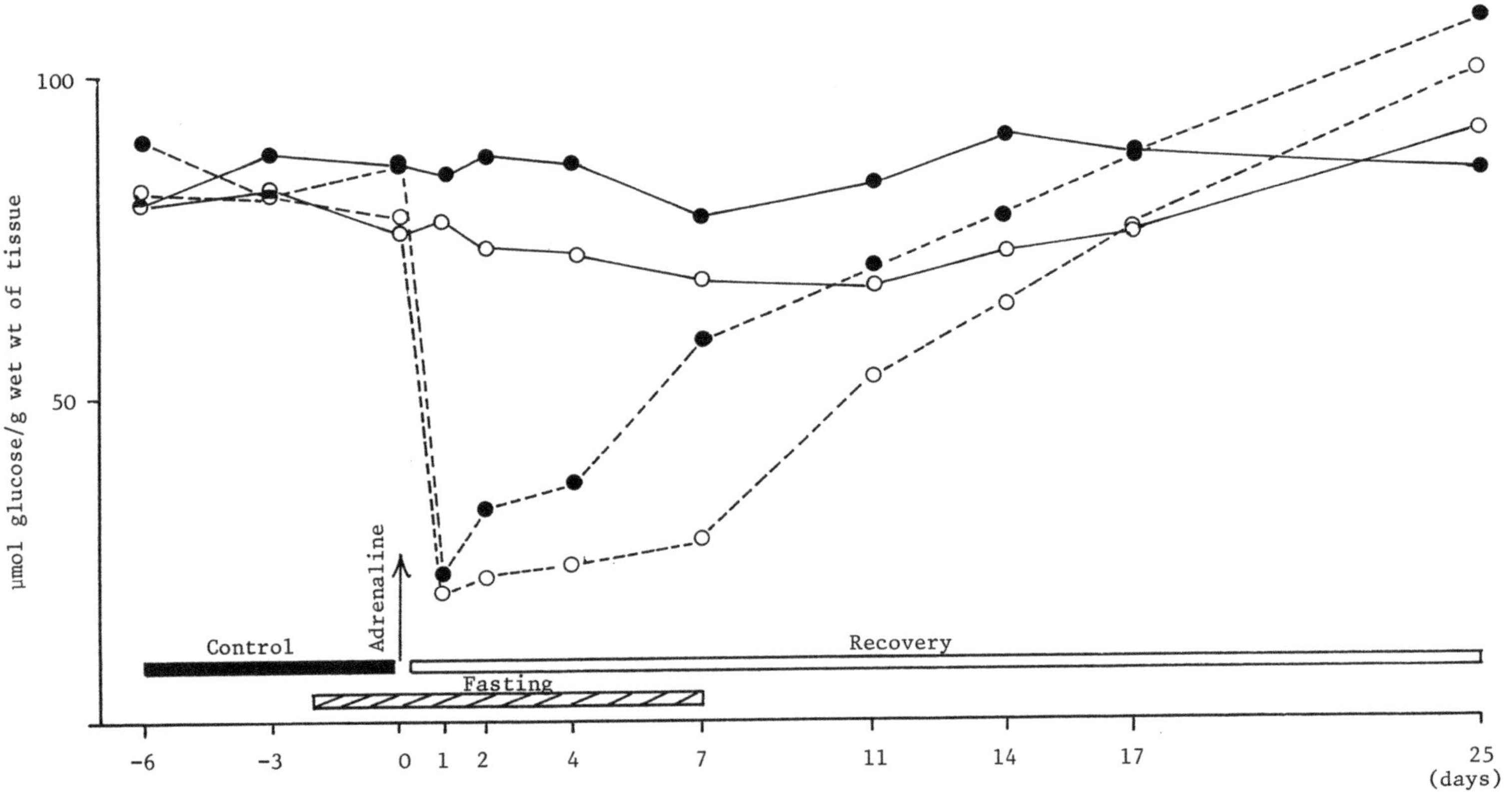

Fig. 1. Glycogen concentration in *M. longissimus dorsi* in adrenaline-treated (----) and untreated (____) hay-fed (●) and fasting (o) heifers. Each of the two fasted groups contained six animals and the fed groups four animals.

Biochemical Assays

Muscle glycogen synthase activity was determined in the whole tissue homogenate in the presence (dependent form) and absence (independent form) of glucose-6-phosphate, by measuring the rate of transfer of C^{14}-glucose from UDPG to glycogen.

Plasma insulin was measured by radioimmuno-assay (Phadebas, Pharmacia) against a porcine insulin standard.

Muscle glycogen and glucose-6-phosphate, blood glucose and plasma creatine kinase (CPK) were determined using standard enzymatic methods. Serum non-esterified fatty acids (NEFA) were measured colorimetrically. Heart rate was measured by stethoscopic examination.

Adrenaline treatment

On day 0, after muscle and blood sampling, adrenaline (1mg/ml Antigen, Ireland) was injected subcutaneously into the shoulder area at a dosage of 0.13 mg/kg liveweight. This dosage was repeated after an interval of approximately 6 hours.

Statistical analysis

An analysis of covariance was carried out between the four experimental groups, adjusting for control values in each animal. Occasionally within-group comparisons were made using Student's t-test for impaired values.

RESULTS

Muscle glycogen metabolism in hay-fed beef heifers

Adrenaline caused a depletion of muscle glycogen from 86.4 μmol glucose/g wet weight of tissue to 23.1 μmol/g (Figure 1). Resynthesis to 71.1 μmol/g took 10 days corresponding to a glycogen repletion rate of 4.8 μmol/g/day.

Glycogen synthase per cent I activity increased from a resting value of 38 per cent of total synthase activity to 68 per cent on day 2, 48 h after the start of adrenaline treatment (Figure 2). During the period of muscle glycogen repletion, glycogen synthase activity remained elevated and only declined slowly throughout the recovery period. By day 25 synthase activity was close to pre-adrenaline levels. The specific activity of glycogen synthase (I+D) was 2.13 ± 0.057 μmole UDPG min/g wet weight of tissue at 30°C and pH 7.8.

The glycogen precursors blood glucose and muscle glucose-6-phosphate are shown in Figure 3 and Table 1 respectively. In group B blood glucose was not significantly below the mean control value during the period of muscle glycogen repletion. Glucose-6-phosphate tended to decrease during this period, but was not significantly below the mean control value (unpaired Student's t-test).

Plasma immunoreactive insulin (Figure 4) increased significantly ($P < 0.01$) from a resting concentration of 15 μU/ml to 82 μU/ml, on day 1, 24 h after the start of adrenaline treatment. Insulin declined to its lowest level (10 μU/ml) on the fourth day after adrenaline treatment ($P < 0.01$) and subsequently (day 7 and afterwards) remained close to the resting value.

Muscle glycogen metabolism in fasted beef heifers

Adrenaline caused depletion of muscle glycogen from 80.8 μmol/g to 20.3 μmol/g (Figure 1). A paired Student's t-test showed that at the termination of the fast (day 7) the muscle glycogen concentration had increased significantly ($P < 0.01$) and was at 29.0 μmol/g. The repletion rate during the fasting period was 1.5 μmol/g/day. In a control group of heifers which were fasted without adrenaline treatment, muscle glycogen declined from a resting value of 79.7 μmol/g to 69.1 μmol/g at the termination of the fast (day 7) ($P < 0.05$).

Glycogen synthase I activity (Figure 2) increased from a resting value of 42 per cent to 64 per cent at 48 h after the first adrenaline injection. Glycogen synthase activity declined slowly during the course of the recovery period. This response

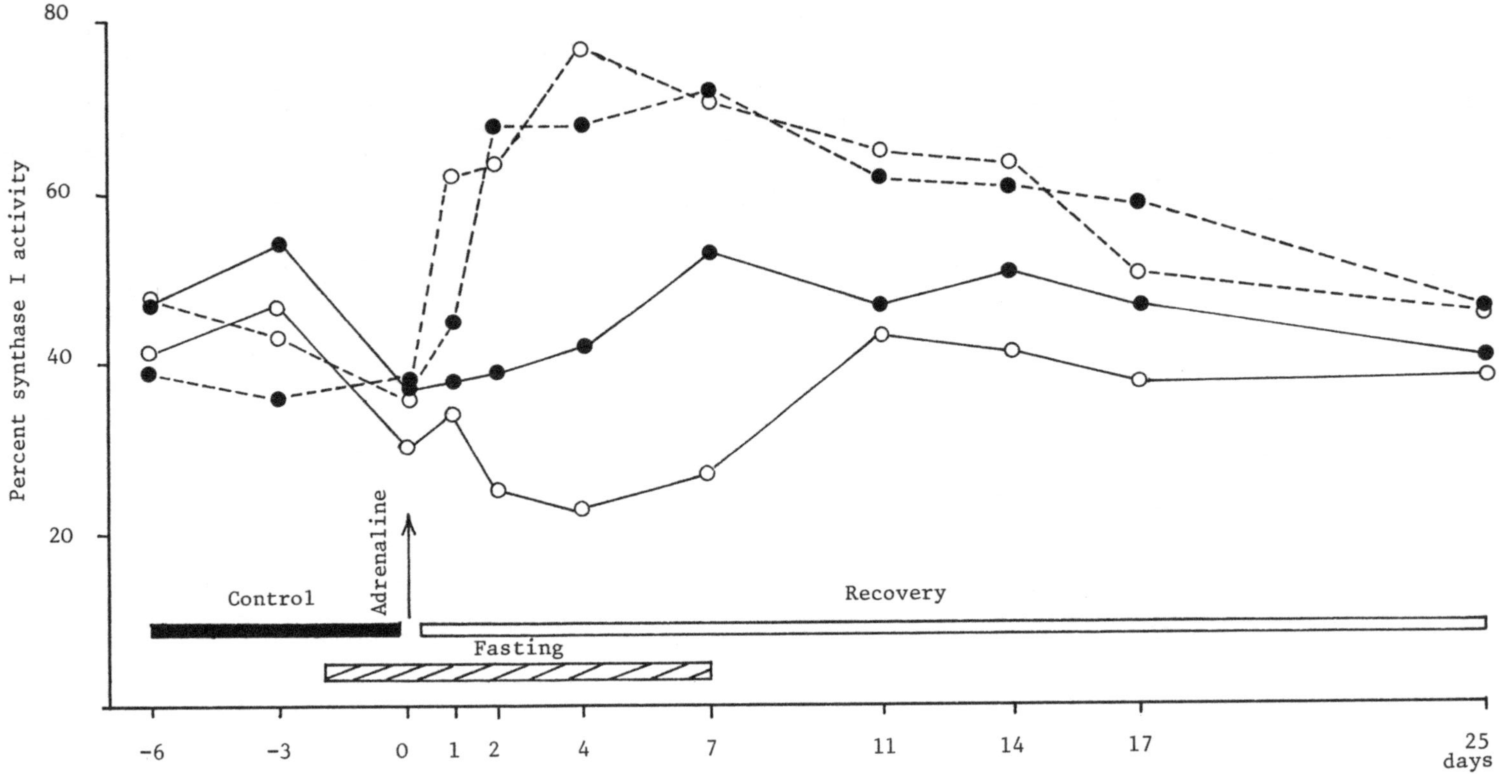

Fig. 2. Glycogen synthase I activity in *M. longissimus dorsi* in adrenaline-treated (----) and untreated (——) hay-fed (●) and fasting (o) beef heifers. Each of the four experimental groups contained two animals.

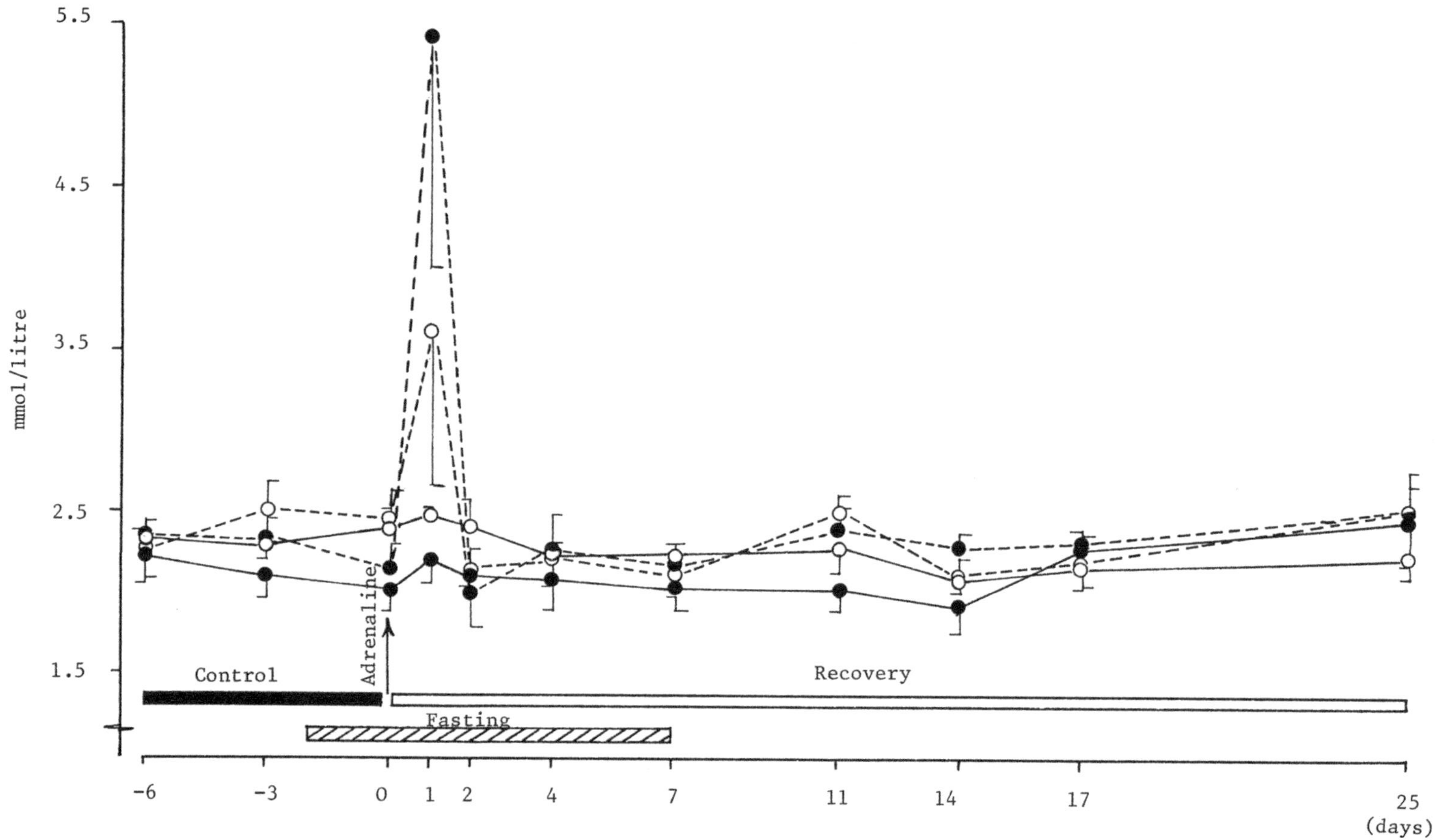

Fig. 3. Blood glucose concentration in adrenaline-treated (----) and untreated (———) hay-fed (●) and fasting (o) beef heifers. Each of the two fasted groups contained six animals and the fed groups four animals.

TABLE 1

MUSCLE GLUCOSE-6-PHOSPHATE CONCENTRATION IN THE *M. longissimus dorsi* OF FOUR GROUPS OF HEREFORD HEIFERS

Day	Fed Control (Group A)	Fed, Adrenaline-Treated (Group B)	Fasted Control (Group C)	Fasted, Adrenaline-Treated (Group D)
-6	1.4 ± 0.22 (3)	1.8 ± 0.27 (3)	2.2 ± 0.29 (5)	1.6 ± 0.58 (4)
-3	1.5 ± 0.23 (3)	2.2 ± 0.58 (3)	1.9 ± 0.34 (5)	2.1 ± 0.52 (5)
0	1.6 ± 0.29 (3)	2.0 ± 0.34 (2)	2.1 ± 0.37 (5)	1.9 ± 0.17 (5)
1	1.8 ± 0.08 (3)	1.6 ± 0.21 (2)	2.3 ± 0.40 (5)	1.0 ± 0.26 (4)
2	1.3 ± 0.31 (3)	1.3 ± 0.11 (2)	1.7 ± 0.52 (4)	1.1 ± 0.25 (5)
4	1.0 ± 0.05 (3)	1.2 ± 0.13 (3)	1.8 ± 0.83 (3)	1.3 ± 0.29 (4)
7	2.4 ± 0.36 (2)	1.6 ± 0.23 (3)	2.8 ± 0.51 (5)	2.3 ± 0.36 (4)
11	2.2 ± 0.27 (3)	1.6 ± 0.50 (2)	2.7 ± 0.49 (4)	1.1 ± 0.11 (3)
14	2.0 ± 0.14 (3)	1.7 ± 0.30 (3)	2.7 ± 0.34 (5)	1.3 ± 0.24 (4)
17	1.9 ± 0.42 (3)	1.6 ± 0.41 (3)	2.3 ± 0.22 (4)	1.3 ± 0.38 (4)
25	2.3 ± 0.31 (2)	2.0 ± 0.00 (2)	2.3 ± 0.32 (2)	2.5 ± 0.45 (2)

Results are expressed as μmol/g wet weight of tissue. Values are given as means, standard errors and numbers of experimental animals in parenthesis.

was similar to that observed in the fed adrenaline-treated heifers. The control group which were fasted without adrenaline treatment showed a decline in glycogen synthase I activity from a resting value of 44 per cent to 27 per cent at the termination of fast (day 7).

The concentrations of the glycogen precursors muscle glucose-6-phosphate (Table 1) and blood glucose (Figure 3) were not significantly affected by fasting (group C). Muscle glucose-6-phosphate concentrations were lower during the period of glycogen repletion compared with the mean control value (group D) (not statistically significant). Blood glucose was slightly lower after glycogen depletion compared to the mean control value (group D) ($P < 0.05$).

Plasma immunoreactive insulin increased from a resting value of 18 μU/ml to 27 μU/ml on day 1, 24 h after the first adrenaline injection (Figure 4). Subsequently it declined to its lowest level (9 μU/ml) on the fourth day after adrenaline ($P < 0.01$). No significant deviations from the mean resting values were observed for the remainder of the recovery period.

The effect of fasting on serum non-esterified fatty acid concentration is shown in Figure 5. Significant elevations occurred in both the adrenaline-treated and untreated animals which persisted for the duration of the fast.

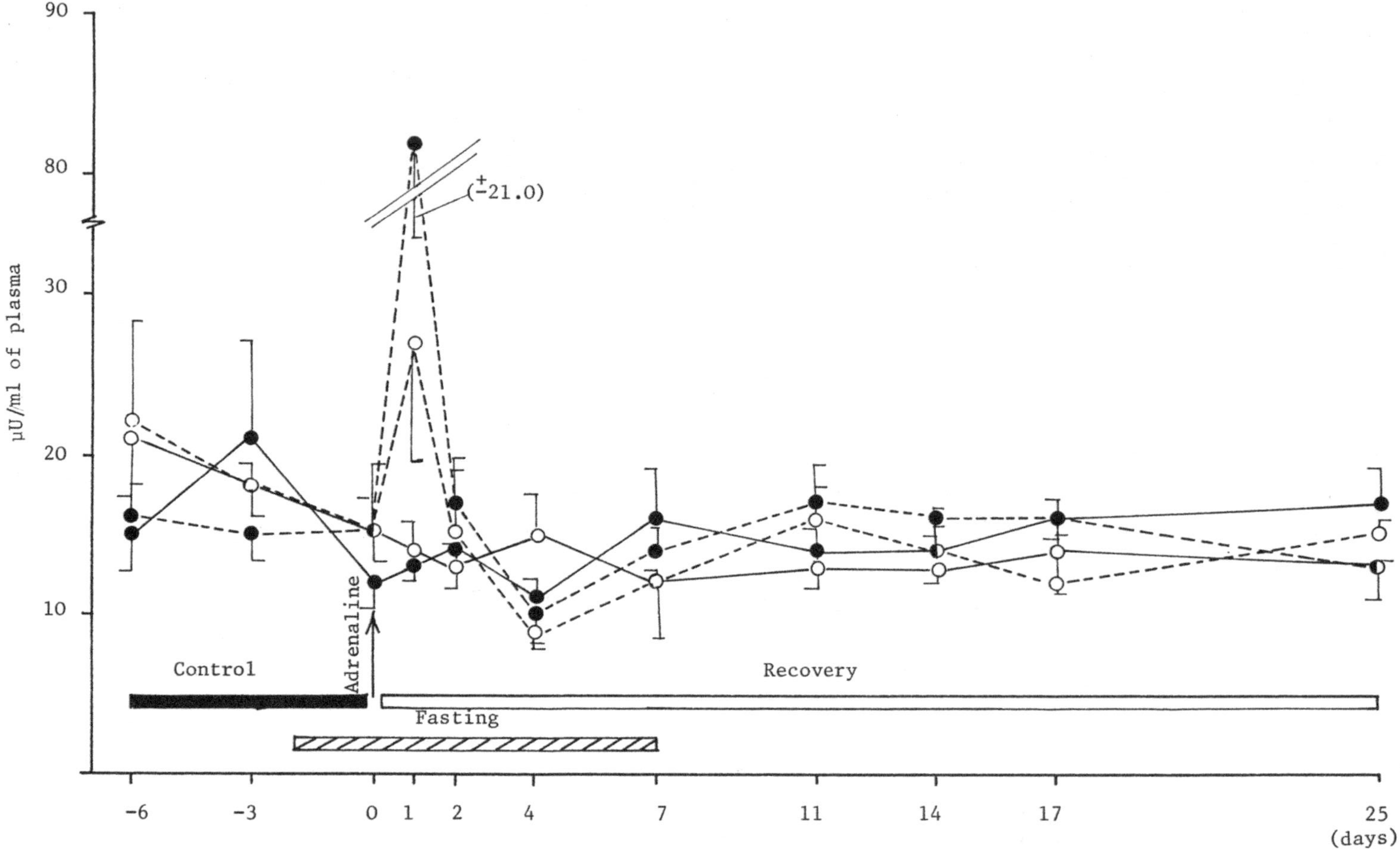

Fig. 4. Plasma immunoreactive insulin concentration in adrenaline-treated (----) and untreated (——) hay-fed (●) and fasting (o) beef heifers. Each of the two fasted groups contained six animals and the fed groups four animals.

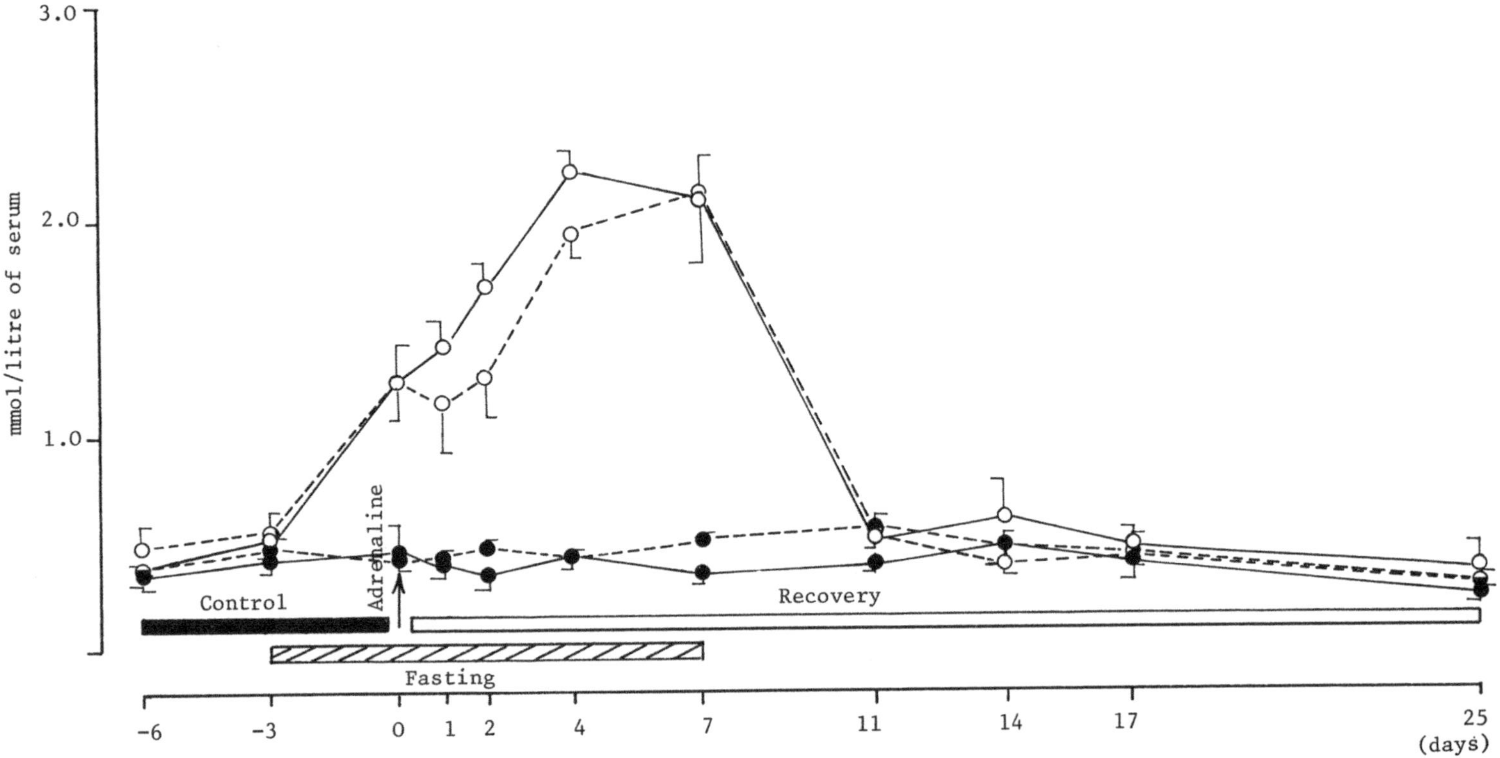

Fig. 5. Serum non-esterified fatty acid concentration in adrenaline-treated (---) and untreated (———) hay-fed (●) and fasting (o) beef heifers. Each of the two fasted groups contained six animals and the fed groups four animals.

CONCLUSIONS

Feed intake has a major effect on replenishment of glycogen in *M. longissimus dorsi* after depletion by adrenaline injection. Recovery is a slow process in hay-fed heifers, and is practically absent during fasting.

Fasting alone, as a stressor, does not cause a substantial loss of muscle glycogen.

A slow rate of muscle glycogen recovery is associated with somewhat lower plasma insulin and muscle glucose-6-phosphate concentrations. Also of importance in this respect may be the low resting blood glucose concentration in both hay-fed and fasting cattle, compared with non-ruminant species.

The specific activity of beef muscle glycogen synthase is similar to that reported for other species. Furthermore, the enzyme is present in the active (I) form when muscle glycogen content is low.

REFERENCE

McVeigh, J.M. and Tarrant, P.V., 1979. The effect of skeletal muscle biopsy on blood constituents, muscle glycogen and heart rate of cattle. Res. Vet. Sci., 27: 325-328.

SOME ODOURS PRODUCED BY BACTERIA ON HIGH pH AND NORMAL BEEF

J.T. Patterson[1,2] and G. Bolton[1]

[1]Agricultural and Food Bacteriology Research Division
Department of Agriculture for Northern Ireland

[2]The Queen's University of Belfast
Newforge Lane, Belfast BT9 5PX.

ABSTRACT

The pHµ values, measured on the cut surfaces of two muscles, (M. longissimus dorsi), varied quite considerably from outer to inner sites. Even though the mean values were different (5.7 and 6.3), site values overlapped, and in general fatty tissues had higher values than lean. Since significant microbial activity occurs at the surface of the meat, probably in a film of exudate, these differences may be important in determining the composition and rate of development of the spoilage association. A method for detecting the components of spoilage odours is described, using both gas chromatography and gas chromatography/mass spectrometry. High pH meat spoiled in air after about 100 h at 15°C, by which time there was a large increase in sulphur compounds in both lean and fat samples. Meat of normal pH had not reached this stage until about 11 days. Degradation of methionine to methanethiol may have occurred.

INTRODUCTION

Pearson (1980) has pointed out that although dark-cutting beef has been a problem to the beef industry for years, its incidence and severity have not declined. From the microbiologist's point of view the differences between spoilage of meat of normal pH and that of meat with a pH value > 6.0 are quite considerable and have only been recognised fairly recently. Nichol et al. (1970) stored beef at 1° - 2°C under low O_2 tension either in gas-impermeable packs or in controlled atmospheres and found that an organism *Ps. Mephitica* (syn. *A. putrefaciens*) produced H_2S when the O_2 tension was about 1 per cent and the pH value of the meat 6.0 or above, resulting in the production of sulphmyoglobin and greening the meat. Bem et al. (1976) found that high pH meat either from bovines or pigs had a poorer keeping quality than normal meat and was unsuitable for vacuum-packaging. Vacuum-packaged meat of normal pH stored at chill temperatures supports the growth of lactic acid bacteria (Sutherland et al., 1975) but if high pH meat is vacuum-packaged some Gram negative groups, more commonly associated with aerobically stored meat may develop, giving a much reduced shelf-life (Taylor and Shaw, 1977).

The work of Gill (1976), Gill and Newton (1977; 1978) Newton and Gill (1978a, b) on the sequence of utilisation of nutrients, when meat is stored aerobically or anaerobically has greatly helped our understanding of meat spoilage. This has shown that although pH, *per se* is important for the multiplication of certain organisms, the preferential utilisation of some low moleular weight compounds, particularly glucose, has important implications for the keeping quality of meat. Patterson and Gibbs (1977) studied the incidence and spoilage potential of isolates from vacuum-packaged beef, pH 6.6, stored for up to 8 weeks at 0° - 2°C. They detected off-odours, probably due to high numbers of Gram negative organisms such as *Proteus, Hafnia, Serratia, Pseudomonas, Aeromonas* and *Alcaligenes*, at the 6 week stage. When sterile pieces of meat of normal pH, (5.4), and intermediate pH, (6.15), were inoculated with representative isolates and stored in air at 4°C and 15°C, 9/12 of the Gram negative organisms gave off-odours on normal meat after 14 days at 4°C, while certain of the Gram positive isolates gave acid, buttery odours. On the higher pH meat, 11/12 of the former gave off-odours after 14 days at 4°C. However, under simulated vacuum-package conditions much less pronounced off-odours were detected. Even after 14 days at 15°C only 7/20 isolates produced objectionable odours.

Although there is a considerable amount of published data on the spoilage aromas of fish, unfortunately comparable data for naturally spoiling beef stored aerobically are not available. The work of Gibbs et al. (1979) and that of Dainty and Hibbert, (1980) describes the production of spoilage volatiles by pure cultures growing axenically. Preliminary attempts to characterise some of these odours for meat allowed to spoil in air at 15°C are described below.

METHODS

Determination of ultimate pH

The pH values of the surfaces of two dry freshly cut defrosted bovine *M. longissimus dorsi*, were measured at various points on both fat and lean sites using an Orion research electrode. The muscles had been boned out in the abbatoir after ca 48 h in chill.

Detection and identification of odours produced during incubation at 15°C.

Slices (100 g) of lean meat or fat layers from the two muscles were placed in an all-glass system with teflon valves which allowed headspace sampling for gas chromatography (GC) or gas chromatography/mass spectrometry (GC/MS). The flask was connected via a 6-way valve to the N_2 carrier gas supply for GC, and helium was used as a carrier gas supply for GC/MS. Before sampling, the flask was heated to 40°C in a water-bath for at least 30 min to allow stabilisation of the headspace components. After sampling the flask was flushed through with compressed air before resealing for further incubation, which was continued until the meat was considered badly spoiled when tested olfactorily.

RESULTS AND DISCUSSION

The pH values measured by the surface electrode (Figure 1) showed considerable variation from the outer surface to the inner in both muscles, with overlapping values, even though the means were quite different (5.7 and 6.3). In general, the fatty tissues had higher pH values than the lean. Tarrant and Sherington (1980) have also recorded considerable pH_u differnces between muscles in a carcass. Since significant microbial activity will occur at the surface of the meat, probably in a film of exudate, these differences may be important in determining the composition and rate of development of the spoilage association. Although the growth rates of pseudomonads, which dominate under aerobic conditions, are unaffected by pH values between 5.5 - 7.0, the development of other components of the flora (*Acinetobacter* spp, *A. putrefaciens*), is pH dependent (Barnes and Impey, 1968; Gill and Newton, 1977).

Some volatile off-odour components detected by GC/MS from normal and high pH *M. longissimus dorsi* lean and fat at spoilage are given in Table 1. The high pH meat was sampled after about 4 days, and the normal after about 11 days at 15°C, the latter period being much longer than expected for the meat to spoil. Some odours appeared only after prolonged incubation, while others disappeared. GC analysis of headspace vapours, carried out daily, showed a large increase in sulphur compounds after about 100 h with the high pH meat, both in fat and lean samples. Decomposition by certain bacteria of methionine to methanethiol, a possible precursor of dimethylsulphide may have occurred (Herbert and Shewan, 1976).

The results confirm the findings of Gill and Newton (1980) that the spoilage of adipose tissue is essentially similar to that of lean meat.

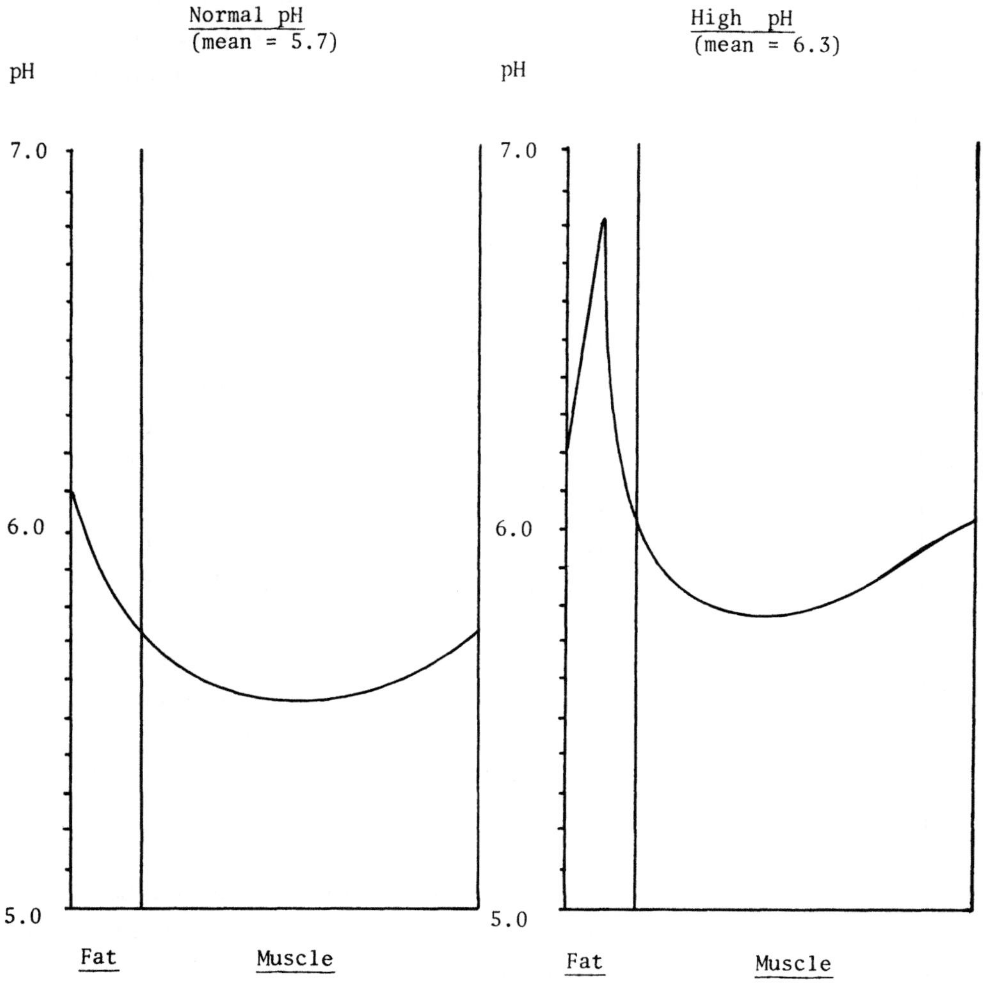

Fig. 1. Ultimate pH values across two bovine *M. longissimus dorsi*.

Further work is being undertaken to identify odours produced at lower temperatures, after aerobic and anaerobic storage of naturally-spoiled beef.

TABLE 1

ODOUR COMPONENTS (MOLECULAR WEIGHT ABOVE 36) FROM SPOILED MEAT AROMA, DETECTED BY GC/MS.

	High pH†		Normal pH‡	
	Lean	Fat	Lean	Fat
Sulphur dioxide	+	+	+	+
Methane thiol	+	+	+	+
Dimethyl sulphide			+	+
Dimethyl disulphide	+	+		+
Ethanol	+	+	+	+
Butan-1-ol			+	+
Butan-2-ol			+	+
Propan-1-ol			P	+
Acetone	+	+	P	
Butan-2-one		+	+	+
Pentan-2-one		+		
Acetic acid		+	+*	+
Ethyl acetate	+			
Ethybutyrate			P	
Ethyl isobutaneoate			+*	
Ethyl propionate				+
Diethyl ether			+*	+
Dichloromethane	+			
Pent-1-ene		+		+
Mw 90			+	

† sampled after 4 days; mean ultimate pH = 6.3

‡ sampled after 11 days; mean ultimate pH = 5.5

+ present when meat spoiled aerobically at 15°C

P detected on prolonged incubation (at 6 weeks)

* absent on prolonged incubation (at 6 weeks)

ACKNOWLEDGEMENT

The authors wish to acknowledge the assistance of Mr. R. Thompson and Dr. D.B. Harper in collecting and interpreting the GC/MS data.

REFERENCES

Barnes, E.M. and Impey, C.S., 1968. Psychrophilic spoilage bacteria of poultry. Journal of Applied Bacteriology, 31, 97-107.

Bem, Z., Helchelmann, H. and Leistner, L., 1976. The bacteriology of DFD meat. Die Fleischwirtschaft 56, 985-987.

Dainty, R.H. and Hibbard, Christine M., 1980. Aerobic metabolism of *Brochothrix thermosphacta* growing on meat surfaces and in laboratory media. Journal of Applied Bacteriology, 48, 387-396.

Gibbs, P.A., Patterson, J.T. and Harper, D.B., 1979. Some characteristics of the spoilage of sterile beef by pure cultures. Journal of the Science of Food and Agriculture, 30, 1109-1110.

Gill, C.O., 1976. Substrate limitation of bacterial growth at meat surfaces. Journal of Applied Bacteriology, 41, 401-410.

Gill, C.O. and Newton, K.G., 1977. The development of aerobic spoilage flora on meat stored at chill temperatures. Journal of Applied Bacteriology, 43, 189-195.

Gill, C.O. and Newton, K.G., 1978. The ecology of bacterial spoilage of fresh meat at chill temperatures. Meat Science, 2, 207-217.

Gill, C.O. and Newton, K.G., 1980. Development of bacterial spoilage at adipose tissue surfaces of fresh meat. Applied and Environmental Microbiology, 39, 1076-1077.

Herbert, R.A. and Shewan, J.M., 1976. Roles played by bacterial and autolytic enzymes in the production of volatile sulphides in spoiling North Sea cod (*Gadus morhua*). Journal of the Science of Food and Agriculture, 27, 89-94.

Newton, K.G. and Gill, C.O., 1978a. The development of the anaerobic spoilage flora of meat stored at chill temperatures. Journal of Applied Bacteriology, 44, 91-95.

Newton, K.G. and Gill, C.O., 1978b. Storage quality of dark, firm, dry meat. Applied and Environmental Microbiology, 36, 375-376.

Nichol, D.J., Shaw, M.K. and Ledward, D.A., 1970. Hydrogen sulphide production by bacteria and sulfmyoglobin formation in prepacked chilled beef. Applied Microbiology, 19, 937-939.

Patterson, J.T. and Gibbs, P.A., 1977. Incidence and spoilage potential of isolates from vacuum-packaged meat of high ph value. Journal of Applied Bacteriology, 43, 25-38.

Pearson, K.M., 1980. What's new in research? The National Provisioner, July 26, 42-47.

Sutherland, J.P., Patterson, J.T. and Murray, 1975. Changes in the microbiology of vacuum-packaged beef. Journal of Applied Bacteriology, 39, 227-237.

Taylor, A.A. and Shaw, B.G., 1977. The effect of meat pH and package permeability on putrefraction and greening in vacuum packed beef. Journal of Food Technology, 12, 515-521.

Tarrant, P.V. and Sherington, J., 1980. An investigation of ultimate pH in the muscles of commercial beef carcasses. Meat Science, 4, 287-297.

THE INCIDENCE OF DARK-CUTTING BEEF IN YOUNG BULLS IN FINLAND

Eero Puolanne and Heljä Aalto[1]
Institute of Meat Technology, University of Helsinki
E-talo, Viikki, 00710 Helsinki 71, Finland.

ABSTRACT

The pH-value of M. longissimus dorsi and information about transport, rest period and carcass characteristics were obtained for each of 6909 young bulls.

The incidence of dark-cutting beef (DFD meat) increased with distance and duration of transport, up to 200 - 250 km, or 5 - 7 h, after which it decreased slightly. When the rest period immediately before slaughter was increased, the incidence of DFD meat first decreased, but increased to an inexplicably high value at 8 - 11 h of rest, and then decreased again after further rest.

Keeping bulls from different farms in open pens (mixed lairage) caused a much higher incidence of DFD meat than bulls individually penned (or tethered).

The difference between the effects of these two modes of lairage increased with increasing duration of lairage. Comparison of different slaughterhouses using single pens (or tethering) showed that other factors, not studied here, also influence the formation of DFD meat.

Carcass characteristics, breed, weight, quality-grade and fatness-grade, showed that large, well-fed (fat) animals are less susceptible to the formation of DFD meat than smaller animals.

[1] Present address: Helsingin Kauppiaat Co.,
Vanha Talvitie 1-3, 00500 Helsinki 50, Finland.

INTRODUCTION

The very high incidence of dark-cutting beef (DFD meat) is a serious problem in Finland. A research group was therefore formed to find methods to reduce the incidence of DFD and to develop useful outlets for DFD meat. Puolanne and Aalto (1980) presented the results of a study on the formation of DFD meat. The present study is based on the same material, but deals only with bulls.

A brief description of beef production in Finland is necessary to facilitate evaluation of this paper.

Beef is a by-product of milk production, though specialised beef production is on the increase. These beef-bulls are almost never castrated. The number of animals per farm is very small and is usually of the order of 30 to 150. The bulls are kept in open fields in summer and tethered in byres during the winter. They are seldom kept permanently free or permanently tethered all year round.

Animals are usually collected from several farms for transport to the slaughterhouse. This practice tends to increase the distance and duration of transport.

The animals are usually kept overnight in the slaughterhouse before slaughter. The most common method has been to keep 4 - 20 bulls, usually from different farms (mixed lairage), in an open pen, but nowadays the use of tethering or single pens for bulls is increasing.

MATERIAL AND METHODS

The study was conducted at 14 slaughterhouses in various parts of Finland during the period March - October, 1979. The total number of animals investigated was 6909 bulls. The following information was collected for each animal:

Date of slaughter	distance of transport
breed	duration of transport
weight	length of rest period
quality-grade	mode of lairage
fatness-grade	pH value

The pH value of *M. longissimus dorsi* adjacent to the 5th and 6th vertebrae was measured 24 h *post mortem*. This measurement was used to estimate the ultimate pH of the meat. Particularly in the case of small, lean carcasses which cool relatively quickly, this may be a source of error. The result may be a tendency to over-estimate the per cent high pH values by a small amount. The pH meter normally used in slaughterhouses was a Knick Portamess 96 (Knick Elektronische Messgeräte, FRG) with an Ingold type 10-404-3041 meat electrode (W. Ingold AG, Switzerland). The pH meters were intercalibrated by the authors with a control pH meter at the time of measurement. The pH measurements were carried out by trained personnel at each slaughterhouse.

In this study pH values below 5.99 indicated normal meat, pH values of 6.00 - 6.39 moderately DFD meat and a pH of 6.40 or above extremely DFD meat.

RESULTS AND DISCUSSION

Carcass weight

The incidence of DFD meat decreased with increase in carcass weight of the bulls (Table 1). This effect was clearly seen both in bulls kept singly in separate pens (A) and in groups in open pens (B). The result suggests that fighting, in which small animals endure greater stress than larger animals (Duchesne, 1978), cannot be the only stress factor for small animals in the slaughterhouse.

Breed

Finncattle bulls were more susceptible to the formation of DFD meat than the other breeds (Table 2).

TABLE 1

THE RELATIONSHIP BETWEEN THE CARCASS WEIGHT OF BULLS AND THE INCIDENCE OF DFD MEAT, AS INDICATED BY pH MEASURED AT 24 h *post mortem.*

Weight (kg)	Number of bulls		Per cent with pH 6.00 - 6.39		Per cent with pH ⩾ 6.40		Total (per cent with pH ⩾ 6.00)
	A	B	A	B	A	B	
< 140	28	222	10.7	32.4	10.7	13.1	43.1
< 160	138	530	13.8	26.0	8.7	14.9	37.6
< 180	406	909	11.1	22.2	5.4	13.3	30.3
< 200	605	895	10.9	20.1	4.3	12.5	25.6
< 240	1021	845	10.7	20.2	2.6	9.9	21.5
< 280	338	180	7.1	17.8	0.3	11.7	14.9
⩾ 280	86	67	9.3	14.9	1.2	7.5	15.7
Total	2624	3655	10.5	22.1	3.5	12.4	26.3

A = individual pens or tethering   B = open pens

TABLE 2

THE INCIDENCE OF DFD MEAT IN BULLS OF SEVERAL BREEDS

Breed	Number of bulls	Per cent with pH 6.00 - 6.39	Per cent with pH ⩾ 6.40	Total (per cent with pH ⩾ 6.00)
AY	3411	18.7	9.3	28.0
FC	269	24.9	17.8	42.7
FR + X	1161	19.6	10.5	30.1
CH + X	147	11.6	8.8	20.4
HE + AA + X	140	15.7	6.4	22.1

AY = Ayshire; FC = Finncattle; FR = Friesian; CH = Charolais;
HE = Hereford; AA = Aberdeen Angus; X = Crossbreed.

Finncattle are smaller than the other breeds listed, and this may be one of the causes of stress in slaughterhouses, especially in open pens.

Table 2 shows that milk breeds have a slightly higher incidence of DFD meat than beef breeds. If this effect really is confirmed, the relatively high proportion of dairy animals in the total beef stock could be one of the reasons for the high incidence of DFD meat in Finland. At the same time Tables 1, 3 and 4 show that large, well-fed animals are less susceptible to the formation of DFD meat. Because dairy breeds are usually smaller, the breed effect could be a combination of several factors.

Quality grade and fatness grade

In the Finnish system carcass quality is determined on the basis of the size, shape and colour of meat, and therefore only large well-developed animals achieve the best quality grade. Table 3 shows an increase in the incidence of DFD meat with decreasing quality grade. With increase in fatness (not desirable in Finland), the incidence of DFD meat is decreased (Table 4). Both the quality characteristics and weight seem to show that large well-fed animals were less susceptible to stress. The question remains whether or not stress-resistance helps the animals to grow large and fat.

TABLE 3

INFLUENCE OF CARCASS QUALITY GRADE ON THE INCIDENCE OF DFD MEAT IN BULLS

Quality grade	Number of carcasses	Per cent with pH 6.00 - 6.39	Per cent with pH $\geq$ 6.40	Total (per cent with pH $\geq$ 6.00)
E + (best)	54	9.3	3.7	13.0
E	598	12.0	4.2	16.2
I +	1943	14.7	7.3	22.0
I	3422	20.1	9.2	29.3
I -	671	21.5	12.5	34.0
II (worst)	56	19.6	17.9	37.5

TABLE 4

INFLUENCE OF CARCASS FATNESS GRADE ON THE INCIDENCE OF DFD MEAT IN BULLS

Fatness grade	Number of carcasses	Per cent with pH 6.00 - 6.39	Per cent with pH $\geq$ 6.40	Total (per cent with pH $\geq$ 6.00)
T (lean)	1018	21.2	10.8	32.0
A	5573	17.5	8.2	25.7
C	141	11.4	6.4	18.0
D x)	12	0	0	0
R x) (extremely fat)	3	0	0	0

x) very seldom found in bulls

Distance and duration of transport

The transport distance sometimes seems to influence the incidence of DFD meat (Nestorov et al., 1972; Puolanne and Aalto, 1980), but this effect is not always apparent (Puolanne and Aalto, 1980). The present study shows that when the distance is increased to 200 - 250 km, the incidence of DFD meat is increased (Table 5). The same increase is naturally seen with the duration of transport, where the maximum incidence is reached at 5 - 7 hours (Table 6). When the distance or duration of transport is high, the incidence seems to decrease. This might be due to adaptation to stress and to subsequent regeneration of glycogen;

however, there was no opportunity to carry out the required biochemical tests to answer such questions.

Length of the rest period

The lairage of animals in slaughterhouse collecting yards (rest period) has been shown to be one of the most important factors in the formation of DFD meat (Nestorov et al. 1972; Duchesne 1978; Augustini et al., 1979). Table 7 shows the effect of the rest-period on tethered animals and on animals in single and open pens. As the length of the rest-period is increased, there is an initial decrease in the incidence of DFD meat, but at 8 - 11 hours there is a marked increase in DFD meat. Scrutiny of the basic material revealed no obvious reason for this increase; the animals were evenly distributed in different groups with respect to transport distances, slaughterhouses, etc. Whether the increase has a physiological cause or is due to some other environmental factor remains unanswered.

After the high incidence at 8 - 11 h, the incidence is decreased again but it is finally increased after a very long rest-period.

Method of lairage

The incidence of DFD meat is presented both for single pens and tethered animals (A) and for open pens (B) in Tables 1, 5, 6 and 7. The average incidence of moderately DFD meat for single pens was less than half that in open pens; correspondingly, the incidence of extremely DFD meat was about one quarter in single pens than in open pens.

This study therefore shows that keeping the animals in open pens causes a considerably higher incidence of DFD meat than keeping them separated. By increasing the rest-period the difference between these two modes of lairage is more evident (Table 7). In this respect, single pens are to be recommended rather than tethering, because some animals are raised free, which leads to difficulties in tethering them and subsequent stress, which might result from this procedure.

TABLE 5

THE INCIDENCE OF DFD MEAT IN BULLS, RELATED TO DISTANCE OF TRANSPORT AND MODE OF LAIRAGE IN SLAUGHTERHOUSES

Distance of transport (km)	Number of animals		Per cent with pH 6.00 - 6.39		Per cent with pH ≥ 6.40		Total (Per cent with pH ≥ 6.00)
	A	B	A	B	A	B	
> 10	22	16	9.1	25.0	0.0	12.5	21.1
> 50	412	733	10.7	20.2	2.4	9.4	23.7
> 100	1034	1422	8.8	20.8	2.4	13.1	24.3
> 150	724	799	10.8	23.9	4.4	10.8	25.4
> 200	204	341	14.2	23.2	5.4	19.7	34.2
> 250	78	100	18.0	30.0	11.5	17.0	39.3
≥ 250	71	91	12.7	25.3	1.4	16.4	29.6
Total	2545	3502	10.5	22.0	3.5	12.6	25.9

A = individual pens or tethering   B = open pens

TABLE 6

THE INCIDENCE OF DFD MEAT IN BULLS, RELATED TO DURATION OF TRANSPORT AND MODE OF LAIRAGE IN SLAUGHTERHOUSES

Duration of transport (h)	Number of animals		Per cent with pH 6.00 - 6.39		Per cent with pH > 6.40		Total (Per cent with pH ≥ 6.00)
	A	B	A	B	A	B	
< 2	385	490	7.8	22.0	1.0	5.7	18.6
< 3	629	594	8.0	21.4	1.6	10.9	20.2
< 4	526	726	10.7	18.7	4.2	12.4	24.5
< 5	361	688	10.3	20.1	2.8	13.4	26.5
< 6	130	285	14.6	28.4	10.0	19.0	39.9
< 7	96	263	18.8	21.7	8.3	19.8	35.7
< 8	108	139	9.3	28.1	0.9	19.4	29.2
≥ 8	293	279	16.0	26.5	6.8	11.5	31.4
Total	2528	3464	10.6	21.9	3.5	12.7	25.9

A = individual pens or tethering B = open pens

TABLE 7

THE INCIDENCE OF DFD MEAT IN BULLS, RELATED TO LENGTH OF REST PERIOD AND METHOD OF LAIRAGE

Rest period (h)	Number of animals		Per cent with pH 6.00 - 6.39		Per cent with pH $\geq$ 6.40		Total (Per cent with pH $\geq$ 6.00)
	A	B	A	B	A	B	
(x	292	437	7.2	21.6	2.4	18.9	28.1)
< 2	39	340	10.3	18.8	7.7	1.5	20.1
< 5	108	441	4.6	10.0	0.0	3.6	11.8
< 8	11	13	9.1	15.4	0.0	0.0	12.5
< 12	79	85	41.8	52.9	16.5	23.5	67.7
< 16	558	700	15.1	24.9	4.8	14.0	30.5
< 20	765	998	9.7	20.3	4.2	15.3	26.2
< 30	554	468	4.9	21.8	1.3	12.6	19.1
< 50	137	97	7.3	37.1	0.0	17.5	26.9
$\geq$ 50	82	105	19.5	47.6	2.4	8.6	41.2
Total	2333	3247	10.9	22.2	3.6	11.6	25.7

x) includes animals slaughtered immediately and those with incomplete information about rest period.

A = individual pens or tethering   B = open pens

TABLE 8

THE INCIDENCE OF DFD MEAT IN BULLS IN DIFFERENT SLAUGHTERHOUSES

Slaughterhouse	Number of animals	Per cent of animals held individually or tethered	Per cent with pH 6.00 - 6.39	Per cent with pH $\geq$ 6.40
1	1099	0.0	14.9	11.8
2	685	50.1	20.4	9.3
3	234	100.0	3.9	1.3
4	87	100.0	26.4	0.0
5	724	87.3	7.0	1.1
6	66	1.5	27.7	9.2
7	380	46.8	12.9	5.0
8	340	48.5	42.4	18.3
9	135	83.0	15.6	3.7
10	317	60.3	16.1	3.8
11	211	30.3	30.1	4.3
12	1221	35.8	13.4	14.5
13	558	0.0	23.4	3.2
14	256	71.9	14.8	13.7

Slaughterhouse

The incidence of DFD meat in different slaughterhouses is shown in Table 8.

In slaughterhouses where the incidence of DFD meat was very high, the animals were kept in large open pens, with 4 - 20 animals per pen. The area per animal was very small and the animals could not lie down to rest. They were in constant physical contact with each other, and when some moved, all had to move. The air in the pen was very bad, especially on hot summer days, because the pens were made of concrete without holes for ventilation.

An improvement has been achieved by building individual pens with good ventilation and water supply, and by increasing the proportion of cattle going for immediate slaughter. This has been shown to be beneficial, especially after a short journey, compared with overnight lairage before slaughter.

On line measurements of the incidence of DFD bulls at a large meat packing plant buying from all parts of Finland are shown in Table 9. The incidence was 10 - 22 per cent at the beginning of 1979. During August three of the important slaughterhouses delivering meat to this packing plant built single-pen lairage systems, resulting in a considerable decrease in the incidence of DFD meat. This is more clearly seen in a particular slaughterhouse, where the incidence fell from 50 per cent to below 10 per cent after the construction of single pens (Table 9).

In conclusion it can be said that the mode of lairage may be the most important factor affecting the formation of DFD meat in Finland. However, the material must be studied using step-by-step regression analysis to clarify the relative importance of the various factors.

TABLE 9

INCIDENCE OF DFD BULL CARCASSES AT A LARGE MEAT PACKING PLANT BUYING CARCASSES FROM ALL PARTS OF FINLAND AND IN ONE OF THE SUPPLYING SLAUGHTER-HOUSES, SHOWING THE EFFECT OF THE INTRODUCTION IN SEPTEMBER 1979 OF SINGLE-PEN LAIRAGE SYSTEMS ON THE INCIDENCE OF DFD

Month	Total bulls at the packing plant		Bulls from one particular slaughterhouse	
	1979	1980	1979	1980
	Per cent with pH ≥ 6.0			
I	-	7.9	-	1.7
II	9.7	6.9	22.9	2.1
III	13.0	9.7	45.3	3.5
IV	15.0	14.4	41.0	5.7
V	25.1	10.8	50.9	5.5
VI	22.0	12.2	56.6	8.8
VII	22.0	14.3	59.0	4.7
VIII	20.6		53.6	
IX	11.3		2.4 x)	
X	13.3		6.0	
XI	12.4		5.1	
XII	13.7		19.3	
TOTAL N	26022	15039	2919	2303

x Single pens were built

REFERENCES

Augustini, Chr., Fischer, K. and Schön, L., 1979. Zum Vorkommen von dark cutting beef unter Praxisbedingungen. Fleischwirtschaft 59, 342-344.

Duchesne, Helen E., 1978. The actiology of dark-cutting beef: a study on the management and behavioural factors that affect meat quality in entire male cattle. Ph.D. Thesis. University of Bristol.

Nestorov, N., Tomov, Tr., Krustov, Ar. and Sedloev, N., 1972. Investigation on the influence of transport upon the appearance, run and ceasing of stress reaction in calves and pigs and its impact on the technological qualities of meat. 18th Meeting of European Meat Research Workers, Guelph, Ontario.

Puolanne, E. and Aalto, Heljä, 1980. Factors bearing on the formation of DFD meat. Proc. of the 26th Eur. Meeting of Meat Res. Workers, Colorado Springs, Colorado, USA, C 7.

THE USE OF FREEZE-DRYING IN INVESTIGATIONS ON THE MICROBIOLOGY OF VACUUM-PACKED DFD BEEF

J.J. Sheridan

Meat Research Department, The Agricultural Institute,
Dunsinea Research Centre, Castleknock, Co. Dublin, Ireland.

ABSTRACT

A method involving freeze-drying of DFD beef steaks was developed to allow the addition, on a weight basis, of glucose or buffers. Initially, a comparison was made between the microflora on DFD steaks and beef of normal pH. After freeze-drying and reconstituting there was an increase in bacterial numbers on DFD beef compared with non-freeze-dried steaks. No difference was found between freeze-dried steaks reconstituted in either water (control) or glucose. Freeze-drying had the effect of delaying the production of H_2S *in vacuum-packs. Reconstituting the steaks in 200 µg/ml (145 - 150 µg/g) glucose solution increased the shelf-life of the vacuum-packs. The method allowed the pH of the meat to be regulated using buffers, without the steaks reverting to their original values within a short time. The pH of the steaks also appeared to influence the production of* H_2S *in the packs.*

INTRODUCTION

In a number of investigations attempts have been made to determine the influence of pH on the putrefaction of DFD beef by the addition of buffers to the surface of the meat and a similar method has also been used with glucose (Newton and Gill, 1980; Sheridan and Lynch, 1980). The latter authors found this method unsatisfactory because the buffering capacity of the meat was such that the meat surface returned to its original pH within a short time and addition of glucose was equally unsatisfactory since it was impossible to measure the amounts added accurately on a weight basis.

The method described below was designed to allow the addition of solutions to meat by freeze-drying and reconstitution in the appropriate solutions. Freeze-drying is known to have a detrimental effect on the survival of some bacteria, particularly gram-negative organisms such as species of *Vibrio* (Fry, 1966). An attempt was made to establish possible changes in the microflora, which is of particular importance in relation to hydrogen sulphide producing organisms on DFD beef.

MATERIALS AND METHODS

Three striploins *(M. longissimus dorsi)* were obtained from cattle slaughtered in an Irish meat export factory. They had the following pH values, 6.65, 6.70 and 6.65, and each was cut into 50 or more steaks, about 4 mm thick, and weighing approximately 15 g. The steaks were weighed and placed 12/plate in a Virtis freeze-drier, (Model USM 15) after freezing overnight (14 - 16 h) at -23°C. In these conditions freezing of the steaks was rapid and would therefore cause least physical damage to the meat (Love, 1966). Drying was at 50 microns (0.05 mm Hg) pressure, with a plate temperature of 27 - 37°C for 12 - 14 h. Dried steaks were reconstituted in (1) 50 μg/ml (35 - 38 μg/g) and (2) 200 μg/ml of glucose

(145 - 150 μg/g) and (3) in sterile distilled water (DFD freeze-dried control). A non-freeze-dried DFD control was also used.

The pH of the freeze-dried steaks was regulated by reconstitution in either (1) 0.1 M citrate buffer, pH 4.8 or (2) a solution of low pH (1.9), specifically recommended for use on meat and meat products (van Kerrebroeck and Herreygers, 1974).

The steaks were vacuum-packed in Ølgaard hydrogen sulphide (H_2S) detector bags (Ølgaard, 1974). This showed the presence of H_2S in the vacuum-packs and the location of H_2S producing organisms on the meat. The packs were stored in duplicate at 4°C and examined daily for the presence of H_2S. After 7 days storage at 4°C one of the packs from each duplicate was transferred to a 22°C incubator and the time for H_2S production observed at 12 h intervals. This test was used to accelerate H_2S production by the bacteria present on the meat and to determine if this process was affected by the different treatments.

At 7 day intervals changes in the microflora were determined. To each vacuum-pack of meat (15 g) 180 ml of 0.1 per cent peptone water was added and the contents agitated in a Colworth stomacher for about 1 min. Aliquots of the solution of macerated meat (0.1 ml) were placed on the surface of different media to determine the following (1) total bacterial numbers on Oxoid Tryptone Glucose Yeast Agar (TGYA), (2) *Brochothrix thermosphacta* on STAA medium (Gardner, 1966), (3) Lactobacilli on Oxoid MRS medium (de Man et al., 1960) and species of *Pseudomonas* on CFC medium (Mead and Adams, 1977). All plates were incubated at 22°C for 3 days.

Where the pH of the meat had been regulated, readings were taken on the meat surface at weekly intervals and the progress of blackening in the packs noted. No microbiological investigations were carried out on this meat.

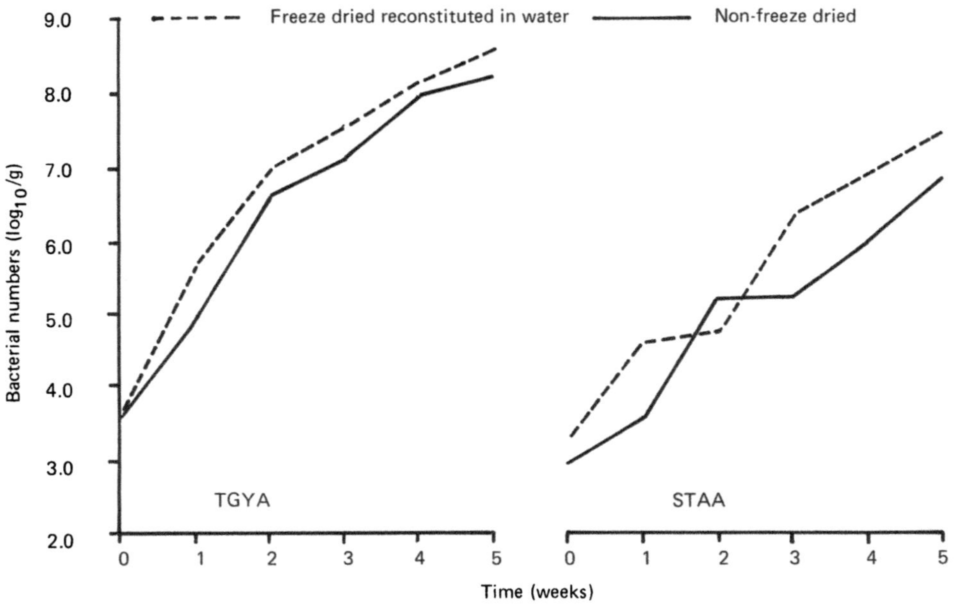

Fig. 1. Bacterial numbers on vacuum packed freeze-dried DFD beef reconstituted in water and in non-freeze-dried steaks stored at 4°C.

When freeze-dried DFD steaks were compared with non-freeze-dried meat, the total bacterial counts were increased as a result of freeze-drying (Figure 1). This was also noted for the lactobacilli, the pseudomonads and *B. thermosphacta* and is shown by the results for STAA. For both the total bacterial numbers and the selective media it was not possible to show a difference in the flora between freeze-dried DFD controls (i.e. reconstituted in water) or either of the glucose treatments, as illustrated in Figure 2 for 200 μg/ml glucose.

The data in Table 1 show that freeze-drying the meat delayed the onset of H_2S production. This confirms the greater sensitivity to freeze-drying of gram-negative organisms (Fry, 1966), although this was not obvious from the results for the pseudomonads (CFC medium).

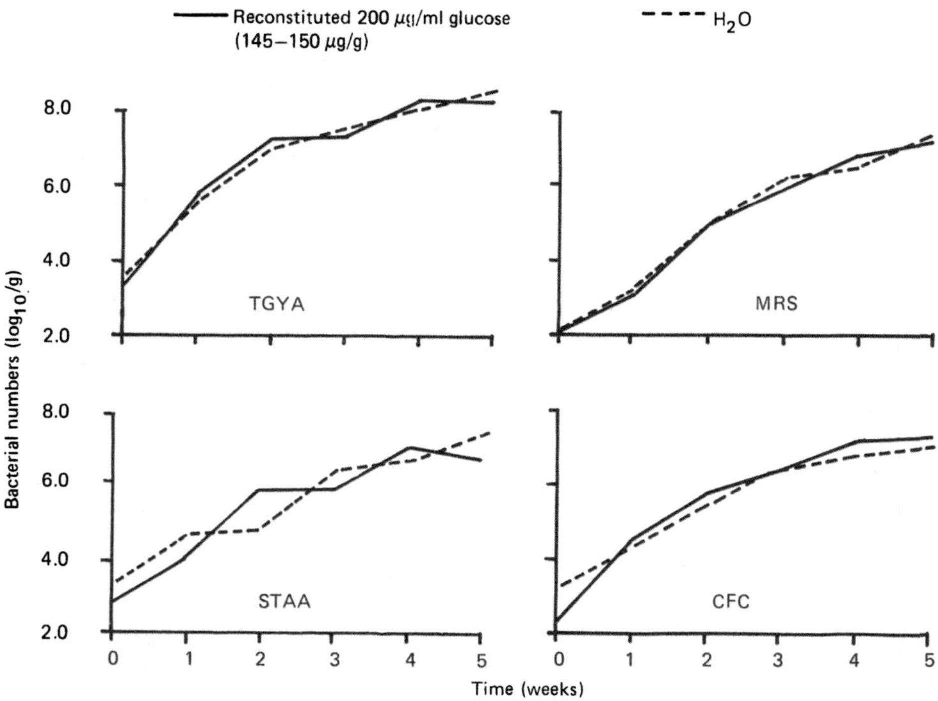

Fig. 2. The effect of glucose on the microflora of freeze-dried DFD beef stored at 4°C, estimated using four media.

Repeated isolations of the organisms responsible for H_2S production in these studies have shown the presence of a species of *Aeromonas*, while a H_2S producing strain of *Alteromonas* has not been found. Although H_2S producing strains of *Aeromonas* have been detected by other workers, their role in greening of DFD meat is considered to be secondary to that of *Alteromonas putrefaciens* (Seelye and Yearbury, 1979).

Newton and Gill (1978) suggested that a lack of free glucose in DFD meat was responsible for the production of H_2S by bacteria present on the meat. It should therefore be possible to delay the onset of 'greening' by addition of glucose to DFD meat at concentrations similar to those present in meat of normal pH, i.e. 100 - 200 μg/g of meat.

TABLE 1

PERCENTAGE DFD STEAKS IN VACUUM PACKS SHOWING BLACKENING (H_2S PRODUCTION) AFTER STORAGE AT 4°C

Storage time (days)	Reconstituted freeze-dried DFD steaks			Non-freeze-dried DFD control
		Glucose		
	H_2O	35 - 38 μg/g	145 - 150 μg/g	
11				73 (22)*
12				82 (22)
14				100 (22)
28			7 (14)	
29	42 (12)		17 (12)	
30	70 (10)	80 (10)	20 (10)	
31	90 (9)	100 (10)	50 (10)	
32	100 (10)		70 (10)	
35			100 (10)	

*Number of packs examined

Table 1 shows that only the higher level of glucose (145 - 150 μg/g) was effective in increasing the shelf-life of the vacuum-packed steaks. Where the microbial growth was accelerated, by incubation at a higher temperature, the effect of the higher concentration of glucose was again in evidence (Table 2). Gill and Newton (1979) and Newton and Gill (1980) added glucose to the surface of vacuum-packed DFD beef at a concentration of 500 μg/g of meat but obtained no delay in the onset of greening. The results obtained in the present work suggest that while it is possible to delay H_2S production by the addition of glucose to DFD meat, surface application is unsatisfactory and the glucose must be present at the appropriate concentration within the cells of the meat.

Using either citrate or pH liquid it was possible to alter the pH of the meat so that it did not revert to its original value within a short time (Table 3). In experiments in which the same buffers were added to the surface of meat it was observed that the pH had returned to its original value within 14 days (Sheridan, 1980). Newton and Gill (1980) also found that citrate buffer at a pH of 4.8 was ineffective in reducing the pH of DFD meat, even at a molarity of 1.9. The results in Table 3 show that the pH of the meat remained low using the pH liquid and after 28 days H_2S production was not observed. With the citrate buffer, the pH of the meat was not lowered as much initially and H_2S production was evident in the packs within 21 days. These results suggest that as well as a glucose effect in DFD meat there may also be one involving pH. With the buffers used, however, it may be that the constituents are being preferentially metabolised by the bacteria present on the meat, in the same way as added glucose.

TABLE 2

TIME (H) TO BLACKENING (H_2S PRODUCTION) IN VACUUM-PACKED DFD STEAKS STORED AT 4°C, AND SUBSEQUENTLY TRANSFERRED TO 22°C

Storage time (days)	Reconstituted freeze-dried DFD steaks			Non-freeze-dried DFD control
		Glucose		
	H_2O(8)+	35 - 38 µg/g(8)	145 - 150 µg/g(8)	
7	48	48	60	24
14	48	36	48	-*
21	36	36	36	-
28	24	24	24	-

*All steaks at 4°C showed blackening

+Number of packs examined

TABLE 3

EFFECT OF RECONSTITUTION IN BUFFERS ON THE pH OF FREEZE-DRIED DFD STEAKS (pH 6.7) STORED AT 4°C

Buffer	pH immediately after reconstitution	Storage time (days) 7	14	21	28
Citrate (pH 4.8) (10)*	5.8	5.7	5.7	5.9**	5.9
pH liquid (pH 1.9) (10)	3.0	4.5	4.7	4.9	5.0

*Numbers of packs examined

**Blackening in all packs

CONCLUSIONS

1. By allowing the addition of different substances on a weight basis, freeze-drying provides a quantitative technique for investigating bacterial spoilage of reconstituted vacuum-packaged beef.

2. Freeze-drying DFD steaks did not appear to influence greatly the microflora.

3. It was not possible to detect any difference in the microflora of freeze-dried DFD beef reconstituted in water or glucose.

4. Freeze-drying DFD beef caused a delay in the onset of H_2S production.

5. Treatment of freeze-dried DFD beef with 200 μg/g of glucose caused a delay in H_2S production in the packs.

6. The pH of freeze-dried DFD steaks could be regulated by reconstitution in buffers.

REFERENCES

de Man, J.C., Rogosa, M. and Sharpe, E.M., 1960. A medium for the cultivation of lactobacilli. J. appl. Bact. 23, 130-135.

Fry, R.M., 1966. Freezing and drying of bacteria. In: Cryobiology (ed. H.T. Meryman), 665-693.

Gardner, G.A., 1966. A selective medium for the enumeration of *Microbacterium thermosphactum* in meat and meat products. J. appl. Bact. 29, 455-460.

Gill, C.O. and Newton, K.G., 1979. Spoilage of vacuum-packaged dark, firm, dry meat at chill temperatures. Appl. Microbiol. 37, 362-364.

Love, R.M., 1966. The freezing of animal tissue. In: Cryobiology (ed. H.T. Meryman), 317-398.

Mead, G.C. and Adams, B.W., 1977. A selective medium for the rapid isolation of Pseudomonads associated with poultry meat spoilage. Br. Poult. Sci. 18, 661-670.

Newton, K.G. and Gill, C.O., 1978. Storage quality of dark, firm, dry meat. Appl. Environ. Microbiol. 36, 375-376.

Newton, K.G. and Gill, C.O., 1980. Control of spoilage in vacuum packaged dark, firm, dry (DFD) meat. J. Fd. Technol. 15, 227-234.

Ølgaard, K., 1974. Technical note: A hydrogen sulphide detector. J. Fd. Technol. 9, 397-398.

Seelye, R.J. and Yearbury, B.J., 1979. Isolation of *Yersenia enterocolitica*-resembling organisms and *Alteromonas putrefaciens* from vacuum-packed chilled beef cuts. J. appl. Bact. 46, 493-499.

Sheridan, J.J. and Lynch, B., 1980. The effect of pH and glucose on the microflora of dark, firm, dry (DFD) beef. Proc. Fd. Sci. Technol. Conf. Univ. College Cork.

Sheridan, J.J., 1980. Unpublished data.

van Kerrebroeck, W.A. and Herreygers, F.V., 1974. The up-to-date meat industry-technology and economics. Organisation 9890 Knesselare, Belgium.

DISCUSSION

J. Wismer-Pedersen *(Denmark)*

Referring to the paper of K. Fischer on the influence of temperature, fasting and transportation on the occurrence of dark-cutting beef, I understand from the Poster that there was an effect only at high temperatures; lower temperatures did not affect the animals as far as increased frequency was concerned. Is that correct?

K. Fischer *(FRG)*

That is not correct. The temperatures investigated had no effect on dark-cutting.

J.J.A. Heffron *(Ireland)*

In Dr. Fischer's 'Conclusions' he states that the incidence of dark-cutting meat in young bulls is not initiated by an accelerated breakdown of ATP as is frequently found with pigs. Nevertheless, the effect of fasting, which was referred to in the statement just prior to that, must ultimately be attributed to ATP hydrolysis in the living animal. Anything which accelerates ATP hydrolysis in the living animal will accelerate the depletion of energy reserves, including muscle glycogen.

K. Fischer

We concluded that there were marked effects on the glycogen level, but not on the actual creatine phosphate or ATP concentrations in the muscles.

C.L. Davey *(New Zealand)*

I would like to make a point about this. With an animal which is just about depleted of its glycogen reserves while it is still on the hoof (almost going into *rigor mortis* on the hoof, if that were possible), if you looked at the ATP levels in that tissue they would be as high as in the resting animal; they would not have been depleted at all. Creatine phosphate levels would probably be about half the resting value, but they are still pretty high. The last thing to disappear is the ATP, after the creatine phosphate. If ATP disappeared *in vivo* the animal would actually achieve *rigor mortis* on the hoof, which is impossible!

J.J.A. Heffron

You cannot say much about the rate of ATP hydrolysis in muscle just by measuring the concentrations of glucose, ATP and creatine phosphate, unless you know what other contributors to the pool of ATP there are, and quantify them.

J. Wismer-Pedersen

If there are no further questions on this poster, we will go on to the paper of Dr. Kousgaard, regarding the development of special feeds for young bulls kept in overnight lairages.

D.E. Hood *(Ireland)*

I would like to ask about the practical application of this procedure by industry.

K. Kousgaard *(Denmark)*

I am not sure that industry is very interested in special feeds, unless in exceptional circumstances such as during an industrial dispute. In that case it is necessary to have a special feed because it must be something that all the animals will eat immediately.

J. Wismer-Pedersen

We will now move on to the paper by A. Lacourt and P.V. Tarrant on 'Selective glycogen depletion and recovery in skeletal muscle fibre types of young bulls'.

C.L. Davey

If you take a muscle and cross-section it and picture a zone magnification, you can see the fibres close to the edge of the muscle. Our experience from glycogen staining is that you get a nice ring of glycogen-rich 'fuzz' around the edge of the muscle itself. Is this your experience? It would suggest that either the glycogen has not been depleted in these areas, perhaps due to aerobic usage of the glycogen, which is much slower than the anaerobic usage and would result in more glycogen in these areas. Alternatively, it may suggest that there are different fibre types at the edge.

P.V. Tarrant *(Ireland)*

Our muscle biopsies were taken from approximately the centre of *M. longissimus dorsi*, at a depth of 3 - 4 cm beneath the hide. Therefore we would not have data relating to the peripheral part of that muscle. Apart from that, I think you are referring to glycogen loss due to thermogenesis, whereas the glycogen loss that we examined was caused by the mixing together of young bulls. Consequently there was a physical type of stress plus a psychological type of stress. There was no element of hypothermia. In fact there was hyperthermia, with the body temperature rising by about 1 - 2°C due to physical activity. If glycogen depletion was different in the peripheral and central parts of the muscle, our technique would not have shown it. We would not have expected to find such a difference in the specific stress situation that we examined.

J. Wismer-Pedersen

Are there any questions on the poster of J.M. McVeigh and P.V. Tarrant?

D.B. Lindsay *(UK)*

I was interested to see the marked change in creatine kinase. Usually it is regarded as an indicator of damage to the muscle. Is this your opinion, that there is damage to the surface of the muscle cell and you have reparative processes as well as glycogenesis?

P.V. Tarrant

We find the increase in blood CPK activity occurs whether we induce stress by adrenaline injection or by mixing young bulls together. When strange animals are mixed together and there is unaccustomed physical activity there may be some damage to muscle cells and, consequently, loss of a muscle enzyme into the blood stream. It is not clear what happens when adrenaline is administered, but it certainly does cause a similar, and sometimes larger, increase in creatine kinase activity in blood. We do not know what the mechanism of loss of creatine kinase is after adrenaline infusion. Perhaps there is some damage to muscle cell membranes, but I am not sure. However, it is a very good indicator of stress.

J. Wismer-Pedersen

We come now to the paper of Eero Puolanne and Heljä Aalto from Finland, on 'The incidence of dark-cutting beef in young bulls in Finland'. Are there any questions?

P.V. Tarrant

I would like to ask Mr. Puolanne to comment on the possible causes of the very high incidence of DFD observed in Finland. I recall, from the survey which I conducted, that it was the highest incidence reported from any of the countries surveyed. I am sure that the reasons for this very high incidence are important to everyone concerned with this problem, particularly because not only young bulls, but cows and heifers are affected. It seems like a very good opportunity to investigate the causative factors.

E. Puolanne *(Finland)*

We use an ultimate pH value of 6.0 as an indicator of DFD. Some researchers use a higher pH value and get an apparently lower incidence. Concerning the causes, the method of lairage at the slaughterhouse is most important. Our country is quite large and the roads are not good, therefore, after heavy transportation stress, there is a rest period overnight in the slaughterhouse. Perhaps the stables in the slaughterhouses leave something to be desired. For example, in one slaughterhouse there was an incidence of about 60 per cent DFD meat in young bulls. When individual pens were built, the incidence decreased to below 10 per cent. But this is only one of very many reasons.

P.V. Tarrant

However, you are emphasising transportation and overnight lairage as being two important factors?

E. Puollane

Yes. If you have individual pens the incidence is smaller. The size of the animals is another important factor. Also, in Finland, the animals are mainly milk breeds; this could be a reason too. With meat breeds the incidence is lower.

Lis Buchter *(Denmark)*

I noticed from your paper that you measured the pH one day after slaughter. Was that exactly 24 h or more or less?

E. Puolanne

It was not 24 h exactly because it was a big field survey with 14 slaughterhouses included in the study. However, it was at least 24 h.

Lis Buchter

I think this may be one reason why you have such a high incidence. If you waited until 2 days after slaughter you might find the numbers reduced depending on killing conditions and many other things; to measure one day *post mortem* can give a somewhat false picture.

E. Dransfield *(UK)*

Can you give us some idea of the importance of young

bulls in beef production in Finland, concerning the types of meat products and whether the meat is consumed within Finland or exported.

E. Puolanne

Bulls are produced in Finland and not exported. As half of the calves are male, 50 per cent of the meat products are from bulls and young bulls.

G. Eikelenboom *(The Netherlands)*

In your grading system, is colour included?

E. Puolanne

There are 20 points but colour represents only 3 points. Grading is done within 2 h after slaughter.

J. Wismer-Pedersen

Did you find a seasonal variation in the DFD occurrence? In Dr. Tarrant's survey, we saw that April and October/November were critical months. Did you find the same thing with your study?

E. Puolanne

No, our survey was only from March to October.

J. Wismer-Pedersen

Thank you. We will turn now to the paper of J.T. Patterson concerning odours produced by bacteria on high pH and normal beef.

J.T. Patterson *(UK)*

May I make a general point about measurement of pH? Both Dr. Sheridan and I use a surface measurement of pH, using a surface probe. A different value can be obtained by inserting the pH meter into the meat. In fact, if you take a section of

M. longissimus dorsi and measure the surface pH at various points there will be a considerable variation, even in a so-called 'high pH' muscle. The pH at the middle may be 5.7, whereas the pH at the surface may be 6.3 or 6.4. If you take the pH of the fat, it may be 6.6, 6.7 or 6.8. There is a lot of variation. From the microbiological point of view, this could be of considerable significance. After all, the micro-organisms tend, initially, to grow on the surface, and probably in a surface zone after that.

C.L. Davey

There is a point which can be extended from what Dr. Patterson has just said. With the surface tissue of the muscle one continues to get aerobic metabolism which continues with something like 18 times the efficiency of the glycolytic process. Though it takes about a day for the inside muscle to go into *rigor mortis*, the surface tissue remains in a pre-*rigor* condition for anything up to 2 or 3 weeks if it can be kept in a reasonably sterile condition. What effect could this have on the type of bacteria growing on the surfaces?

J.T. Patterson

I wish I knew! There are obviously a number of surface effects. These are the pH, Eh, water activity, competition and ecological effects. So there will be a number of interacting factors insofar as the micro-organisms are concerned. Of course there is also the availability of nutrients. However, I believe Dr. Gill has shown that the nutrient aspect is not so important, but there will be these interacting factors which are quite important. Another factor is that some of these organisms have shorter lag phases than others. For example, we think that *Pseudomonas* may have a shorter lag phase than, for example, certain of the psychrotrophic aerobes. When the pH is under about 5.8 the pseudomonads, because of their shorter lag phase, will dominate. But when the pH goes above 6.0, some of the psychrotrophic aerobes will begin to dominate because they can grow more rapidly under those pH conditions, possibly overcoming their longer lag phase. Therefore, the situation is rather complex; one result is obtained with sterile meat innoculated with a pure culture. Another result is obtained with naturally spoiling meat. There would probably be a third result if one worked with two cultures growing together - or three cultures. It is a very complex situation and, as microbiologists, we are only beginning to scrape the surface as it were!

D.E. Hood *(Ireland)*

There have been various attempts today to classify DFD meat on the basis of pH. I would like to ask Dr. Patterson and, perhaps, the other microbiologists among us how they would classify it in terms of keeping quality? How would they define DFD meat in terms of pH?

J.T. Patterson

Again, this is a bit subjective. I think that microbiologists differ as do others present here today. From a purely microbiological point of view, meat is normal up to about pH 5.8; from 5.8 to 6.1 would be intermediate pH meat; 6.2 upwards, I would be inclined to call high pH. There is a fairly important dividing line around 6.0 insofar as some organisms are concerned, particularly *Alteromonas putrefaciens* (if one is lucky enough to find it). It seems to me that there is a 'normal', an 'intermediate', and then a 'high' pH insofar as micro-organisms are concerned. I am talking about meat surface pH values.

J. Wismer-Pedersen

I think we have reached a most important point. After all, the keeping quality of beef is extremely important, and is especially influenced by sensitivity to stress in animals. It is most important to the trade and to the consumer.

C.L. Davey

Some microbiologists, and New Zealand workers in particular, have found that fatty tissue spoils just as quickly as lean tissue. This was something I was unaware of until quite recently when we tried it for ourselves. We are not dealing here with a lipolytic type of spoilage, we are dealing with attack on amino acids. We must be grateful to the New Zealand workers for pointing this thing out.

SUMMARY

D.E. Hood
Meat Research Department, The Agricultural Institute, Castleknock, Co. Dublin, Ireland.

The objective of this seminar has been to scrutinise the problem of dark-cutting in beef in all its various aspects in order to achieve a better understanding of the condition which will allow practical recommendations to be made to industry and also indicate where more research work is needed. We have attempted to identify the occurrence and assess the incidence of the condition; to define its biochemical and physiological aetiology; to deal with the microbiological hazards associated with high pH; to establish methods of early identification; to compare its physical properties and eating quality with normal beef and to exploit as far as possible any advantages which it has for processing. Scientists from a wide range of backgrounds and representing many basic disciplines have attended the seminar, making it possible to have a widely based scientific study of the problem. Meat scientists do not often have the opportunity to discuss problems of meat quality with animal welfare experts, veterinarians, ethologists and specialists in carbohydrate biochemistry all at the same time. The diversity of interest of the participating scientists has contributed significantly to the success of the seminar. By broadening the scope and scientific base of our discussion, we have increased the practical usefulness and results of our work.

Early in the seminar M. Dumont indicated the important change towards a greater homogeneity in quality required in the market place with modern beef marketing systems. Problems of meat quality including dark-cutting become more serious as the carcass is cut into smaller units and where the emphasis is on retail marketing of standard products. Where large numbers of meat cuts are displayed for sale together, the consumer demand is for homogeneous presentation and standard appearance. In the past the role of the traditional butcher helped to minimise differences and lack of consistency in meat cuts.

Although it is difficult to define in precise terms, the problem of dark-cutting is well understood. There is an inherent difficulty in quantifying exactly what we describe as dark-cutting beef and also in quantifying the incidence of the problem because of its rather spasmodic appearance. Dr. Davey listed the important aspects of the problem to be causes, incidence, alleviation, effect on quality, economic consequences and measurement and all of these have been covered in a comprehensive way.

There is general agreement about the immediate cause of dark-cutting beef. It occurs as a direct result of a low muscle glycogen store when the animal is slaughtered, leading to a high ultimate pH in meat. Glycogen deficiency may result from physiological stress caused by physical activity or emotional excitement, both of which conditions are commonly encountered by meat animals in the immediate pre-slaughter period.

Both from the survey data presented by Dr. Tarrant and the results reported by authors at the meeting, dark-cutting is confirmed as a persistent condition, occurring in all categories of cattle, but in some more frequently than others. Young bulls are agreed to have the highest incidence. In these animals dark-cutting does not necessarily indicate ill-treatment before slaughter since they are of a naturally excitable temperament which is likely to be accentuated by the circumstances immediately preceding slaughter, including exposure to a strange environment, and mixing with strange animals. On the other hand, the incidence in cows may be indicative of lower standards of care before slaughter, including starvation.

Reported incidences were most frequently put at 1 - 5 per cent for steers and heifers, 6 - 10 per cent for cows and 11 - 15 per cent for young bulls in Dr. Tarrant's survey and other results would seem to support these figures. The incidence reported in Finland is much higher than these, representing over 20 per cent for all categories of cattle and over 25 per cent for young bulls. *M. longissimus dorsi* is generally adjudged to be the muscle most badly affected by the condition. However, no single muscle is adequate to predict accurately the pH status of the carcass as a whole.

We need to have more fundamental information about differences between individual muscles which lead to major differences in meat quality. Muscles exhibit a wide range of metabolic activities and are accordingly influenced to varying extents by stress. It is only through fundamental study of the underlying biochemical processes occurring within the muscle cell that a full understanding of muscle quality differences will emerge. In this respect we have had the most up-to-date information available relevant to dark-cutting, in the areas of carbohydrate metabolism, energy supply and glycolytic enzyme control mechanisms, as well as new research on muscle fibre differentiation in metabolic activity. The usefulness of biopsy sampling coupled with histochemical staining techniques in elucidating glycolytic breakdown and recovery patterns in individual fibres following stress has been demonstrated. A specific problem identified for further study is the interaction of insulin with the glycogen synthase kinases in the control of glycogen synthesis. Another concerns the relative importance of long chain fatty acids and glucose as sources of energy in ruminant muscle.

There is good agreement, in general, about how dark-cutting beef can be avoided, but again, exact recommendations are not always so easily defined. Thus it is clear that animals destined for slaughter must be treated carefully and without inducing stress. Pre-slaughter handling of young bulls in particular should receive special consideration. Time in transport to the slaughterhouse should be as short as possible and the animals should be slaughtered without delay. Prior mixing with strange animals should be avoided. On the other hand it is difficult to put precise limits on transport time to the slaughterhouse or on the period spent in the lairage. Perhaps it is time that these and other questions should be considered in detail by a working group composed of animal husbandry experts, animal welfare people, ethologists, veterinarians, meat technologists and muscle physiologists. The objective would be to examine the various steps in pre-slaughter handling from the farm to the abattoir and to make specific recommendations on how each should be carried out. There are some contentious areas, disagreement on feeding for example and differences of opinion about resting before slaughter. The general consensus at the seminar regarding resting is that it is undesirable from both an animal welfare and a meat quality point of view. This is because restful conditions cannot readily be achieved in a slaughterhouse lairage and, in practice, holding of animals often results in further stress. Certain regulations are in existence and regulatory agencies must take heed of recommendations made in the light of current scientific knowledge and practice. More information is needed to ensure that proposals are soundly based. There will be some variation in requirement depending on the category of animal to be dealt with, whether it is a steer, young bull, culled cow or whatever.

In this respect the science of ethology might provide some useful answers. We have heard the value of animal behaviour studies in relation to improving farming systems. Development of these techniques could be equally rewarding in finding the best systems of pre-slaughter treatment. The meat industry is likely to face greater constraints in the future on the ways in which animals are handled and transported. We will need agreement between animal welfare and meat quality objectives. As far as dark-cutting is concerned these objectives of course agree very well; animals need to be handled carefully and the avoidance of stress is paramount in order to produce good quality meat.

Apart from the well-known quality defects affecting colour, pH and keeping quality, other aspects of quality of dark-cutting beef have been considered during the seminar, including tenderness and flavour. We may conclude that DFD beef is markedly more tender than normal beef but at the same time flavour is not so good and meat of high pH may be preferred less for this reason. A beneficial quality attribute of DFD beef is its high water-holding capacity which is a significant advantage in meat processing. On the other hand its poor keeping quality can be very troublesome. Some of the worst spoilage effects of DFD meat may be reduced by application of some simple preventive treatments. A small quantity of glucose has been found to inhibit early aerobic spoilage. Anaerobic spoilage on the other hand can be retarded by the addition of a small amount of citrate buffer before vacuum-packaging.

Reliable methods of monitoring the DFD condition are increasingly sought by industry. These may range from a subjective measure of colour to pH determinations by pH meter or by indicator strip. Glucose may also be measured using an indicator strip. The latter methods have the merit of being simple and are suitable for use by unskilled staff. Early prediction of the DFD condition in carcasses may be achieved by freeze-thaw pH determinations on pre-*rigor* muscle. These values are closely correlated with true ultimate pH values and the technique may be extended to *ante mortem* identification. Colour evaluation by means of a fibre optic probe shows promise as a non-destructive method for assessing dark-cutting. This instrument, which measures the back scatter of light transmitted into the meat, showed a doubling of the light scattering coefficient Sy in beef from pH_u of 6.8 to 5.7.

A dark-cutting carcass inevitably results in some financial loss, the actual amount depending on marketing conditions and the uses to which the meat will be put. As we have seen the problem becomes increasingly significant as the carcass is divided into smaller cuts or units. Thus a high pH muscle in a vacuum-pack presents a much greater marketing problem than it does in a carcass, and the cut must accept a correspondingly greater penalty in price. On the other hand the difficulty may be minimised (and the high water-holding capacity advantage exploited) if an appropriate processing outlet for the high pH meat is available. M. Sornay estimated the financial loss of a dark-cutting carcass in France to be 25 - 30 per cent of the value of a normal carcass. The survey data indicated a somewhat lower loss for most responding countries. Dr. Puolanne quoted a figure of 5 - 10 per cent for Finland. Whatever the exact figure the economic consequences of any increase in incidence are real and must be guarded against.

Double-muscled cattle are reported to be more sensitive to stress than normal animals which could have serious implications for cattle breeding in relation to meat quality. Sensitivity to stress has been associated with meat quality defects, particularly in pigs and for this reason beef quality from meaty beef animals should be carefully monitored. At this stage it is not clear whether increased stress sensitivity is a major factor in producing inferior beef. There is a need for more information on genetic aspects of meat quality in cattle, including data on breed comparisons and heritability. A marker gene such as the 'Halothane gene' in pigs has not been found in cattle.

Finally, we returned again to the difficulty of giving a precise definition for DFD beef in terms of pH or colour or a combination of both these parameters. As Dr. McGloughlin indicated, a bench-mark would be of great practical advantage. However, no clear recommendation seems possible in the light of the variations and interactions which occur within muscles and carcasses and between different animals and categories of beef. Nevertheless the recognition of this fact and the realisation that care is required in interpreting pH and other quality data provides a worthwhile caveat in a commercial situation. In the absence of a single pH value it is worth recalling Dr. Tarrant's suggested scale for pH in *M. longissimus dorsi* which appears to be acceptable to everyone. Beef quality deteriorates when the ultimate pH is equal to or above 5.8; within the range 5.8 to 6.3 the precise value at which a carcass is deemed to be 'dark-cutting' depends on processing and marketing factors and on the category of beef; values above 6.3 are always associated with an unacceptable degree of DFD in beef.

This brief account of some of the major points that have emerged during the course of this seminar is far from complete and does not do justice to the research work done nor to the individual effort of the many scientists who have taken part in it. The papers presented during the plenary and poster sessions and the general discussions we have had on the many questions raised, together make a substantial contribution to the current scientific knowledge about the problem of dark-cutting in beef. In this respect at least the seminar has fulfilled its objective and I feel sure you will agree that the effort has been well worthwhile.

LIST OF PARTICIPANTS

BELGIUM

Dr. M. Casteels	Rijksstation voor Veevoeding Scheldeweg 68 B-9231 Melle Gontrode
Dr. J. Connell	Commission of the European Communities DG VI 200 rue de la Loi Brussels

DENMARK

Mrs. Lis Buchter	Slagteriernes Forskningsinstitut Maglegardsvej 2 DK-4000 Roskilde
Mr. K. Kousgaard	Slagteriernes Forskningsinstitut Maglegardsvej 2 DK-4000 Roskilde
Dr. J. Wismer-Pedersen	Dept. of Meat Science and Technology Royal Veterinary and Agricultural University Howitzvej 11 DK-2000 Copenhagen F

FEDERAL REPUBLIC OF GERMANY

Dr. Chr. Augustini	Bundesanstalt für Fleischforschung E.-C. Baumann Strasse 20 D-8650 Kulmbach
Dr. Christina Fischer	Bundesanstalt für Fleischforschung E.-C. Baumann Strasse 20 D-8650 Kulmbach
Mr. K. Fischer	Bundesanstalt für Fleischforschung E.-C. Baumann Strasse 20 D-8650 Kulmbach
Prof. Dr. E. Kallweit	Institut für Tierzucht und Tierverhalten Mariensee D-3057 Neustadt 1
Prof. Dr. L. Schön	Bundesanstalt für Fleischforschung E.-C. Baumann Strasse 20 D-8650 Kulmbach

FINLAND

Mr. E. Puolanne	University of Helsinki Institute of Meat Technology 00710 Helsinki 71

FRANCE

Dr. Marie-France Bouissou	INRA Station de Physiologie de la Reproduction 37380 Nouzilly
Dr. B.L. Dumont	INRA Laboratoire de Recherches sur la Viande CNRZ 78350 Jouy-en-Josas
Dr. A. Lacourt	INRA Station de Recherches sur la Viande CRVZ de Theix 63110 Beaumont
Dr. Jeanne Fourneau	INRA Laboratoire de Recherches sur la Viande CNRZ 78350 Jouy-en-Josas
Dr. G. Monin	INRA Station de Recherches sur la Viande CRVZ de Theix 63110 Beaumont
Dr. M.J. Sornay	ITEB Route d'Epinay 14310 Villers Bocage

IRELAND

Dr. J.J.A. Heffron	Department of Biochemistry University College Cork
Dr. D.E. Hood	Meat Research Department The Agricultural Institute Dunsinea Research Centre Castleknock Co. Dublin
Dr. Patricia McGloughlin	Animal Breeding and Genetics Department The Agricultural Institute Dunsinea Research Centre Castleknock Co. Dublin
Mr. J. McVeigh	Meat Research Department The Agricultural Institute Dunsinea Research Centre Castleknock Co. Dublin

Dr. J.J. Sheridan	Meat Research Department The Agricultural Institute Dunsinea Research Centre Castleknock Co. Dublin
Dr. P.V. Tarrant	Meat Research Department The Agricultural Institute Dunsinea Research Centre Castleknock Co. Dublin

ITALY

Dr. E. Cosentino	Istituto di Produzione animale dell'Università di Napoli Facoltà di Agraria 80055 Portici
Prof. A. Romita	Istituto Sperimentale per la Zootecnia di Roma Via O. Panvinio 11 1 Rome

THE NETHERLANDS

Dr. G. Eikelenboom	Instituut voor Veeteelkundig Onderzoek 'Schoonoord' PO Box 501 3700 AM Zeist
Prof. G. van Logtestijn	Utrecht University Veterinary Department VVDO Biltstraat 172 Utrecht

NEW ZEALAND

Dr. B. Chrystall	Meat Industry Research Institute of New Zealand Hamilton PO Box 617 North Island
Dr. C.L. Davey	Meat Industry Research Institute of New Zealand Hamilton PO Box 617 North Island

SWEDEN

Dr. H. Ruderus	Swedish Meat Research Institute S-24400 Kavlinge

UNITED KINGDOM

Miss. S.V. Danes	Janssen Services 33a High Street Chislehurst Kent BR7 5AE
Dr. E. Dransfield	ARC Meat Research Institute Langford Bristol BS18 7DY
Mr. S.E.W. Hallam	Janssen Services 33a High Street Chislehurst Kent BR7 5AE
Dr. J.T. Patterson	Department of Agriculture for Northern Ireland and The Queen's University Newforge Lane Belfast BT9 5PX
Dr. D.B. Lindsay	ARC Institute of Animal Physiology Babraham Cambridge CB2 4AT
Dr. D. Lister	ARC Meat Research Institute Langford Bristol BS18 7DY
Dr. D.B. MacDougall	ARC Meat Research Institute Langford Bristol BS18 7DY
Dr. R. Moss	MAFF Hook Rise South Tolworth Surbiton Surrey

UNITED STATES

Dr. T.R. Dutson	Texas A & M University Meats and Muscle Biology College of Agriculture College Station Texas 77843
Prof. H.B. Hedrick	University of Missouri Department of Food Science and Nutrition College of Agriculture 21 Agriculture Building Columbia Missouri 65211

Manuscript prepared by:

JANSSEN SERVICES, 33a High Street, Chislehurst, Kent BR7 5AE, UK.

GPSR Compliance

The European Union's (EU) General Product Safety Regulation (GPSR) is a set of rules that requires consumer products to be safe and our obligations to ensure this.

If you have any concerns about our products, you can contact us on ProductSafety@springernature.com

In case Publisher is established outside the EU, the EU authorized representative is:

Springer Nature Customer Service Center GmbH
Europaplatz 3
69115 Heidelberg, Germany

Batch number: 10620143

Printed by Printforce, the Netherlands